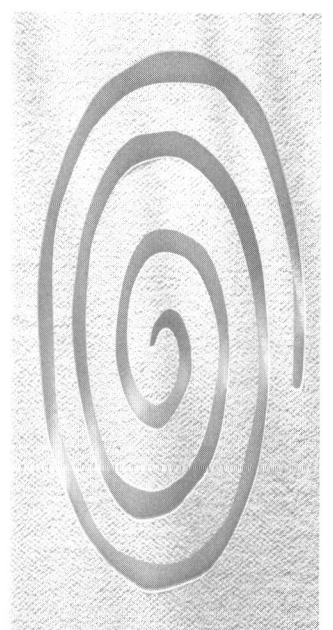

Community Health

Academic Editor
Shelley Wilkerson Smith
St. Joseph Memorial Hospital

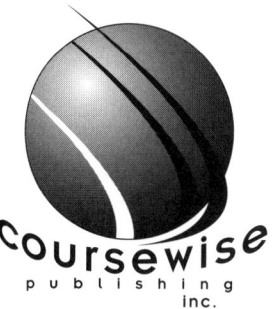

coursewise
publishing
inc.

Bellevue • Boulder • Dubuque • Madison • St. Paul

Our mission at **Coursewise** is to help students make connections—linking theory to practice and the classroom to the outside world. Learners are motivated to synthesize ideas when course materials are placed in a context they recognize. By providing gateways to contemporary and enduring issues, **Coursewise** publications will expand students' awareness of and context for the course subject.

For more information on **Coursewise,** visit us at our web site: http://www.coursewise.com

To order an examination copy, contact: Houghton Mifflin Sixth Floor Media: 800-565-6247 (voice); 800-565-6236 (fax).

Coursewise Publishing Editorial Staff

Thomas Doran, ceo/publisher: Environmental Science/Geography/Journalism/Marketing/Speech
Edgar Laube, publisher: Political Science/Psychology/Sociology
Linda Meehan Avenarius, publisher: **Courselinks**™
Sue Pulvermacher-Alt, publisher: Education/Health/Gender Studies
Victoria Putman, publisher: Anthropology/Philosophy/Religion
Tom Romaniak, publisher: Business/Criminal Justice/Economics
Kathleen Schmitt, publishing assistant
Gail Hodge, executive producer

Coursewise Publishing Production Staff

Lori A. Blosch, permissions coordinator
Mary Monner, production coordinator
Victoria Putman, production manager

Note: Readings in this book appear exactly as they were published.
Thus, inconsistencies in style and usage among the different
readings are likely.

Library of Congress Catalog Card Number: 99-64793

ISBN 0-395-97322-8

Printed in the United States of America by Coursewise Publishing, Inc.
7 North Pinckney Street, Suite 346, Madison, WI 53703

10 9 8 7 6 5 4 3 2 1

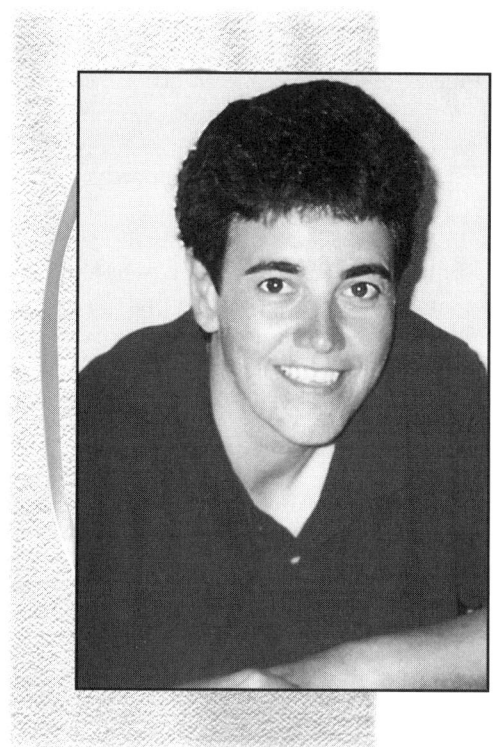

from the
Publisher

Sue Pulvermacher–Alt

Coursewise Publishing

ME As the Basis for WE

I put myself first. When it comes to my personal health, I can be very selfish. I take the time I need to exercise regularly, enjoy a variety of foods, watch my weight, drink alcohol in moderation, monitor my stress, practice my faith, and nourish my relationships. I have friends who put all other needs before their own. They're so involved with taking care of others (spouses, children, parents, colleagues) that they don't have time to take care of themselves. I imagine they think they're making a larger contribution to community health than I am. I think they're wrong. I'm selfish and I'm proud of it.

To me, good personal health habits are the foundation of my contribution to community health. If I take care of myself, I just might have the energy to help others. If I watch what I eat, I just might persuade my son to pay attention to nutrition labels. If I enjoy exercise, I just might convince the kids I coach that exercise is fun. If I question my health insurance statement, I just might save my colleague a buck on a prescription. If I don't drink and drive, I just might take home my softball buddy and keep another drunk driver off the road. If I ask my doctor questions, I just might help my dad understand his antidepressant medication better. If I speak up about our society's unhealthy obsession with thinness, I just might keep my daughter from a future battle with anorexia. The way I see it—community health starts with me.

And it starts with you. Understanding community health means understanding all aspects of a capital "C" community. Throughout this *Perspectives: Community Health* volume, you'll find readings that will help you understand the larger "Community" of health, including worksite health promotion, school-based programming, community health promotion, and health care–based programming. In addition, you'll find web sites that we hope will expand your understanding of the issues. The R.E.A.L. sites you'll find throughout this reader and at the **Courselinks**™ web site for Community Health have been chosen because they are particularly useful sites.

I invite you to be selfish as you use our materials. Read the articles with an eye toward using the information to help you get a better grade or to be better prepared for a health promotion career. Skim our R.E.A.L. web site annotations and decide if the site is worth visiting. Do the activities so you can get to know the site better. Search our **Courselinks** site by key topic and find the information you need. You'll contribute more to your Community if you take care of yourself first.

In putting this material together, I got to work with Shelley Wilkerson Smith. Shelley is the Academic Editor and **Courselinks** Editor for Community Health. Take a look at her bio (see page v) and see how she has experienced Community Health in its many contexts. Shelley has many balls to juggle in her life; I selfishly made sure mine was the bright red one that stayed in the air. Our Editorial Board members—who collectively represent health care, worksite, academia, and school health promotion—helped us make wise decisions. They offered critical feedback and posed interesting challenges. My thanks to Shelley and the entire Editorial Board.

Do you want to learn how to improve the health of others in your Community? Be selfish and improve your health first. Then you can turn to your Community. If along the way you want to help me, let me know what you think of these materials. What worked and what didn't work in this *Perspectives: Community Health* volume and the accompanying **Courselinks** site? Don't be selfish. . . . Let me know what you think.

Sue Pulvermacher-Alt, Publisher
suepa@coursewise.com

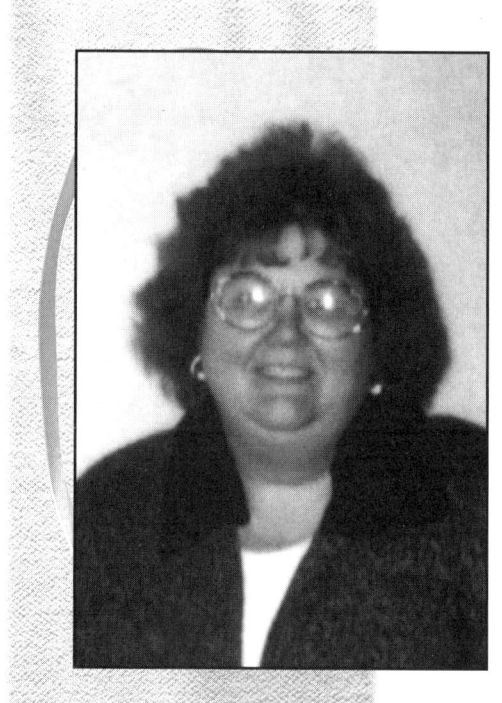

Shelley Wilkerson Smith received both her bachelor of science (1983) and master of science (1986) in education from Southern Illinois University at Carbondale. Her undergraduate emphasis was health education with a secondary teacher certification, and her graduate degree was in school health. She is also CHES certified.

Since 1995, Shelley has been employed by Southern Illinois Healthcare (SIH) as a community health educator for St. Joseph Memorial Hospital. She brings over ten years of experience in health education and prevention programming at schools, in communities, at worksites, and in health care facilities to this volume. She is actively involved in a variety of community-based programs, including comprehensive school health curriculums, support group facilitations, worksite health promotion and screenings, diabetes programs for both adults and youth, and community coalitions on racism, domestic violence, and maternal and child health, to name a few.

Prior to her employment with SIH, Shelley served on the adjunct faculty at John A. Logan College for over ten years. Her teaching responsibilities included health, first aid, and CPR. She was also co-coordinator of the campus substance awareness campaign.

from the
Academic Editor

Shelley Wilkerson Smith
St. Joseph Memorial Hospital

When the average person hears the words *community health,* his or her thoughts often jump to local public health departments or national nonprofit organizations aimed at reducing or eliminating specific diseases. In this volume, we work to expand the concept of community health.

Perspectives: Community Health examines issues surrounding the larger "community" of health, including school-based programming, worksite health promotion, community health promotion, and health care–based programming.

The readings in this volume were selected in conjunction with an outstanding Editorial Board, whose members gave of their time and talents to make this project happen. Members of the Editorial Board are individuals representing academia, health care, worksite, and school health promotion.

Having spent my entire professional life as a "community health educator" with experience in every arena that the title implies, I was elated at the challenge of serving as the Academic Editor of this publication. The books opens with an introduction that covers such topics as Americans' opinions on public health, cultural sensitivity, health education as a profession, and the current state of America's health. The next four sections address the four arenas of community health—school-based programming, worksite health promotion, community health promotion, and hospital/health care–based programming. The final section of the book highlights some truly notable collaborative projects. In an age of budget restraints and downsizing, solving America's health problems requires a collaboration of dedicated individuals and industry with a common goal.

Creating healthier communities, one step at a time.

Editorial Board

We wish to thank the following instructors for their assistance. Their many suggestions not only contributed to the construction of this volume, but also to the ongoing development of our Community Health web site.

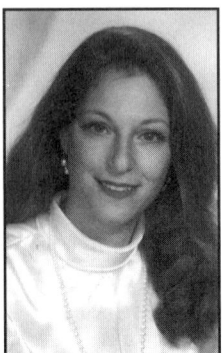
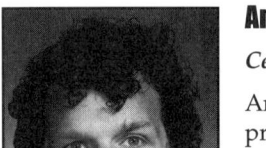

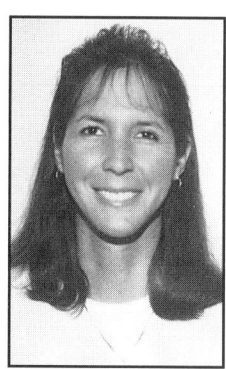
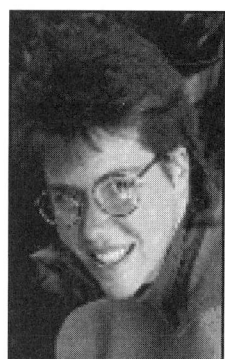

WiseGuide Introduction

Question Authority

Critical Thinking and Bumper Stickers

The bumper sticker said: Question Authority. This is a simple directive that goes straight to the heart of critical thinking. The issue is not whether the authority is right or wrong; it's the questioning process that's important. Questioning helps you develop awareness and a clearer sense of what you think. That's critical thinking.

Critical thinking is a new label for an old approach to learning—that of challenging all ideas, hypotheses, and assumptions. In the physical and life sciences, systematic questioning and testing methods (known as the scientific method) help verify information, and objectivity is the benchmark on which all knowledge is pursued. In the social sciences, however, where the goal is to study people and their behavior, things get fuzzy. It's one thing for the chemistry experiment to work out as predicted, or for the petri dish to yield a certain result. It's quite another matter, however, in the social sciences, where the subject is ourselves. Objectivity is harder to achieve.

Although you'll hear critical thinking defined in many different ways, it really boils down to analyzing the ideas and messages that you receive. What are you being asked to think or believe? Does it make sense, objectively? Using the same facts and considerations, could you reasonably come up with a different conclusion? And, why does this matter in the first place? As the bumper sticker urged, question authority. Authority can be a textbook, a politician, a boss, a big sister, or an ad on television. Whatever the message, learning to question it appropriately is a habit that will serve you well for a lifetime. And in the meantime, thinking critically will certainly help you be course wise.

Getting Connected

This reader is a tool for connected learning. This means that the readings and other learning aids explained here will help you to link classroom theory to real-world issues. They will help you to think critically and to make long-lasting learning connections. Feedback from both instructors and students has helped us to develop some suggestions on how you can wisely use this connected learning tool.

WiseGuide Pedagogy

A wise reader is better able to be a critical reader. Therefore, we want to help you get wise about the articles in this reader. Each section of *Perspectives* has three tools to help you: the WiseGuide Intro, the WiseGuide Wrap-Up, and the Putting It in *Perspectives* review form.

WiseGuide Intro

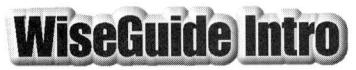

In the WiseGuide Intro, the Academic Editor introduces the section, gives you an overview of the topics covered, and explains why particular articles were selected and what's important about them.

Also in the WiseGuide Intro, you'll find several key points or learning objectives that highlight the most important things to remember from this section. These will help you to focus your study of section topics.

At the end of the WiseGuide Intro, you'll find questions designed to stimulate critical thinking. Wise students will keep these questions in mind as they read an article (we repeat the questions at the start of the articles as a reminder). When you finish each article, check your understanding. Can you answer the questions? If not, go back and reread the article. The Academic Editor has written sample responses for many of the questions, and you'll find these online at the **Courselinks**™ site for this course. More about **Courselinks** in a minute. . . .

WiseGuide Wrap-Up

Be course wise and develop a thorough understanding of the topics covered in this course. The WiseGuide Wrap-Up at the end of each section will help you do just that with concluding comments or summary points that repeat what's most important to understand from the section you just read.

In addition, we try to get you wired up by providing a list of select Internet resources—what we call R.E.A.L. web sites because they're **R**elevant, **E**nhanced, **A**pproved, and **L**inked. The information at these web sites will enhance your understanding of a topic. (Remember to use your Passport and start at http://www.courselinks.com so that if any of these sites have changed, you'll have the latest link.)

Putting It in *Perspectives* Review Form

At the end of the book is the Putting It in *Perspectives* review form. Your instructor may ask you to complete this form as an assignment or for extra credit. If nothing else, consider doing it on your own to help you critically think about the reading.

Prompts at the end of each article encourage you to complete this review form. Feel free to copy the form and use it as needed.

The Courselinks™ Site

The **Courselinks** Passport is your ticket to a wonderful world of integrated web resources designed to help you with your course work. These resources are found at the **Courselinks** site for your course area. This is where the readings in this book and the key topics of your course are linked to an exciting array of online learning tools. Here you will find carefully selected readings, web links, quizzes, worksheets, and more, tailored to your course and approved as connected learning tools. The ever-changing, always interesting **Courselinks** site features a number of carefully integrated resources designed to help you be course wise. These include:

- **R.E.A.L. Sites** At the core of a **Courselinks** site is the list of R.E.A.L. sites. This is a select group of web sites for studying, not surfing. Like the readings in this book, these sites have been selected, reviewed, and approved by the Academic Editor and the Editorial Board. The R.E.A.L. sites are arranged by topic and are annotated with short descriptions and key words to make them easier for you to use for reference or research. With R.E.A.L. sites, you're studying approved resources within seconds—and not wasting precious time surfing unproven sites.

- **Editor's Choice** Here you'll find updates on news related to your course, with links to the actual online sources. This is also where we'll tell you about changes to the site and about online events.

http://www.courselinks.com

- **Course Overview** This is a general description of the typical course in this area of study. While your instructor will provide specific course objectives, this overview helps you place the course in a generic context and offers you an additional reference point.

- **www.orksheet** Focus your trip to a R.E.A.L. site with the www.orksheet. Each of the 10 to 15 questions will prompt you to take in the best that site has to offer. Use this tool for self-study, or if required, email it to your instructor.

- **Course Quiz** The questions on this self-scoring quiz are related to articles in the reader, information at R.E.A.L. sites, and other course topics, and will help you pinpoint areas you need to study. Only you will know your score—it's an easy, risk-free way to keep pace!

- **Topic Key** The online Topic Key is a listing of the main topics in your course, and it correlates with the Topic Key that appears in this reader. This handy reference tool also links directly to those R.E.A.L. sites that are especially appropriate to each topic, bringing you integrated online resources within seconds!

- **Web Savvy Student Site** If you're new to the Internet or want to brush up, stop by the Web Savvy Student site. This unique supplement is a complete **Courselinks** site unto itself. Here, you'll find basic information on using the Internet, creating a web page, communicating on the web, and more. Quizzes and Web Savvy Worksheets test your web knowledge, and the R.E.A.L. sites listed here will further enhance your understanding of the web.

- **Student Lounge** Drop by the Student Lounge to chat with other students taking the same course or to learn more about careers in your major. You'll find links to resources for scholarships, financial aid, internships, professional associations, and jobs. Take a look around the Student Lounge and give us your feedback. We're open to remodeling the Lounge per your suggestions.

Building Better Perspectives!

Please tell us what you think of this *Perspectives* volume so we can improve the next one. Here's how you can help:

1. Visit our **Coursewise** site at: http://www.coursewise.com

2. Click on *Perspectives*. Then select the Building Better *Perspectives* Form for your book.

3. Forms and instructions for submission are available online.

Tell us what you think—did the readings and online materials help you make some learning connections? Were some materials more helpful than others? Thanks in advance for helping us build better *Perspectives*.

Student Internships

If you enjoy evaluating these articles or would like to help us evaluate the **Courselinks** site for this course, check out the **Coursewise** Student Internship Program. For more information, visit:

http://www.coursewise.com/intern.html

Brief Contents

Contents

At **Coursewise,** we're publishing connected learning tools. That means that the book you are holding is only a part of this publication. You'll also want to harness the integrated resources that **Coursewise** has developed at the fun and highly useful **Courselinks**™ web site for *Perspectives: Community Health.* If you purchased this book new, use the Passport that was shrink-wrapped to this volume to obtain site access. If you purchased a used copy of this book, then you need to buy a stand-alone Passport. If your bookstore doesn't stock Passports to **Courselinks** sites, visit http://www.courselinks.com for ordering information.

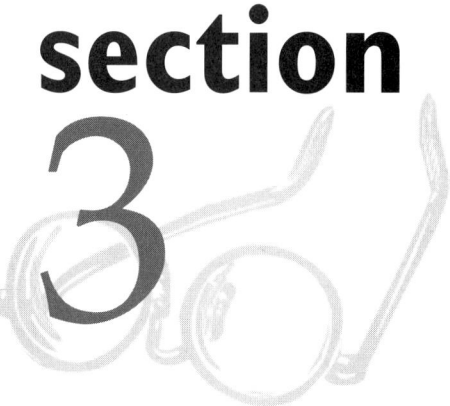

section
2

School-Based Programming

section
3

Worksite Health Promotion

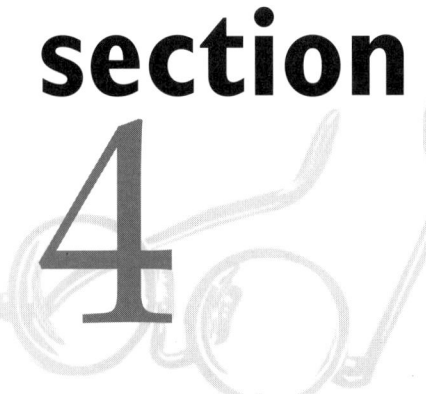

section

4

Community Health Promotion

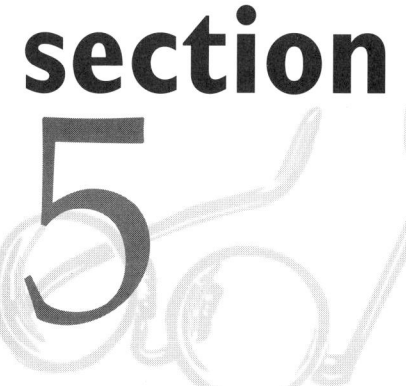

section

5

Hospital/Health Care–Based Programming

section

6

Collaborative Projects

Topic Key

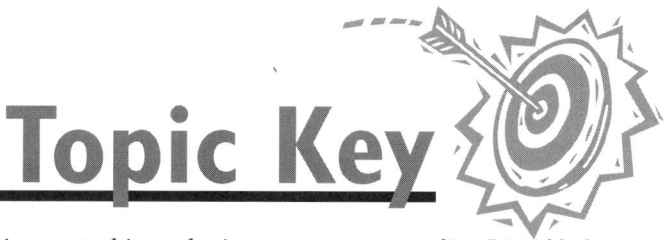

This Topic Key is an important tool for learning. It will help you integrate this reader into your course studies. Listed below, in alphabetical order, are important topics covered in this volume. Below each topic you'll find the reading numbers and titles, and R.E.A.L. web site addresses, relating to that topic. Note that the Topic Key might not include every topic your instructor chooses to emphasize. If you don't find the topic you're looking for in the Topic Key, check the index or the online topic key at the **Courselinks**™ site.

Access
27 Removing Barriers and Improving Choices: A Case Study in Reproductive Health Services and Managed Care

Assessment
18 From Measuring to Improving Public Health Practice
24 Community Assessment: A Model "How-To" Based on Two Communities' Experience

Community Profiler
http://207.87.15.154/commpro/

Community Health Needs Assessment/Managing Change
http://wchd.neobright.net/

ATOD (Alcohol, Tobacco, and Other Drugs)
8 Peer Helping/Involvement: An Efficacious Way to Meet the Challenge of Reducing Alcohol, Tobacco, and Other Drug Use among Youth?
21 Community-Based Approaches for the Prevention of Alcohol, Tobacco, and Other Drug Use

Collaboration
29 The HERO Study on Risks and Costs: Research Findings
30 Premises, Promises, and Potential Payoffs of Responsible Health Education
31 Creating a Districtwide Social Development Project
32 Five Years of Collaboration: Baton Rouge Health Forum Focuses on Community Needs

The Cochrane Collaboration
http://www.cochrane.de/

WHO Collaboration
http://www.wits.ac.za/wits/fac/med/
    comhealth/collabor.htm

Cultural Sensitivity
7 Becoming Culturally Sensitive: Preparing for Service As a Health Educator in a Multicultural World
12 Dealing with the Health Crisis in Our Schools: Clarion University's Health Education Model for Elementary and Early Childhood Education Majors
31 Creating a Districtwide Social Development Project

Multi-Cultural Health Communication Service
http://mhcs.health.nsw.gov.au/

Employee Assistance Programs
16 Costs of Employee Assistance Programs: Findings from a National Survey

Epidemiology
22 The Use of Prevalence Data to Unite the Community in Prevention Programs

Globalization
4 The Globalization of Public Health, I: Threats and Opportunities
5 The Globalization of Public Health, II: The Convergence of Self-Interest and Altruism

Health (Status)
1 How Healthy Are We?

The Michigan Electronic Library: Health Information Resources
http://mel.lib.mi.us/health/health-statistics.
    html

Community Profiler
http://207.87.15.154/commpro/

Community Health Needs Assessment/
    Managing Change
http://wchd.neobright.net/

Health Resource Links
http://www.whitehouse.gov/WH/pointers/
    html/health.html

Health Departments
18 From Measuring to Improving Public Health Practice
19 Assessing the Impact of Medicaid Managed Care on TB Activities in Local Health Departments
20 Impact of Medicaid Resources on Core Public Health Responsibilities of Local Health Departments in Illinois

Health Education (Profession)
2 The Future of Health Education: The Knowledge to Practice Paradox
6 Creating the Future of Public Health: Values, Vision, and Leadership
7 Becoming Culturally Sensitive: Preparing for Service As a Health Educator in a Multicultural World
12 Dealing with the Health Crisis in Our Schools: Clarion University's Health Education Model for Elementary and Early Childhood Education Majors
30 Premises, Promises, and Potential Payoffs of Responsible Health Education

The National Commission for Health Education Credentialing, Inc.
http://www.nchec.org

Health Screenings
14 Worksite Health Promotion Programs in the U.S.: Factors Associated with Availability and Participation
26 Community Health Initiative Uses Casefinding, Intervention to Boost Prevention and Revenues

section

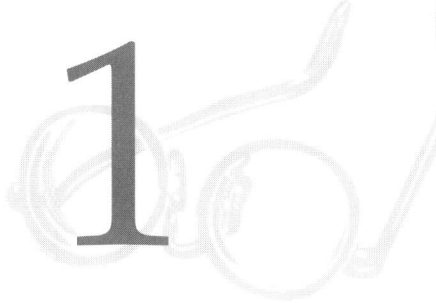

1

Learning Objectives

- To learn Americans' thoughts on health

- To examine health education as a profession

- To review public opinion about public health

- To gain insight into the global issues of public health

- To examine the values, vision, and leadership of public health

- To become culturally sensitive to health education in a multicultural world

Introduction

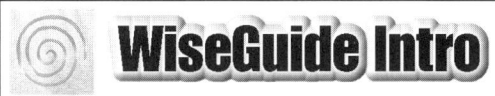

WiseGuide Intro

Webster defines *community* as all of the people living in a particular district, city, and so on. *Health* is defined as physical and mental well-being and freedom from disease, pain, or defect. Based on these definitions, we can conclude that community health is the total well-being of any group of individuals.

Community health educators, as a profession, assist individuals and communities in choosing more healthful behaviors and lifestyles and work for healthier environments. Community health educators are prepared to work in a variety of communities and address a broad range of social, behavioral, environmental, political, and economic factors that influence public health.

As an introduction to issues surrounding the larger "community" of health, we will examine the current state of America's health, the public perception of public health, the role of health education as a profession, the globalization of public health, and the need for cultural sensitivity.

Mark Clements and Dianne Hales, in a 1997 *Parade Magazine* feature, present "How Healthy Are We?" This national survey, prepared by the independent research firm of Mark Clements, explores America's opinion of health—what defines it, how to make it last, and how to pay for it. It also includes the leading killers, what we fear the most, and how closely we follow our doctors' advice.

Gary M. English, Ithaca College, and Donna M. Videto, State University of New York at Cortland, present an in-depth look at the profession of health education. "The Future of Health Education: The Knowledge to Practice Paradox" highlights the establishment of national objectives, a professional credentialing process, and national standards. They maintain that the profession of health education is positioned for success. Additionally, they report that there is a need to unify the profession to reduce fragmentation and replication of professional services and to maximize the potential for professional growth.

The Centers for Disease Control and Prevention *Morbidity and Mortality Weekly Report* presents "Public Opinion about Public Heath—California and the United States." This report summarizes surveys conducted by two organizations, one a public health center in California and the other a national opinion polling firm, to measure support for public health activities. The findings indicate widespread support for community-oriented disease-prevention and health-promotion activities.

Derek Yach and Douglas Bettcher, both with the World Health Organization, Geneva, Switzerland, present a two-part feature on the globalization of public health. "The Globalization of Public Health, I: Threats and Opportunities" identifies the major threats and opportunities presented by the process of globalization and emphasizes the need for transnational public health approaches to take advantage of the positive aspects of global changes and to minimize the negative ones.

"The Globalization of Public Health, II: The Convergence of Self-Interest and Altruism" discusses the transnationalization of disease and health risks that will require global awareness, analysis, and action. It further indicates a need for global cooperation. A strong case can be made that enlightened self-interest and altruism will converge in the increasingly interdependent world being shaped by the process of globalization.

Barry S. Levy, director of Barry S. Levy Associates, presents the 1997 American Public Health Association Presidential Address, "Creating the Future of Public Health: Values, Vision, and Leadership." This address answers the following questions: What is public health? What are the trends? What do we need to do? Who do we need to be?

Martha Loustaunau, New Mexico State University, presents a very timely topic. "Becoming Culturally Sensitive: Preparing for Service As a Health Educator in a Multicultural World" examines a world of cultural diversity and mobile populations. Loustaunau reports that due to an increasing cultural mix of teachers and learners, health educators will be challenged to have the skills needed to bridge the culture gap and convey a culturally sensitive, caring, meaningful, and effective message.

❓ Questions ❓

Reading 1. _____ is the third most common disease reported by the survey respondents. According to Dr. Claude Lenfant, director of the National Heart, Lung and Blood Institute, "Americans are living longer, but they aren't living healthier." Explain this statement.

Reading 2. The Planned Approach to Community Health (PATCH) model emphasizes the principles of _____ in the development of health interventions. In 1991, the Joint Committee on Health Education Terminology defined community health education as _____.

Reading 3. According to respondents, the three top-priority public health services are _____. Opinion polling is used extensively as an adjunct to or in assessing contemporary public policy. Why is polling helpful?

Reading 4. Define _globalization_. Describe the health benefits of globalization for developing countries.

Reading 5. Globalization of public health means _____. In order to effectively address the transnationalization of health risks and diseases, what must be done?

Reading 6. What is public health? Explain how the ten trends that Levy identifies can be both dangers and opportunities.

Reading 7. Meeting the challenge of cultural sensitivity will require what? Define and describe _cultural relativity_.

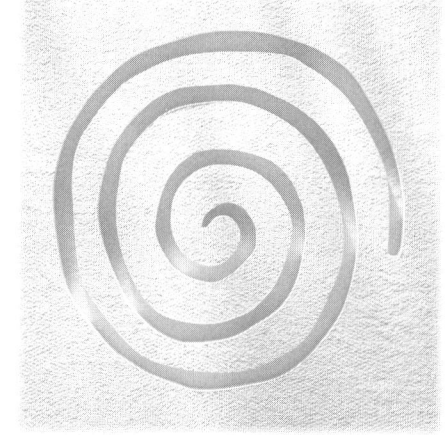

_____ is the third most common disease reported by the survey respondents. According to Dr. Claude Lenfant, director of the National Heart, Lung and Blood Institute, "Americans are living longer, but they aren't living healthier." Explain this statement.

How Healthy Are We?

Mark Clements and Dianne Hales

Health—what defines it, how to make it last and, increasingly, how to pay for it—has become a major concern for Americans. What are the leading killers? How closely do we follow what our doctors advise?

To learn more about Americans' thoughts on health, Parade surveyed a nationally representative sample of 1752 men and women, ages 18 and older.

Here is what we found:

Americans are feeling good about their health. Two-thirds of our survey respondents, in fact, told us that they're in "excellent" or "good" physical health. That's the good news.

The not-so-good-news is that many of us could be taking better care of ourselves—and we know it: 57% of our respondents describe themselves as overweight, 52% don't exercise, 26% smoke, and 39% do not get annual checkups. Yet 90% agree with the statement: "My physical well-being is in my hands."

"Americans are living longer, but they aren't living healthier," says Dr. Claude Lenfant, director of the National Heart, Lung and Blood Institute

in Bethesda, Md. "This is a country of free spirits. It's hard to get people to make changes now for the sake of how they'll feel in the future. Even though Americans feel fine now, if they don't take steps to reduce risk factors like obesity and high blood pressure, one of every two of us will develop heart disease in the future."

Our Top 10 Health Problems

Our findings may surprise you. The most common health problem cited by our survey respondents is *arthritis:* 25% of those surveyed say they have it. Women suffer from arthritis more than men (31% vs. 20%), and the likelihood rises with age, to 54% of those 65 and older. *High blood pressure* comes next, affecting 23%. Both sexes are equally affected, and it also increases with age, from 8% of those aged 18–34 to 49% of those 65 and older.

Depression is the third most common disease reported by our survey respondents; 14% say they became depressed in the last year (17% of the women and 10% of the men). In this case, the incidence is lowest among those 65 and older.

Asthma affects 9% of our survey respondents—more women (11%) than men (7%). Next comes *cancer.* About 8% of those surveyed—equal numbers of men and women—report having had some form of the disease other than skin cancer. The incidence of cancer also increases with age, from 2% of those aged 18–34 to 23% of those 65 and older.

Seven percent of our respondents have *heart disease,* with slightly more women (8%) reporting this problem than men (6%). The incidence of heart disease rises from less than 1% of those aged 18–34 to 22% of those 65 and older.

Six percent of the respondents have *diabetes,* which affects both sexes equally. And 5% report that they suffer from an *anxiety disorder,* with the rate higher among women (7%) than men (4%).

Finally, 4% of the respondents have had *skin cancer,* and 4% cite *alcoholism* as a personal health problem.

Who Are Healthier— Men or Women?

Backaches, colds and the flu affect both sexes equally. But women report higher rates of heartburn, arthritic pain, allergy,

Reprinted with permission from *Parade,* copyright © 1997, and from the authors, Dianne Hales and Mark Clements of Mark Clements Research, Inc.

- **Two-thirds of Americans** surveyed say they are in "excellent" or "good" health, yet one in five is afraid to go to the doctor.

- **The majority** (66%) say they would prefer to change their diets to treat a health problem, rather than to take medication.

- **Almost two-thirds** of us (64%) currently take medications, with 49% taking prescription drugs and 30% using over-the-counter medications.

- **Half of Americans** do *not* exercise—but 87% of us say that we should.

- **92% of those surveyed** have medical insurance. For 57%, it's managed care.

- **Sterilization** is the most popular form of birth control, chosen by 29%.

- **More women** than men go to doctors.

- **Assisted suicide** is supported by two-thirds of those surveyed.

- **16% have sought help** from mental-health professionals, but 59% of us have no faith in them.

- **We are most concerned** with having enough money or insurance to pay for a major illness or operation (49%) or for long-term care (46%).

- **43% of us self-medicate** to avoid paying for a visit to the doctor.

What We're Taking

More than six in 10 survey respondents say they currently take medications: 49% take prescription drugs, and 30% take over-the-counter preparations; 89% maintain that they "always follow the recommended dosage." More women (54%) than men (43%) use prescription drugs, and those aged 65 and older use the highest proportion of prescription drugs (76%).

Sixty percent of the survey respondents say, "If possible, I avoid taking any kind of medication." And 66% say they would prefer to change their diet to treat a medical problem, rather than to take medication.

Half of those surveyed take vitamins or supplements. Older respondents are much more likely to take vitamins: 59% of those 65 and older report taking vitamins or supplements, compared with 47% of those 18 to 34 years of age.

A third of the respondents say they get annual flu shots—but this figure more than doubles to 69% for those 65 and older.

acne, depression, bronchitis and urinary-tract problems. Women also are much more prone to headaches, with 61% (compared with 45% of the men) reporting that they had at least one headache in the last year. In fact, men are not significantly more likely than women to suffer from any of the top 10 health problems except one—alcoholism, with men outnumbering women 6% to 1%.

More men than women consider themselves healthy and fit. However, more women exercise regularly and say they have improved their eating behaviors. Yet, even though women pay more attention to what they eat, they are much more unhappy with their weight than men: 57% (compared with 45% of men) say they're very or somewhat dissatisfied with how much they weigh. Twice as many women as men have dieted to lose weight in the last 12 months.

Women use more health services than men. More women have a primary-care physician and go for a medical checkup every year. More than half of the women have been to a gynecologist in the last 12 months; 40% have had mammograms. Women use more home-testing kits—mostly for pregnancy—and take more prescription drugs (54%) than men (43%). And 70% of the women respondents examine their breasts, while just 28% of the men examine their testes.

"I'm not sure that if you looked at how men and women stack up in terms of health, you'd see any real differences," says Dr. Nancy W. Dickey, president-elect of the American Medical Association. "But there is a difference in awareness. Women are the caregivers and the managers of health information in the home. They're so ac-

customed to looking at their family and checking if they're not feeling well that they tune in to the same things in themselves. They also see doctors more for regular Pap smears, which is the perfect opportunity to check on other problems. What we need is the equivalent of an annual Pap smear for men to bring them into doctors' offices."

Our Greatest Fears

Weight is our No. 1 health concern—for the *present*, that is, and with good reason. Half of the survey respondents say they're dissatisfied with their weight (84% of those in poor health feel this way). On average, survey participants who describe themselves as overweight estimate that they are carrying 28 extra pounds.

"Obesity is this country's No. 1 public health problem," says Dr. Lenfant. "Americans may be watching what they eat, but the real issue is controlling the amount of food they put on their plates and becoming more active."

When asked, "What is your greatest personal health concern for the *future*?" the largest number of respondents (16%) say cancer, 15% say "heart problems," and 12% say "weight."

Are We Pushing Our Luck?

Americans have taken some steps toward healthier lifestyles, our survey finds. More than half of our respondents say they have changed to healthier eating habits, avoiding fats and eating more fruits and vegetables. But we still have a way to go. Consider:

About a quarter of the respondents (26%) smoke, averaging 1.1 packs of cigarettes a day. (Of those who currently smoke, 74% say they have tried to quit.) Young adults between 18 and 34 years of age who answered our survey are much more likely to smoke (30%) than those 65 and older (13%). More men (28%) than women (23%) smoke. And 12% of the respondents (21% of men and 3% of women) say they smoke cigars occasionally or regularly.

More than half of the respondents (56%) drink alcohol—although there are differences in the gender, age and marital status of those who do. The survey respondents most likely to drink are male

(65% drink), under age 35 (68%), and single (65%).

Half (50%) do not exercise, and nearly nine in 10 (87%) say they should exercise more than they do. Men aged 35 to 64 exercise less than younger and older men. Why don't we exercise more? The top reasons given by the sedentary respondents: "not enough time," "I'm lazy," and "I don't enjoy it." (For more on the survey and exercise, see "Parade's Guide to Better Fitness" on page 8.)*

About seven in 10 respondents (71%) say getting a tan is not worth the risk of skin cancer. However, only 34% proudly report, "I never go out in the sun without using sunscreen."

In terms of awareness and knowing about good health, I'd give Americans an A– or B+. But in terms of doing what we know we should, most of us—myself included—only deserve a C or C–."

—Dr. Nancy W. Dickey,
President-elect of the American
Medical Association

*Not included in this publication.

Almost half of the respondents (49%) say they are "very concerned" about being able to pay for a major illness or operation. Almost as many (46%) worry about the costs of long-term nursing care or in-home care. Says one survey participant, Andrew Mitrano, 62, a real-estate agent in Rochester, N.Y.: "Nobody should work all their life and then have an illness wipe out all their savings. I'm very happy with our healthcare system, but that's one thing that needs to be fixed." Nine out of 10 respondents have health insurance: 57% belong to a managed-care plan.

Older and Wiser

Eating and health habits improve with age: 77% of those 65 and older describe their eating habits

as "excellent" or "good," compared with 53% of those between 18 and 34.

Older Americans are less stressed and have made more changes to improve or maintain their health: Of those 65 and older, 71% say they are eating a healthy diet, 65% aren't smoking, and 37% are trying to relieve stress. And 59% take vitamins (compared with 47% of those aged 18 to 34). More than 80% of those 65 and older have a primary-care physician and go for a medical checkup every year.

Getting Help— and Paying for It

Nearly eight people in 10 (77%) have a primary-care physician whom they consider to be their main doctor: 83% are satisfied

with the care that the physician provides. Among the respondents who've been to each type of specialist, patients are most satisfied with their gynecologists, ophthalmologists, and cardiologists. More than one person in five (22%) has used an alternative-treatment method (most often chiropractic services) in the last three years.

More than half of the respondents (57%) participate in a managed-care plan: 17% have a "nonmanaged" health-care plan; and the others are covered by Medicare, Medicaid or another government health plan. About half are restricted to physicians available through their insurance provider, must get a referral from their primary physician before seeing a specialist and must meet a deductible. Of the respondents with health coverage, 65% obtain insurance through their employer, 18% through the government, 14% on their own, 4% through a union, and 3% through other group insurance plans.

When Your Health Is Good, So Is Your Sex Life

More than two-thirds of those surveyed (68%) are sexually active (74% of the men and 61% of women). And 77% of those who consider their health to be "excellent" are currently sexually active, compared with 50% of those in poor health. Among those 18 to 34 years old, 84% are sexually active. Among those aged 35 to 49, the percentage is almost as high—82%. But sexual activity drops off after age 50: Among those 50 to 64 years old, 58% are sexually active; among those 65 and older, only 28% are active.

Should Your Doctor Help You Die?

As we increasingly recognize the limitations of medicine, most of us believe we should be allowed to take things into our own hands, our survey indicates. Two-thirds of the respondents (66%) feel doctors should be allowed to help terminally ill patients die with dignity. The higher their income, the more likely the respondents are to feel this way: 76% among those earning $75,000 a year or more favor doctor-assisted deaths, compared with 59% of those earning less than $25,000. Men and women 65 and older are less likely to support this view. (About 53% do, compared with 69% of those aged 18 to 34.)

Eight in 10 respondents (80%) say that doctors should be allowed to withhold life support. But only about half (52%) think physicians should provide patients with the means to end their own lives, while 44% say doctors should administer the lethal medications.

Seven in 10 of those surveyed say they use birth control, with unmarried respondents (80%) more likely to use contraceptives than married ones (69%). Single respondents who have never married are most likely to use condoms and practice safe sex (58%). The birth-control pill is the contraceptive of choice for 17%, and the condom is also used by 17%. But the most popular option is sterilization—chosen by 29% overall (and by 36% of the married respondents).

Our Mental Health

More than eight in 10 respondents (85%) describe their mental health as "excellent" or "good." Yet anxiety and depression are not uncommon: 18% report that they often suffer from anxiety, while 14% say they've suffered from depression in the last year.

More than half of the respondents (56%) say there no longer is a stigma attached to seeking help for a mental problem. About 16% of the respondents have seen a mental-health professional for medical problems, family problems, problems with a partner or other troubles. Eight in 10 say that if insurance provided equal coverage for mental illness, more people would seek help for mental disorders. Yet nearly six in 10 respondents (59%) disagree with the statement. "I have faith in a mental-health professional's ability to solve my problems."

More than four in 10 respondents (43%) report experiencing stress often. The employed are much more stressed than the retired (49% vs. 20%). Nearly half (46%) say they are trying to relieve stress. And 91% agree that mental stress can cause physical ailments, with 70% saying that mental stress wears them out more than physical activity.

Nearly half (49%) of those who suffer from stress, a third (31%) of those with anxiety and a quarter (25%) of those with depression identified the major cause of their distress as "financial concerns." This was followed by "family problems." Overall, talking with friends is the most common way that our respondents deal with stress, but there are gender and age differences in the way people cope: Secondary to talking with friends as a coping measure, women say they talk with family; younger respondents (aged 18 to 34) say they listen to music; and men say they watch TV to relieve stress. Older respondents (over 50) are the least likely to talk with friends, preferring to watch TV.

When We're Hurting

Do we run to the doctor, reach for the medicine cabinet—or tough it out? The top three ailments for which we consult a doctor are eye problems (83% of respondents did so), bronchitis (78%) and urinary-tract problems (76%). To treat other ailments, our respondents often self-medicate. (See "Our Most Common Complaints . . . And How We Handle Them," on page 5.)*

"With the exception of headaches, which can have multiple causes, the health problems generally are self-limiting and do not go on to progress to more serious or life-threatening illnesses," says Dr. Laurel Dawson, an assistant clinical professor in the medical department of the University of California at San Francisco.

Overall, 43% of respondents say they self-medicate "to avoid paying for a visit to the doctor."

*Not included in this publication.

Parade's survey was conducted in February 1997 by the independent research firm of Mark Clements Research, Inc. The overall sample was selected to conform to the latest available U.S. Census data for men and women aged 18 and older. Of the 2568 questionnaires mailed out, 1752 were completed and returned, representing a response rate of 68.2%. The results are accurate to within plus or minus 2.4% at the 95% level of confidence. This report was prepared with the assistance of and additional reporting by Dianne Hales and with data analysis by Maria DeFrino.

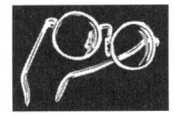 **Article Review Form at end of book.**

The Planned Approach to Community Health (PATCH) model emphasizes the principles of _____ in the development of health interventions. In 1991, the Joint Committee on Health Education Terminology defined community health education as _____.

The Future of Health Education:

The Knowledge to Practice Paradox

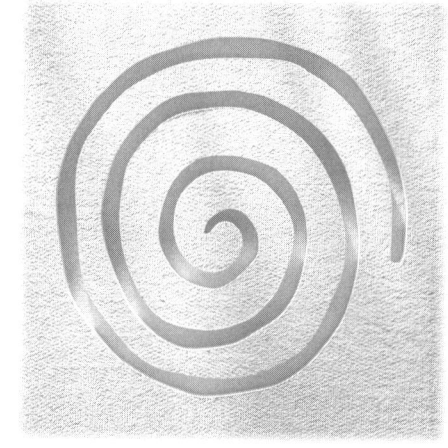

Gary M. English
and Donna M. Videto

Gary M. English is with Ithaca College, Ithaca, NY 14850. Donna M. Videto is with State University of New York at Cortland, Cortland, NY 13045.

Abstract

The challenge before us is to put into practice what the profession has known and professed for years. Regardless of our place of practice, our ability to identify and meet the needs of our local communities and neighborhoods is likely to be the measure that will determine our success as health educators. Social, demographic, political, and economic changes will force the way we deliver health education programming to change. Time, energy, and resources that are currently being directed to our site(s) of operation, i.e., schools, worksite, etc. are likely to diminish as the concept of "healthy communities" gains favor. With the establishment of national objectives, a professional credentialing process, and national standards, the profession is positioned to achieve great success. The collaborative efforts of our professional organizations have positioned the profession to move into the next century. In addition to these efforts, there is also a need to unify the profession to reduce the fragmentation and replication of professional services and to maximize the potential for professional growth.

For years a cry has been heard from a number of dedicated individuals working in the health promotion and education profession for clarity and focus to strengthen what, at times, appears to be a fragmented and categorical profession defined more by site of operation than by universal standards or theories. Recently, three nationally significant events have occurred that hold the potential to provide the profession with this clarity and unity. These events include publication of the document *Healthy People: National Health Promotion and Disease Prevention Objectives for the year 2000* (1991), establishment of the National Commission for Health Education Credentialing and the CHES credentialing process, and the recently released *National Health Education Standards: Achieving Health Literacy* (1995).

With these documents and adoption of entry level standards providing a vision of where we need to go, what prevents the health profession from reaching new heights, from achieving success in programming and promotional efforts, from seeing the sought after outcomes? The clarity, vision, and recommendations for the profession to move forward exist. Unfortunately, there is a tendency for health educators to have difficulty putting into practice what research indicates is needed. While the profession continues to "get its act together," a number of social and political changes are either occurring, or are about to occur, that will force health professionals to alter the way in which business is conducted. Population and demographic changes will impact

This article is reprinted with permission from the *JOURNAL OF HEALTH EDUCATION,* January/February, 1997, pages 4–8. The *JOURNAL OF HEALTH EDUCATION* is a publication of the American Alliance for Health, Physical Education, Recreation and Dance, 1900 Association Drive, Reston, Virginia 20191.

clientele and communities; movement in the political structure may limit future funding and shift discretionary power to state and localities; demands for accountability to justify program funding and continuation are being heard; and economic trends that result in demand for tax relief are being realized. Promoted as a return to the "basics," many of these trends have tended to put programming such as health education in a vulnerable and, at times, losing position.

In health education there tends to be the belief that knowledge leads to practice. As a profession, we know what has to be done to enhance the probability for programs to be successful. Ironically, much like the gap between knowledge and practice, we have either chosen to ignore this information or have simply failed to act upon it. In addition to addressing trends that are likely to have an impact on the profession, this article will revisit recommendations that have existed largely in the literature and less in practice, many of which can no longer be ignored.

Research to Practice

Recent literature often refers to the concept of grassroots or community efforts. The PRECEDE planning model (Green, 1986) and the Planned Approach To Community Health (PATCH) (Kreuter, 1992) clearly identify community involvement as the key to successful programming. Yet, all too often programs continue to be planned and implemented, ignoring the principle of community involvement.

In 1991, the Joint Committee on Health Education Terminology defined community health educa-

tion as "The application of a variety of methods that result in the education and mobilization of community members in actions for resolving health issues and problems which affect the community. These methods include, but are not limited to group process, mass media, communication, community organization, organization development, strategic planning, skills training, legislation, policy making, and advocacy" (p. 181). According to this definition, community health education should not focus on a single disease, i.e., AIDS or a single event, i.e., child immunizations, but emerge as a collaborative process intended to promote health and prevent disease through a combination of educational, political, organizational, and environmental changes as determined by members of the local community. This definition, although relatively new, contains information that has been in the literature for decades.

The concept of comprehensive school health education and the importance of parent and community involvement in the model has been discussed in professional journals since the mid 80s. Single or categorical programs alone, such as in the case of traditional school health, have demonstrated limited success in changing behavior, which is often stated as one of the primary goals of school health programming. However, when categorical efforts are combined with a community-wide approach, health interventions have been shown to have a greater impact on long-term behavior change (Flynn, Worden, Seckler-Walker, et al. 1992; Vartiainen, Fallonen, McAlister, et al., 1990).

As noted in the document *National Health Education Stan-*

dards: Achieving Health Literacy (Joint Committee on National Health Education Standards, 1995), the future of school health education requires a broader approach than the present model. In fact, the call for collaborative planning is a high priority in both the education and community standards presented in this document. Traditionally, school health education has been perceived as the focal point of health education, mainly because of the accessibility to children and the potential for effective prevention programming. However, the calls to integrate school and community health promotion efforts have largely been ignored by educators and the local public health community (Iverson, 1981). In 1988, Green stated that those working in the domain of public health viewed the schools as a channel of information transfer rather than an active partner in "community health" with the schools resisting the responsibilities and accountability that would come with that partnership (p. 1149). For whatever reason, "turf" lines often exist which prevent health educators from forming collaborative relationships. The time has come to address these barriers and create a stronger support base for a more comprehensive health education/ promotion community (Luebke & Bohnenblust, 1994).

Hits and Misses

As we approach the year 2000, there is little doubt that we will be successful in attaining a number of the objectives established by the document *Healthy People 2000* (1991). Clearly, the voluntary health agencies such as Heart, Lung, and Cancer have demonstrated the value of their efforts for the middle class population. School health programs, when provided with adequate resources and support, may also demonstrate success. However, we also need to consider the segments of the community that are not the mainstream middle class. In 1990, Mason stated that children, minorities, the economically disadvantaged, and the elderly need to be the main targets of health promotion endeavors, as the potential for health improvement is the greatest for these groups, and it is not possible to achieve our national goals without raising their health status. Identifying and promoting the value of targeting these groups is only the first step toward altering the quality of life for the underserved.

Many have held the perception of the United States as a "melting pot" where each individual would share similar language, values, and beliefs, which is clearly not the case. What has emerged is a society that expects each of us to acknowledge and respect the cultural norms of the diverse sub-populations that reflect contemporary society. Further, a number of health programs have been developed with the assumptions that everyone has at least a high school education, speaks English fluently, can read a newspaper, and is under the age of 60. Unfortunately this isn't the case. Hence, traditional programs often are not meeting the diverse needs of our society. As our profession prepares for the future, we must be cognizant of the dramatic changes that lie on the horizon and be ready to address the challenges associated with these changes.

From a sociocultural point of view, the literature points out that we have consistently missed the mark in meeting the needs of underserved populations. For example, school based health programs often are viewed as the primary avenue for educating our country's youth and the resulting adult population. It is estimated that only 20 percent of the American population is enrolled in public and private schools (O'Rourke, 1995). Yet, 80 percent of the American population is not being served by school based programming, and a segment of our young people which includes dropouts, homeless, and runaways do not have access to sorely needed programming. Other population groups such as immigrants and refugees may come to this country as adults and are beyond the reach or abilities of the schools. This problem of access is not limited to the schools; in the area of worksite health promotion, a relatively new area for health programming, already there are criticisms emerging that programs are not reaching the people who need them most (Edmunson, 1995).

Along with these changes the profession must consider the larger picture that will emerge as a result of additional demographic shifts. It is predicted that by the year 2000, through immigration alone, the U.S. population will increase by up to six million people with more than 25 percent of the U.S. population consisting of minorities, and that by 2080 approximately 51 percent of the population will consist of those who belonged to non-dominant groups (Andrews, 1992). In addition to this influx of new citizens, our aging population is also likely to impact our society and our profession. By the year 2030, it is estimated that there will be 55 million people over the age of 65. This will represent about 18 percent of the population compared with 11 percent in 1980 (NCHS, 1990). As outlined in *Healthy People 2000*, one priority for the nation's health is increasing the proportion of people age 65 and older who had the opportunity to participate in at least one organized health promotion program in a setting that serves older adults. We have known this and still have ignored the health needs and educational concerns of this population.

As these demographic changes occur, the profession must explore different, and more creative, approaches to providing health education and programming to the growing segments of minorities, underserved, and aging populations. A more diverse society will want, and expect, a different mix of programs, services, and support activities. To accomplish this, it is essential that active involvement from the stakeholders is sought throughout the planning and implementation process so that programs are appealing to those groups we are hoping to reach.

In addition to programmatic changes, the settings in which programs occur must also be considered. While computer and media technologies are quickly becoming more practical modes for information transfer, we cannot overlook the available, but less utilized, settings to reach these underserved populations. Settings such as churches, community centers, restaurants, and even airports offer avenues for reaching those considered difficult to reach. In reality we are limited only by our own creativity to identify ways to get information into the hands of those who need it most.

Program Advocacy

In addition to these changes in demography, we are experiencing political turbulence that is likely to impact funding and other avenues of support. House Republicans are expected to propose additional cuts in education spending in an attempt to trim the budget, and plans are to package many, if not most, education programs into one or several block grants (*Education Week*, 1995). If this approach is adopted, State governments will, at their discretion, distribute funds in ways that either help or hurt health education programs.

Historically, funding reductions have negatively affected programming such as health education, which often have been perceived as "extras" or "frills." To be recognized in the current political climate, it is vital that we advocate for our programs and successes at local, state, and national levels. Further, advocacy efforts are likely to require a unified voice which means not only coming together professionally, but also crossing sites of practice and working with school, community, public, and worksite health promotion programs. It is also likely that it will be necessary to recruit support from the larger pool of health professionals such as nurses, counselors, and physicians who share the prevention philosophy and are willing to assist us as we state our case.

Additionally, advocacy efforts must not overlook the aging segment of our population. With only 23 percent of adults having children in schools, educational leaders may no longer expect the public support they had when 60 to 70 percent of the population had school-aged children (Usdan,

1990). Yet, according to a 1994 study, nearly 84 percent of the population appear to support the concept of comprehensive school health education (Seffrin, 1994). Despite this popularity, school health programs easily become "political footballs." Because health, like athletics in most districts, is popular, it may be included with items that are considered "expendable" in hopes that voters will support these other, less popular, budget items included with health. The risk of a failed budget may result in the elimination or reduction of health education programming, or services in the schools.

Finally, as we advocate, it is important to keep in mind that we seek to improve the health status of all Americans. Unfortunately, but understandably, when jobs are being threatened there is a tendency to ask others to support mandates or other forms of legislation that are designed, primarily, to keep us employed. If we are able to objectively show the value of our programs and adopt the attitude that our proven results are deserving of merit, chances are that we will fare much better than if we continue the call for protection through mandated programs.

Community Empowerment

In a discussion of the origins of PATCH, Kreuter (1992) describes the principle of community participation in development of health interventions as embodying the concept of empowerment. If health promotion is the process of enabling people to increase control over and improve their health status, empowerment in some form is being stressed. But

empowerment of whom? Given the changes we face, communities must make decisions based on the assessments of health needs and resources in their respective environments. At present community based efforts, though well intended, often do not meet the needs as perceived by the target population. There have been criticisms that community based programs have been developed, and services provided, from the agency perspective and then offered to the community. When this occurs the community may need and use the service; however, it is not really empowered. This problem is not unique to community based programs and can be observed in nearly all health settings.

As health educators we are familiar and comfortable with the models and theories associated with program planning and evaluation. Unfortunately, we sometimes forget to come to the planning process with open minds. Rather than leading the process and listening to the needs as described by the populations we claim to serve we willingly assume a passive role during the planning process, or perhaps worst yet, in our quest to do what is "right," we implement programs based on personal knowledge or experiences.

To enhance this planning process, a paradigm shift in how site-specific health promotion/intervention programs operate may be necessary. In this model schools, community health agencies, workplace health promotion programs, and treatment facilities will have to put aside "turf" issues and expand their collaborative partnerships if they expect to continue to exist in the current economic and political climate. When a community chooses to address their health concerns, the process they adopt is likely to be quite different, from an urban inner city to a rural or suburban district, from a labor intensive worksite to a highly technological workplace, each program must be constructed and tailored to meet the individual needs of their particular community. Regardless of the health education delivery agent, or the community receiving the intervention, the primary focus should be one that results in an improvement of the health status of the community. In fact, it is possible that the only clear outcome that will be consistent from one community to the next is the outcome of improved health status.

The Role of Credentialing

Although there is a need to share leadership and decision making with the community we are attempting to empower, there is also a need for competent and committed leadership. Without committed leadership, programs may lack cohesion, direction, and outcome. The skills needed to accomplish these outcomes are not new to health educators, in fact they are identified in the entry level responsibilities for health educators as described by the National Commission for Health Education Credentialing.

If it is our desire to have others recognize the value of what we do, we need to assume leadership roles in the planning, implementation, and evaluation of health education programs. To create this recognition we need to embrace the concept of credentialing to assure those outside the profession that those who do hold the credential possess the knowl-edge and skills needed to apply the research into their practice.

The areas of responsibilities established by the National Commission for Health Education Credentialing clearly establish that content is not the sole focus of what we do. Unfortunately, health educators, particularly school based educators, perceive the dissemination of content as the "process of health education." Too often the focus has been on health content; i.e., sex and drug education, nutrition, physical fitness. When addressing the controversial and crisis-oriented topics associated with health education, it is easy to get caught up in "doing health education." Each of these issues are important aspects of health that should not be ignored. However, how many other professions can lay legitimate claim to these content areas? Nurses, substance abuse counselors, physical educators, and even law enforcement officers presenting content in any one of these areas are suddenly labeled and perceived to be health educators. Although this perception of others as health educators is bothersome to some, the reality is that the content being addressed truly is interdisciplinary in nature.

Clearly there is a need for school based practitioners to recognize the skills outlined in the responsibilities for entry level certification. Too often school health practitioners view teaching certification as the only credential important to their profession. In a random sample selected from the list of 3,400 CHES individuals certified as of September 1991, less than 15 percent of the respondents worked in the schools; the majority worked in community and medical care settings (Birch & Pearson, 1995). Not surprisingly, as we consider the documented effectiveness of school site programs, they pale in comparison to the success claimed by many of the high profile community based programs. Several studies have provided examples of effective community based approaches, such as the North Karelia Project (Puska et al., 1985), the Stanford Three-Community Study (Farquhar et al., 1977; Flora, Maibach, and Maccoby, 1985), the Stanford Five City Study (Farquhar et al., 1985), the Minnesota Heart Health Program (Mittlemark et al., 1986) and the Pawtucket Heart Health Program (Lansater et al., 1984). The findings from these community-based approaches generally have been positive. The common element in all of these programs appears to be related to the emphasis on community participation in all aspects of the projects.

Luebke and Bohnenblust describe how the discipline will be strengthened by a comprehensive training of future practitioners that prepares health educators without a distinction between practice settings (1994). Professional preparation programs need to focus upon the commonalties within the different sites of practice in order for health educators to deliver comprehensive, collaborative services with the potential to meet the needs of a changing society. Results of such preparation would provide the health educator with more options for selecting a work setting and for movement between those settings (Luebke & Bohnenblust, 1994). This approach to professional preparation could help eliminate some turf battles and thus bridge the existing gap between community and schoolsite health.

Conclusion

In 1990 O'Rourke described the need for the profession to grow and diversify. "In order to achieve our mission, we should continue to expand to meet the needs of health educators and promote health education in diverse settings. These include not only the K–12 schools, but also college/ university, public/agency, and community settings; clinical/ medical care, patient and business settings" (p. 4).

Since the 1980s, nearly all of our professional organizations have become less competitive and more cooperative. Although professional allegiances are strong and philosophical differences exist, health education needs to emerge with a unified voice. In order for us to achieve our mission, all health educators regardless of site of practice, must feel represented by a unified professional organization. The work of each professional organization has been quite good. However, the works that have been the most meaningful and have received the most acclaim are the projects where collaboration was clearly evident. Success of this cooperation is evident in projects such as establishment of National Standards, The Healthy Communities Project, and the CHES credentialing process via the Role Delineation Project.

It is imperative that we begin to provide meaningful opportunities for local involvement with the intent to hear and shape health education. Open forums, focus groups, key informant interviews, and stake holder involvement on advisory boards are but a few of the strategies that can make that happen. Only by hearing and using what our clients have to say can we truly provide the leadership needed to make our work, and ultimately our profession, successful.

If we are to enhance the image of our profession, gain credibility, achieve a stronger voice, and be awarded the respect given the treatment side of health care, professional collaboration and unification is essential. Together we can move to develop curricula and programs based on research aimed at meeting the needs of a diverse and changing society. Our success, and our future as a profession, will likely be reflected in how well we put research into practice.

Andrews, M. M. (1992). Cultural perspectives on nursing in the 21st century. *Journal of Professional Nursing, 8,* 7–15.

Birch, D. A., & Pearson, V. M. (1995). Continuing education interests of certified health education specialists. *Journal of Health Education 26*(3), 167–172.

Edmunson, J. M. (1995). Special populations in worksite health promotion: Focusing on underserved employees. In D. D. Dejoy, & M. G. Wilson (Eds.), Critical issues in worksite health promotion. Needham Heights, MA: Allyn & Bacon, p. 222.

Education Week. (April 5, 1995). Volume 14(28) pp. 1, 34–35.

Farquhar, L., Maccoby, N., Wood, P. D., Alexander, J. K, Breitrose, L., Brown, B. W., Haskell, W. L., McAlister, A. L., Meyer, A. J., Nash, J. D., & Stern, M. P. (1977). Community education for cardiovascular health. *Lancet, 1,* 1192–1195.

Farquhar, L., Fortmann, N. C., Maccoby, D. L., Haskell, W. L., Williams, P. T., Flora, J. A., Taylor, C. B., Brown, B. W., Soloman, D. S., & Hulley, S. B., (1985). Stanford five-city project: Design and methods. *American Journal of Epidemiology, 122,* 323–334.

Flynn, B. S., Worden, J. K., Seckler-Walker, R. H., et al. (1992). Prevention of cigarette smoking through mass media intervention and school programs. *American Journal of Public Health 82*(6), 827–834.

Green, L. W., Kreuter, M. W., Deeds, S. G., & Partridge, K. B., (1980). *Health education planning: A diagnostic approach.* Palo Alto, CA: Mayfield.

Green, L. W. (1988). Bridging the gap between community health and school health. Editorial in the *American Journal of Public Health, 78*(9), p. 1149.

Hayden, J. (1992). Prepared for Certification: Senior health education majors' perceived competencies. *Journal of Health Education, 23*(6), 341–343.

Iverson, D. C., (1981). Promoting health through the schools: A challenge for the eighties. *Health Education Quarterly, 8,* 6–10.

Joint Committee on Health Education Terminology. (1991), *Journal of Health Education, 22*(3), 175–183.

Joint Committee on National Health Education Standards, (1995). *National health education standards achieving health literacy.* American Cancer Society, Publication 95-50M, No 2027.

Kreuter, M. W., (1992). PATCH: Its origin, basic concepts, and links to contemporary public health policy. *Journal of Health Education, 23*(3), 135–139.

Luebke J. K., & Bohnenblust, S. E. (1994). Responsibilities and competencies: Implications for health education professional preparation programs. *Journal of Health Education 25*(4), 227–229.

Mason, J. O., (1990). A prevention policy framework for the nation. *Health Affairs 9*(2), p. 26.

Mittlemark, M. B., Luepker, R. V., Jacobs, D. R., Bracht, N. F., Carlow, R. W., Crow, R. S., Finnegan, J. G., Grimm, R. H., Jeffery, R. W., & Kline, F. G. (1986). Community-wide prevention of cardiovascular disease: Education strategies of the Minnesota health program. *Preventive Medicine, 15,* 1–17.

National Center for Health Statistics. (1991). Health, United States, 1990 (DHHS Publication No. PHS 91-1232). Hayattsville, MD: Public Health Service.

O'Rourke, T. W. (1990). Challenges, opportunities, and future directions: Constancy and change. *Health Education, 21*(3), 4–5.

O'Rourke, T. W. (1995). Creating Capacity: A research agenda for school health education, *Journal of School Health, 65*(1), 33–37.

Puska, P., Salonen, J. T., Nissinen, A., Tuomilehto, J., Koskela, K., McAlister, A., Kottic, T. E., & Maccoby, N. (1985), The community-based strategy to prevent coronary heart disease: Conclusions from the 10 years of the North Karelia project. *Annual Review of Public Health,* 1990. Palo Alto, CA: Annual Reviews, Inc. 6, 147–193.

Seffrin, J. A. (1994). Americans interest in comprehensive school health education. *Journal of School Health 64*(10), 397–399.

Usdan, M. D. (1990). Restructuring American educational systems and programs to accommodate a new health agenda for youth. *Journal of School Health, 60*(4), 139–141.

U.S. Department of Health and Human Services. (1991). *Healthy people 2000: National health promotion and disease prevention objectives.* Washington, DC, DHHS Pub. 91-50212.

Vartiainen, E., Fallonen, U., McAlister, A. L., et al. (1990). Eight-year follow-up results of an adolescent smoking prevention program: The North Karelia youth project. *American Journal of Public Health, 80*(1), 78–79.

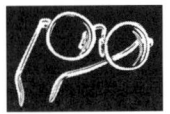

Article Review Form at end of book.

According to respondents, the three top-priority public health services are _____ . Opinion polling is used extensively as an adjunct to or in assessing contemporary public policy. Why is polling helpful?

Public Opinion about Public Health—California and the United States, 1996

Reported by K. Bodenhorn, MPH, California Center for Health Improvement, Woodland Hills, California. H. Taylor, Louis Harris and Associates, Inc., New York. Office of the Director, Public Health Practice Program Office, Centers for Disease Control.

Despite widespread belief that public support is critical to the success of public health programs and agencies, systematic efforts to measure public opinion about public health have been limited. This report summarizes surveys conducted by two organizations—one a public policy center in California, the other a national opinion polling firm—to measure support for public health activities. The findings indicate widespread support for community-oriented disease-prevention and health-promotion activities.

California Survey

From September 30 through November 5, 1996, the Field Institute of San Francisco (with consultation by Louis Harris and Associates, Inc.) conducted a random-digit-dialed telephone survey of California residents aged ≥18 years; the survey was commissioned by the nonprofit California Center for Health Improvement and was funded by The California Wellness Foundation.[1] A representative sample of 4803 persons was interviewed. The standard error associated with the results of this survey was ±2% at the 95% confidence level.

The percentage of respondents who reported that selected public health services were "top priority" ranged from 29% (for collecting community health data) to 84% (for ensuring safe drinking water). The percentage who reported delivery of these services as "very effective"

ranged from 18% (for providing community education and counseling services about improving health) to 37% (for minimizing the spread of disease carried by insects or animals) (Table 1). Selected local and state fees or tax increases were supported by substantial proportions of respondents if funds were needed to pay for what the survey instrument termed as "adequate programs" (Table 2). Most respondents preferred that funds for public health services be raised at the state level instead of at the local level (Table 2). The sources of revenue for those services that were most supported by respondents were increases in state taxes on alcoholic beverages and tobacco. Most respondents opposed state surtaxes on health insurance premiums (72%), local residential property taxes (64%), and local sales taxes (57%). Respondents supported the existing state requirements that nonprofit health-care providers fund community

From *Morbidity and Mortality Weekly Report,* February 6, 1998 (Vol. 47, No. 4), pp. 69–73.

| Table I | Percentage of Survey Respondents Who Reported That Selected Public Health Services Were "Top Priority," and Percentage Who Reported Delivery of These Services As "Very Effective"—California, 1996* |

	% Respondents	
Public Health Service	**Top Priority**	**Very Effective**
Ensuring safe drinking water	84	34
Ensuring that foods are free from contamination (e.g., through restaurant and produce inspections)	77	33
Protecting the public from exposure to toxic chemicals and other hazardous materials (e.g., monitoring the disposal of industrial and medical wastes and after oil spills)	75	29
Protecting the public from the spread of communicable diseases (e.g., AIDS, hepatitis, and tuberculosis)	74	22
Helping treat disease and injury after natural disasters (e.g., earthquakes, wildfires, and floods)	65	30
Providing community education and counseling services about improving health (e.g., through nutrition education programs, alcohol- and drug-abuse programs, and tobacco prevention programs)	53	18
Minimizing the spread of disease carried by insects or animals (e.g., rabies)	49	37
Collecting community health data (e.g., registering births, determining causes of deaths, and monitoring health trends)	29	19

*Results of a random-digit-dialed telephone survey of California residents aged ≥18 years (n = 4803 respondents) (1). The survey was conducted by the Field Institute of San Francisco, with consultation by Louis Harris and Associates, Inc.; the survey was commissioned by the nonprofit California Center for Health Improvement and was funded by The California Wellness Foundation. The standard error was ±2% at the 95% confidence level.

health programs (84%) and that nonprofit health-care providers that convert to for-profit status be required to dedicate funds to promote health (82%). In addition, most respondents indicated support for a statewide initiative for a 63¢ per pack increase in cigarette tax (i.e., 72% strongly or somewhat favored the increase).

National Survey

During December 12–16, 1996, Louis Harris and Associates, Inc., conducted a national-digit-dialed telephone survey of 1004 U.S. residents aged ≥18 years (2). This survey was conducted for the Harris Poll column, which is syndicated to the media but is not commissioned by any one client. The standard error associated with the survey was ±3% at the 95% confidence level. The response rate was 62%.

Respondents were asked to rank the importance of eight services "to improve the health of the public" on a five-point scale (i.e., very important, somewhat important, not very important, not at all important, or did not know). The percentage of respondents who rated specific public health services as very important ranged from 56% (for helping persons cope with stress) to 93% (for preventing the spread of infectious diseases) (Table 3).

Respondents also were asked "Who do you think should be mainly responsible for the performance of prevention rather than the treatment of disease." Most (57%) respondents indicated that government should be responsible for this service; and

Table 2 Preferred Sources of Revenue for Improving Community Health Promotion and Disease and Injury Prevention Programs and Environmental Health Services, by Percentage of Survey Respondents—California, 1996*

Source of Revenue	% Respondents		
	Favor	Oppose	Did Not Know
Increasing state taxes on tobacco products	81	18	1
Increasing state taxes on beer, wine, and other alcoholic beverages	78	21	1
Expanding tax deductions for contributions to charities and other nonprofit organizations	72	24	4
Increasing state income taxes for persons earning >$200,000 per year	68	29	2
Increasing city developer fees on builders of new homes	59	38	3
Increasing local taxes on business property	53	43	4
Increasing local sales taxes	41	57	2
Increasing local taxes on residential property	33	64	3
Charging a surtax on health insurance premiums paid by businesses and persons	24	72	4

*Results of a random-digit-dialed telephone survey of California residents aged ≥18 years (n = 4803 respondents) (1). The survey was conducted by the Field Institute of San Francisco, with consultation by Louis Harris and Associates, Inc.; the survey was commissioned by the nonprofit California Center for Health Improvement and was funded by The California Wellness Foundation. The standard error was ±2% at the 95% confidence level.

Table 3 Percentage of Survey Respondents Who Reported That Selected Public Health Services Were "Very Important" or "Somewhat Important"—United States, 1996*

Public Health Service	% Respondents	
	Very Important	Somewhat Important
Preventing the spread of infectious diseases (e.g., tuberculosis, measles, influenza, and AIDS)	93	7
Vaccinating to prevent diseases	90	9
Delivering medical care to ill patients by doctors and hospitals	85	13
Improving the quality of education and employment	83	14
Ensuring persons are not exposed to unsafe water supply, dangerous air pollution, or toxic waste	82	15
Conducting medical research on the causes and prevention of disease	82	15
Encouraging persons to live healthier lifestyles (e.g., eat well, exercise, and not to smoke)	72	24
Helping persons cope with stress from the problems of daily living and work	56	34

*Results of a random-digit-dialed telephone survey of U.S. residents aged ≥18 years (n = 1004 respondents) (2) conducted by Louis Harris and Associates, Inc., for the Harris Poll column, which is syndicated to the media but is not commissioned by any one client. The standard error was ±3% at the 95% confidence level.

40%, that "someone else" should be responsible. Of those persons who responded that government should provide this service, 53% stated that the federal government should do so; 32%, the state government; and 13%, city and local governments.

When asked the open-ended question, "What do the words 'public health' mean to you?," <4% of respondents gave answers corresponding to what the Harris Poll considered "generally . . . regarded as referring to public health" (i.e., health education/ healthier lifestyles, prevention of infectious diseases, immunization, and medical research).[2] Eighty-three percent of respondents identified one or more of the following: general physical health, mental health, and well-being of the public; the health-care system; welfare programs; universal health care; health assurance; health insurance; and Medicaid and Medicare.

Editorial Note: Opinion polling is used extensively as an adjunct to or in assessing contemporary public policy. Polling can help to clarify the perceived importance of issues and the impact of advocacy campaigns and other factors on public support for, or opposition to, policies. The survey conducted in California identified 1) substantial support for public health services and 2) substantial support for taxes, if necessary, to achieve more effective public health programs and services. Although findings from the national survey were consistent with findings from the California survey about support for public health services, the national survey did not address financial concerns.

The findings in this report are subject to several limitations. First, the results of the two surveys were not directly comparable because the samples were drawn from different populations, the questions differed, and the results were reported in different formats. Second, each survey gauged public opinion at a specific point in time; therefore, the reported opinions could not be linked to contextual, secular events. Other limitations associated with survey methodology (e.g., refusals to be interviewed, wording and order of questions, and interviewer bias) also apply to the results of these two surveys.

Interest in marketing public health has been stimulated by perceived low public support for public health activities, limited financial resources, and the impact of extensive restructuring in the health-care sector. The findings in this report indicate

substantial public support for public health services and suggest the need to determine the extent to which this support is consistent across jurisdictions and whether it can be translated into policy. Finally, these findings suggest the need for strengthened methods to improve the polling of opinion about public health, including clarifications of the distinction between clinical care and community- or population-oriented disease and injury prevention, and the practical meanings of "public health," "community health," and other key terms.

References

1. California Center for Health Improvement. Spending for health: Californians speak out about priorities for health spending. Sacramento: California Center for Health Improvement, 1997.
2. Louis Harris and Associates, Inc. 'Public health': two words few people understand even though almost everyone thinks public health functions are very important. New York: Louis Harris and Associates, Inc., 1997.

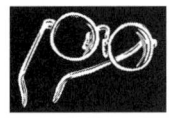 **Article Review Form at end of book.**

Define *globalization*. Describe the health benefits of globalization of developing countries.

The Globalization of Public Health, I:

Threats and Opportunities

Derek Yach, MPH, MBChB, and Douglas Bettcher, MD, PhD, MSc

The authors are with the World Health Organization, Geneva, Switzerland.

Abstract

The globalization of public health poses new threats to health but also holds important opportunities in the coming century. This commentary identifies the major threats and opportunities presented by the process of globalization and emphasizes the need for transnational public health approaches to take advantage of the positive aspects of global change and to minimize the negative ones. Transnational public health issues are areas of mutual concern for the foreign policies of all countries. These trends indicate a need for cross-national comparisons (e.g., in the areas of health financing and policy development) and for the development of a transnational research agenda in public health. (Am J Public Health. 1998;88:735–738)

A web of trade, investment, diplomacy, grassroots action and telecommunications is forging a global village from which our sense of commitment to the other half is strengthened.[1]

Globalization and liberalisation are a fast, new express train and countries have been told that all they need to do was to get on aboard. . . . Those that fail to get aboard will find themselves marginalised in the world community and in the world economy.[2]

The double face of globalization, one promising and the other threatening, is a fact of life as humanity is being catapulted into a more interdependent future and a new millennium. Globalization not only refers to economic processes or the development of global institutions but also describes the interconnection between "individual life" and "global futures."[3] More specifically, globalization is defined as the process of increasing economic, political, and social interdependence and global integration that takes place as capital, traded goods, persons, concepts, images, ideas, and values diffuse across state boundaries.[4] The roots of globalization can be traced back to the industrial revolution and the laissez-faire eco-

nomic policies of the 19th century. However, the globalization of the late 20th century is assuming a magnitude—and taking on patterns—unprecedented in world history.[5,6] It not only embraces the liberalization of financial markets and trade but encompasses transboundary problems such as destruction of the ozone layer.[7]

The link between the lives of individuals and the global context of development is evident in another face of globalization, an often forgotten one: global health futures are directly or indirectly associated with the transnational economic, social, and technological changes taking place in the world. As a result, the domestic and international spheres of public health policy are becoming more intertwined and inseparable.

Since the achievement and maintenance of the health of populations is an integral part of sustainable development, the health impacts of globalization, both positive and negative, are key policy issues. Health development in the 21st century must take advantage of the opportunities afforded by global change and, at the same time, minimize the risks and

Reprinted by permission from Derek Yach and Douglas Bettcher, Tobacco Free Initiative, World Health Organization, 20 Ave Appia, Geneva 27 CH-1211, Switzerland.

threats associated with globalization so that the dramatic improvements in the health of the world's population achieved in this century can be maintained and advanced in the next one. The main theme of this paper is that the challenges posed by globalization make collective action imperative and mutually beneficial.

The Globalization of Public Health

The health benefits to developing countries of increased trade, diffusion of appropriate technologies, and acceptance of human rights throughout the world were emphasized by Roemer and Roemer in 1990.[8] According to the Roemers' analysis, cross-national exchanges have facilitated the diffusion of technological innovations such as effective methods of contraception, techniques for obtaining safe drinking water, low-cost refrigeration, efficient transport and communication technologies, and new therapeutic agents that can effectively treat leprosy, schistosomiasis, trachoma, onchocerciasis (river blindness), and many other diseases. Nevertheless, the Roemers also recognized some of the negative aspects of trade liberalization for health, such as the U.S. threat of trade sanctions against 4 Asian countries in the 1980s if American cigarette companies were not given free access.[8]

The perception of the world has shifted a great deal in the few years since the Roemers' important commentary. The end of the Cold War and of a world characterized by 2 competing social/political systems has unleashed massive global changes. With these changes, our health development paradigm—in other words, our road map for seeing the world—must also shift. This trans-

formed world is characterized by increased competition for market share, liberalization of trade and finance, and global communications. In the health sector, for example, the liberalization of health services under the provisions of the General Agreement on Trade in Services has the potential to blur the boundaries between national and "globalized" health sectors. (The General Agreement on Trade in Services is the first set of multilateral rules governing fair and nondiscriminatory trade in services. It was one of the major components of the Uruguay Round package.) Transformations such as these are generating "powerful transnational dynamics" and suggest that we are on the verge of a "global health village" in which some health problems primarily concern particular countries, while others are of common concern.[9] Moreover, national health systems are becoming transnationalized: the ease and rapidity of communications have facilitated the diffusion of ideas, ideologies, and policy concerns relating to health care (as well as diseases), thereby fostering a global culture of reform.[10]

The domain of globalization includes many interconnected phenomena and risks that affect the sustainability of health systems and the well-being of the populations of both developing and industrialized countries. Although not intended to be a complete list, the transnationalization of health risks and disease is depicted in Table 1. (Refer to a recent article by John Last[11] that evaluates the quality of evidence for various health-related features of global change.)

At the same time, it should not be assumed that the implications of globalization for public health are all negative. Seriously addressing the risks and negative

aspects of increasing global interdependence could help to sustain the process of economic and political globalization. Many of the risks cited in Table 1 could be turned into opportunities for improving our global health future. For instance, if modern information technologies are accessible and affordable to developing countries, the potential benefits are extensive: the uses of modern information technology in health include telemedicine, interactive health networks, communication services between health workers, human resource development and continuing education, and distance learning.[12] However, making these technologies available in the poorest communities of the world may require special government incentives, including incentives that could be at odds with norms governing liberalization of trade and removal of special subsidies.[13]

Adoption of proactive policies that protect essential health system functions from downsizing and privatization would ensure that core components of national health systems are protected as a matter of public safety. Another positive intervention would involve the global media, which could play a major role in health promotion in terms of preventing a portion of the estimated 10 million deaths per year (70% in developing countries) that are expected to occur from smoking-related diseases in year 2020.[14] The global media could also help to reverse the disastrous effects that smoking-related deaths will have on the health and economies of both developing and industrialized countries.

Policy Implications

The policy implications of globalization and transnational trends were one of the major themes of

Table 1 Health and Global Change

Global Transnational Factor	Consequences and Probable Impact on Health Status
Macroeconomic prescriptions	
Structural adjustment policies and downsizing	Marginalization, poverty, inadequate decreased social safety nets,[a]
Structural and chronic unemployment[20]	Higher morbidity and mortality rates[b]
Trade	
Tobacco, alcohol, and psychoactive drugs	Increased marketing, availability, and use[b]
Dumping of unsafe or ineffective pharmaceuticals	Ineffective or harmful therapy[b]
Trade of contaminated foodstuffs/feed	Spread of infectious diseases across borders[b]
Travel	
More than 1 million persons crossing borders/day	Infectious disease transmission and export of harmful lifestyles (e.g., high-risk sexual behavior)[c]
Migration and demographic	
Increased refugee populations and rapid population growth	Ethnic and civil conflict and environmental degradation[c]
Food security	
Increased demand for food in rapidly growing economies, for example, countries in Asia	Structural food shortages as less food aid is available and the poorest countries of the world are unable to pay hard currency[b]
Increase in global food trade continuing to outstrip increases in food production, and food aid continuing to decline[21]	Food shortages in marginalized areas of the world; increased migration and civil unrest[a]
Environmental degradation and unsustainable consumption patterns	
Resource depletion, especially access to fresh water	Global and local environmental health impact[b]
Water and air pollution	Epidemics and potential violence within and between countries (water wars)
Ozone depletion and increases in ultraviolet radiation	Introduction of toxins into human food chain and respiratory disorders
Accumulation of greenhouse gases and global warming	Immunosuppression, skin cancers, and cataracts[22]
	Major shifts in infectious disease patterns and vector distribution (e.g., malaria), death from heat waves, increased trauma due to floods and storms, and worsening food shortages and malnutrition in many regions of the world[22]
Technology	
Patent protection of new technologies under the trade-related aspects of intellectual property rights agreement	Benefits of new technologies developed in the global market are unaffordable to the poor[c]
Communications and media	
Global marketing of harmful commodities such as tobacco	Active promotion of health-damaging practices[b]
Foreign policies based on national self-interest, xenophobia, and protectionism	Threat to multilateralism and global cooperation required to address shared transnational health concerns[c]

[a]Possible short-term problem that could reverse in time.
[b]Long-term negative impact.
[c]Great uncertainty.

last year's Denver Summit of the Eight (G-8). The leaders of the major industrialized countries observed the following:

The process of globalization, a major factor underlying the growth of world prosperity in the last fifty years, is now advancing rapidly and broadly. More openness and integration across the global economy create opportunities for increased prosperity. . . . At the same time, globalization may create new challenges. The increasing openness and interdependence of our economies, with deep trade linkages and ever greater flows of private capital, means that problems in one country can spill over more easily to affect the rest.[15]

The G-8 summit stressed that countries must collaborate in confronting shared problems such as climate changes, environmental health issues, the spread of infectious diseases, trafficking in illicit drugs, and ethical issues surrounding technological developments such as cloning. Unilateral efforts will not be successful.

As the world becomes more interdependent, the objectives of national foreign policies will need to be reexamined; traditional concepts of national security based on the ability to resist armed aggression are being supplemented by notions of "shared human security."[16] For instance, the control and surveillance of communicable diseases has become a matter of preventive diplomacy.[17] In a similar vein, World Health

Organization Director-General Hiroshi Nakajima notes that

foreign policies based on narrow interests of isolationism and protectionism will reduce the creative spirit of international scientific investigation. . . . The global [health] development strategies needed to address these complex and inter-related problems will require innovative, intersectoral interventions, involving a high degree of international cooperation and political will.[18]

As part of renewing the health-for-all policy for the 21st century, the World Health Organization proposes that governments will need to work together to develop a broader base for international relations and collaborative strategies that will place greater emphasis on international health security. A draft of a new policy being developed by the organization emphasizes that addressing the threats to health security should include the health consequences of trade in commodities harmful to health, violations of human rights, transnational disease threats, environmental degradation, migration and population growth, and inequities between and within countries.[19]

These shared areas of foreign policy concern must be translated into well-defined strategies. The following are needed to deal with the major transnational health issues[6,19]:

- Global intersectoral action through transnational cooperation and partnerships, for example, between the health sector and trade/finance sectors both within countries and at the international level.

- An enhanced role for international legal instruments, standard setting, and global norms.

- More comprehensive forms of global vigilance, research, monitoring, and assessment. Information on health status and the global determinants of health is vital for defining future actions in a rapidly changing policy environment.

- Global research programs that concentrate on developing cost-effective technologies to improve the status of the poor.

- Human resource development in certain underdeveloped areas (e.g., public health law).

- Ongoing comparative assessments and cross fertilization of experiences regarding health system reform.

In conclusion, national health systems are increasingly being influenced by global factors that transcend state borders. These trends call for cross-national comparisons of health systems; this will allow for the sharing of information and the development of a transnational research agenda. Moreover, the globalization of public health will act as a strong impetus for global actions to address these areas of shared concern.

References

1. Speth JG. Europe provides a guide to shrinking the world's rich-poor gap. *International Herald Tribune.* February 3, 1997:6.
2. Corea G. Globalization—the opportunities and dangers for Sri Lanka. *Daily News* (Colombo, Sri Lanka). December 11, 1996:8.
3. Giddens A. Anthony Giddens on globalization. *UNRISD News.* 1997; 15:4–5.
4. Hurrell A, Woods N. Globalization and inequality. *Millennium J Int Stud.* 1995;24(3):447–470.
5. Ruggie R. At home abroad, abroad at home—international liberalization and domestic stability in the new world economy. *Millennium J Int Stud.* 1995;24(3):507–526.
6. Bettcher D. *Think and Act Globally and Intersectorally to Protect National Health.* Geneva, Switzerland: World Health Organization; 1997. WHO document PPE/PAC/97.2
7. Bonvin J. Globalization and linkages: challenges for development policy. *Development.* 1997;20(2):39–42.
8. Roemer M, Roemer R. Global health, national development, and the role of government. *Am J Public Health.* 1990;80:1188–1192.
9. Chen L, Bell D, Bates L. World health and institutional change. In: *Pocantico Retreat, Enhancing the Performance of International Health Institutions.* New York, NY: Rockefeller Foundation; 1996:9–21.
10. Altenstetter C, Björkman JW. Globalized concepts and localized practice: convergence and divergence in national health policy reforms. In: Altenstetter C, Björkman JW, eds. *Health Policy Reform, National Variations and Globalization.* London, England: Macmillan; 1997:1–16.
11. Las, JM. Human health in a changing world. In: *Public Health and Human Ecology.* 2nd ed. Stamford, Conn: Appleton & Lange; 1998:395–425.
12. *Health Informatics and Telemedicine.* Geneva, Switzerland: World Health Organization; 1997. WHO document EB99/INF.DOC./9.
13. Adams O. *International Trade in Health Services: Some Key Issues.* Geneva, Switzerland: World Health Organization; 1997.
14. *Tobacco Alert: The Tobacco Epidemic, a Global Public Health Emergency.* Geneva, Switzerland: World Health Organization; 1996.
15. *Final Communique of the Denver Summit of the Eight.* Denver, Colo.: Group of Eight Countries; 1997.
16. Alleyne G. Health and national security. *Bull Pan Am Health Organ.* 1996;30:158–163.
17. O'Brien E. The diplomatic implications of emerging diseases. In: Cahill KM, ed. *Preventive Diplomacy.* New York, NY: Basic Books; 1996:244–268.
18. Nakajima H. Global health threats and foreign policy. *Brown J World Aff.* 1997;IV:319–332.
19. *Health for All in the 21st Century.* Geneva, Switzerland: World Health Organization; 1998, WHO document EB101/8.
20. Martikainen P, Valkonen T. Excess mortality of unemployed men and women during a period of increasing unemployment. *Lancet* 1996;348:909–912.
21. *Food Security Assessment.* Rome, Italy: Food and Agricultural Organization; 1996. FAO document WFS 96/TECH/7.
22. McMichael AJ, Haines A, Sloof R, Kovats S, eds. *Climate Change and Human Health—An Assessment Prepared by a Task Group on Behalf of the WHO, WMO and UNEP.* Geneva, Switzerland: World Health Organization; 1996.

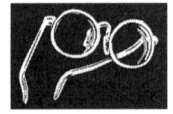 **Article Review Form at end of book.**

Globalization of public health means _____ . In order to effectively address the transnationalization of health risks and diseases, what must be done?

The Globalization of Public Health, II:

The Convergence of Self-Interest and Altruism

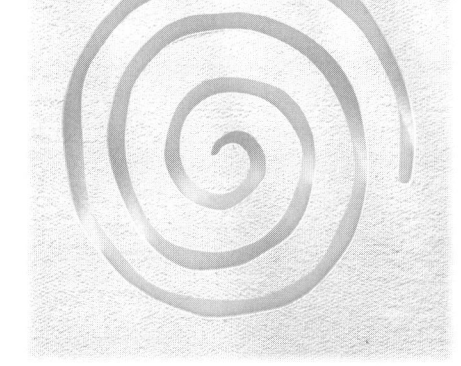

Derek Yach, MPH, MBChB, and Douglas Bettcher, MD, PhD, MSc

The authors are with the World Health Organization, Geneva, Switzerland.

Abstract

The transnationalization of disease and health risks will require global awareness, analysis, and action and indicates a need for global cooperation. Transnational actions must be built on firm local and national foundations, but they also require new forms of transnational collaboration in order to minimize risks and build on opportunities. In a world characterized by the globalization of public health, countries and communities will need to look beyond their narrow self-interests in defining and confronting the shared problems that are emerging. In fact, a strong case can be made that enlightened self-interest and altruism will converge in the increasingly interdependent world being shaped by the process of globalization. (Am J Public Health. 1998;88:738–741)

Introduction

The globalization of public health means that global awareness, analysis, and action must be improved in the coming century. It also means that charting a different course of development for the coming century is an ethical imperative, for this and future generations. Addressing future health challenges will require coordinated responses at many levels: individual, family, community, national, and global.[1]

The development of transnational actions will need to be supported by a strengthened educational and research capacity extending to schools of public health, health sciences faculties, and research bodies. At the global level, influential nations such as the United States should use their strengths to build partnerships for health for the 21st century in key areas of global concern. This will require that countries and communities go beyond narrow self-interests in order to address the problems and take advantage of the opportunities of globalization.

Although national action remains vital, transnational action needs to complement "domestic" initiatives. However, this will not happen if states cloak themselves in policies that attempt to insulate and shield them from transnational threats.

The Need for Global Awareness, Analysis, and Action

The spread of bovine spongiform encephalopathy (BSE, or "mad cow disease") to cattle herds in many European countries in exported feedstuffs and the risk that this agent may pass through the food chain to humans provide an important lesson of what may happen when international vigilance, cooperation, and action fail. When international vigilance and action break down, as in the case of BSE, governments may find themselves in a de facto quarantine.[2] Moreover, the BSE experience demonstrates that in an interdependent world, international strategies are needed for promoting health. The following

Reprinted by permission from Derek Yach and Douglas Bettcher, Tobacco Free Initiative, World Health Organization, 20 Ave Appia, Geneva 27 CH-1211, Switzerland.

analysis maps out a global strategy for avoiding such unfortunate errors.

Awareness

There is a need for all health professionals and the general public to receive information regularly about the health consequences (both positive and negative) of globalization in order to promote awareness of the transnational dimensions of health. This information should be based on sound empirical analysis. Particular attention needs to be given to understanding the consequences of national policies and actions for health in "far-off" lands. Koop's[3] statement concerning the United States' use of Section 301 of the 1974 trade act provides a good example of such action at a distance:

The inconsistency between U.S. tobacco trade policy and U.S. health policy increasingly is obvious and denounced in the international health community. . . . At a time when we are pleading with foreign governments to stop the export of cocaine, it is the height of hypocrisy for the U.S. to export tobacco.

Prospects for effective global health advocacy have profoundly improved with the development of new communications technologies and the growth of the global media. These opportunities have yet to be fully harnessed. Modern communication information networks can provide a vehicle for developing world public opinion concerning, for instance, environmental issues, trade and health problems, and the health repercussions of "downsizing" and health system reform. The global media can help to illuminate health concerns that have not been given sufficient attention.

However, the media's attention span is very limited. Therefore, mechanisms need to be developed to translate awareness of global health problems and advocacy for change into long-term action. Specifically, an independent transnational organization, a "global health watch," could be established as a tool for advancing global health awareness and vigilance. Such an organization could also monitor and assess, on a regular basis, how well governments, United Nations agencies, nongovernmental agencies, and even the private sector fulfill their health development commitments.[4]

Action

In order to effectively address the transnationalization of health risks and diseases, efficient information and surveillance systems are a top priority. Although monitoring and surveillance require and are dependent upon strong local and national systems, global capacity is also essential. For many health threats such as infectious diseases, international risk assessment of the cross-border food trade, and trade of harmful commodities, monitoring systems are already evolving. In the area of infectious diseases, the World Health Organization is in the process of strengthening its global monitoring and alert systems, which will link together specialized laboratories and disease surveillance systems from all countries via electronic and printed media.[5] More specifically, in the case of foodborne diseases, collaboration between European countries in the Salm-Net project provides a shared mechanism for laboratory surveillance of *Salmonella*, thereby alerting member countries about food safety problems transcending state borders.[6] In this regard, however, it is important that global early warning systems exist that are not confined to a small group of industrialized countries.[7]

In other areas, such as the monitoring of health risks associated with tobacco use, a critical mass of data is being collected. For example, the *1997 Tobacco or Health: Global Status Report*[8] compiled, for the first time, economic, social, legal, and other health information from 190 countries pertaining to the tobacco epidemic. Nevertheless, available data concerning the dynamics of the tobacco trade and the potential effects of trade liberalization on the global burden of disease associated with tobacco use are poorly documented.[9] In other areas of trade, such as trade in health services, data are scant.[10] Important areas of transnational action such as these pave the way for a shared global research program and implementation strategy for public health in the coming century.

The tools of surveillance and research must be augmented by international instruments (i.e., norms and standards). Although it is generally recognized that the need for "global norms and commitments (sometimes reflected in legally binding instruments)" will become more important as global interdependence accelerates,[11] it is ironic that international public health law instruments are so poorly developed and that educational capacity is at only a rudimentary stage of development.[12] International legal experts have observed that better use of international legal instruments in public health would encourage the development of national health legislation, thereby helping to achieve improved global health outcomes in the 21st century.[13]

Various international legal instruments (in addition to existing/proposed public health law;

Table 1 Examples of International Public Health Law

International Instrument	Purpose	Obligation of Signatory States	Executing Body	State of Development
International health regulations	International control of communicable diseases	Binding international instrument	WHO	Adopted by WHA in 1948
Codex codes of practice and guidelines	Standards and recommendations for countries on food safety	Standards binding on acceptance by countries; recommendations nonbinding	FAO/WHO Codex Alimentarius Commission	Codex program established in 1962
International code on marketing of breast milk substitutes	Promotion of breast-feeding and regulation of marketing of breast milk substitutes	Nonbinding recommendations	WHO	Adopted by the WHA in 1981
Framework tobacco convention	Facilitation of national and international tobacco control strategies	Binding multilateral convention on ratification	WHO	Proposed in Resolution WHA49.17 and now in the planning stages

Note: WHO = World Health Organization; WHA = World Health Assembly; FAO = Food and Agricultural Organization.

Table 1[14,15]) encompassing multilateral treaties, specific health conventions, international/world health charters, international codes and standards, regional arrangements incorporated into a legal regime over a period of time, and/or the incorporation of disease control strategies as an international human rights issue[16] could be used to address the problems associated with globalization. Moreover, international agreements such as the United Nations Convention on the Rights of the Child have proven to be an invaluable advocacy tool for advancing the health needs of the world's children.

The public health community could learn a great deal from those involved in international environmental law, an area where the development of legal instruments to protect the global common good is gathering momentum. For instance, Global Legislators for a Balanced Environment (GLOBE) comprises 300 parliamentarians who aim to create a "web of global governance" for environmental protection.[17] Legal instruments and regulatory principles, such as the "polluter pays" principle and

"imposition of nondiscriminatory charges, taxes (e.g., carbon taxes), and various economic incentives" to encourage consumers and producers to conform with environmental standards,[18] have been placed on the international policy agenda, even if international compliance cannot yet be assured.

Moreover, the environmental sector has been more successful than the health sector in getting environment issues onto the World Trade Organization policy agenda. In particular, the Uruguay Round negotiations committed to a widened scope to deal with issues not included in previous trade negotiations; trade and environment issues were placed at the top of this list. The Marrakesh ministerial declaration confirmed the establishment of the World Trade Organization Committee on Trade and the Environment, which was commissioned to examine issues including the export of domestically prohibited goods, the relation between the General Agreement on Tariffs and Trade dispute settlement system and international environmental agreements, environmental measures having an impact on trade, and the relation

between the environment and market access.[19] No such recognition of the health sector was made, and no World Trade Organization committee on trade and health exists.

It is unrealistic to assume that global norms and legal instruments in health (or, for that matter, in any other policy domain) will develop into an extensive body of enforced norms and principles as in domestic law. Rather, the globalization of law will likely be confined to "a narrow, limited set of specialized phenomena."[20] The reform of the international legal system will be confined to shared areas of concern that "generate globally parallel legal responses."[20] This does not, however, mean that enforceable public health instruments are not possible at the global level. Already, "globally common and enforceable rules are beginning to emerge."[20] A circumscribed area of relevant global public health law is a practical, obtainable, and desirable goal.

Vigilance

The 3 approaches discussed here need to be seen as operating simultaneously. Anticipation should be based on systems of constant vigilance over the key determinants of health and their influence on health status. Health monitoring and active surveillance systems need to be expanded worldwide to include economic, trade, agricultural, climatic, and other data in order to provide better predictions of future threats to populations. Governments have a vital role in creating an enabling environment for these intersectoral links to occur. Similar sentiments were expressed recently by British Prime Minister Tony Blair, who called on the member states of the European Union to focus on "issues that matter to people [such as] public health, fraud and the environment."[21] The "knee-jerk political responses"[21] in Europe to the BSE problem underscore that the public health community needs to prioritize multisectoral approaches that focus more on the "risk factors associated with diseases and determinants of health."[21] These strategies require that a global public health workforce be educated to meet new interdisciplinary challenges.

Why Should Countries Think Beyond Their Own Self-Interests?

One of the crucial questions remaining unanswered is the following: Why should powerful countries such as the United States look beyond their own narrow self-interests with regard to transnational public health policy?

The Institute of Medicine's recently published report *America's Vital Interest in Global Health*[22] provides an extensive overview of transnational health problems and argues that the "direct interests" of the American people are served when the United States promotes world health. The institute bases its arguments for a more extensive engagement in world health on 3 key U.S. interests: protecting America's population, enhancing the economy, and advancing America's international interests. The report concludes that the United States should lead from its "unsurpassed" position of strength in the health sector. In partnership with other countries and international organizations, the United States can lend a great deal in the areas of research and development, surveillance, education and training, and coordination and leadership.

The importance of international engagement in a globalized world has also been emphasized in other countries, such as Canada. According to a recent report, *Connecting with the World: Priorities for Canadian Internationalism in the 21st Century*,[23] "withdrawal and disengagement make no sense in this age of global markets; global pollution and climate change; changes to the role of the nation-state; of refugees, ethnic hostility, violence, and mass migration; and the growing poverty and intractable disease that does not respect international borders." In this transnational context, it is concluded that Canada's foreign policy is only an enlargement of "national" policy issues, and thus, investment in transnational partnerships to address these issues is in the country's self-interest.[23] Similarly, in developing countries such as South Africa, the economic value of supporting health and development initiatives in other areas is appreciated. In this case, healthy populations will be able to trade more vigorously with South Africa, thereby allowing for industrial development in areas of Africa currently beset with disease

and malnutrition. Similar motivations were behind the U.S. support for malaria control and for development of the yellow fever vaccine so necessary for Central American development projects.[24]

There is also a strong case to be made that the rationale for countries to become engaged in world health development is not only reducible to enlightened self-interest. In an increasingly interdependent world, it can be argued that "altruism" and enlightened self-interest converge. For instance, continued wealth in industrialized countries is not sustainable against a backdrop of poverty, disease, and warfare in many of the world's poorest countries.[23] These problems will have spillover effects for the richest countries. Therefore, in a world of shared global problems, the moral imperatives of addressing these problems also bring mutual benefits. The urgent need to forge knowledge partnerships between rich and poor countries so as to develop an effective, affordable malaria vaccine, which would primarily benefit the poorest areas of the world, is an example of such an "altruistic" project. President Clinton's recent resolve to launch a global research campaign to develop an AIDS vaccine within 10 years is a good example of public health optimism. Another positive step is reflected by the current commitment of the United States to shift its foreign policy to place more emphasis on crucial global issues such as environment, science, and technology.[25]

Our Global Health Future

The common health challenges facing the world community have the potential to enhance international cooperation in a community of sovereign states. This is because international cooperation strengthens the political will of governments by bringing to bear on health problems the power of the international community. We as public health practitioners and policymakers must respond in a timely manner or we will be left in the dust of these sweeping changes. Figure 1* provides one possible vision of a rejuvenated public health for the 21st century. Issues of shared global security (mutually assured progress) need to replace the pessimism of the mutually assured destruction of the darkest Cold War days. In this development scenario, fortresses of military independence are replaced by a shared interest in building human and social capital and reducing cross national disparities in terms of health and disease risk.

In the future, if humanity is to maintain and improve upon the unparalleled gains of the 20th century, we will have to accept the following:

We are increasingly confronted, whether we like it or not, with more and more problems which affect mankind as a whole, so that the solutions to these problems are inevitably internationalised. The globalization of dangers and challenges—war, chaos, self-destruction—calls for a domestic policy which goes beyond parochial or even national items. Yet, this is happening at a snail's pace.[26]

Soon we will begin a new millennium. To ensure the health and well-being of future generations, it is ethically imperative that present generations not continue to address transnational policy issues at a "snail's pace."

*Figure not included in this publication.

References

1. Susser M, Susser E. Choosing a future for epidemiology: eras and paradigms. *Am J Public Health.* 1996;86:668–673.
2. McKee M. Deregulating health: policy lessons from the BSE affair. *J R Soc Med.* 1996; 89:424–426.
3. Koop E. *Tobacco Colonialism Threatening Thailand.* Bangkok, Thailand: Moh-Chao Ban Publishing House; 1990.
4. *A New Global Health Policy—An NGO Perspective.* Geneva, Switzerland. World Health Organization; 1997. WHO document WHO/PPE/PAC/97.3.
5. Nakajima H. Global health threats and foreign policy. *Brown J World Aff.* 1997;IV(1):319–322.
6. Käferstein FK, Motarjemi Y, Bettcher DW. Foodborne disease control—a transnational challenge. *Emerg Infect Dis.* 1997;3:503–510.
7. *Food Safety Considerations in the Revision of the International Health Regulations (IHR).* Geneva, Switzerland: World Health Organization; 1997.
8. *1997 Tobacco or Health: Global Status Report.* Geneva, Switzerland: World Health Organization; 1997.
9. Yach D. Settlement in the USA; benchmark or global sell out? Presented at the Fourth International Conference on Preventive Cardiology, June–July 1997, Montreal, Quebec, Canada.
10. United Nations Conference on Trade and Development. Issues to be considered for inclusion in the proposal for UNCTAD-WHO collaboration. Presented at the World Health Organization Interagency Consultation on the New Global Health Policy, July 1997, Geneva, Switzerland.
11. *The Nordic UN Reform Project: The United Nations in Development—Strengthening the UN through Change: Fulfilling Its Economic and Social Mandate.* Oslo, Norway: Nordic UN Reform Project; 1996.
12. L'hirondel A, Yach D. Develop and strengthen public health law. *World Health Stat Q.* In press.
13. Shattuck HF, Roemer R, Connor S, Curran WJ. American Bar Association report (recommendations and reports): World Health Organization. *Int Lawyer,* 1996;30:686–695.
14. Fluss S. International public health law: an overview. In: Detels R., Holland WW, McEwen J, Omenn GS, eds. *Oxford Textbook of Public Health,* 3rd ed. Oxford, England: Oxford University Press Inc: 1996:371–389.
15. *International Framework Convention for Tobacco Control. Resolution WHA49.17.* Geneva, Switzerland: World Health Organization; 1996.
16. Fidler D. Globalization, international law, and emerging infectious diseases. *Emerg Infect Dis.* 1996;2(2):77–84.
17. *Home from Sophia—The Environment for Europe Process after the Latest Ministerial Conference.* Brussels, Belgium: Globe European Network; 1996.
18. Delbruck J. Globalization of law, politics, and markets: the implications for domestic law: a European perspective. *Global Leg Stud J.* 1993;1:9–36.
19. Schott J, Buurman J. *The Uruguay Round—An Assessment.* Washington, DC: Institute for Health Economics; 1994.
20. Shapiro M. The globalization of law. *Global Leg Stud J.* 1993;1:37–64.
21. Belcher P, Mossialos E. Health priorities for the European intergovernmental conference—long term, multisectoral issues rather than knee jerk political responses. *BMJ.* 1997;314:1637–1638.
22. Institute of Medicine. *America's Vital Interest in Global Health—Protecting Our People, Enhancing Our Economy, and Advancing Our International Interests.* Washington, DC: National Academy Press; 1997.
23. Strong MF, Austin J, Brodhead T, et al. *Connecting with the World. Priorities for Canadian Internationalism in the 21st Century.* Ottawa, Ontario, Canada: International Development Research Centre; 1996.
24. Yach D. Addressing Africa's health needs: time for strong South African involvement. *S Afr Med J.* 1998;88:127–129.
25. Wirth T. Science, technology, and foreign policy. *Science.* 1997;277:1185–1186.
26. Brandt W, The Independent Commission on International Development Issues. *North-South: A Programme for Survival, Report of the Independent Commission on International Development Issues.* London, England: Pan Books; 1981.

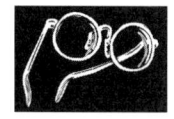 **Article Review Form at end of book.**

What is public health? Explain how the ten trends that Levy identifies can be both dangers and opportunities.

Creating the Future of Public Health:
Values, Vision, and Leadership

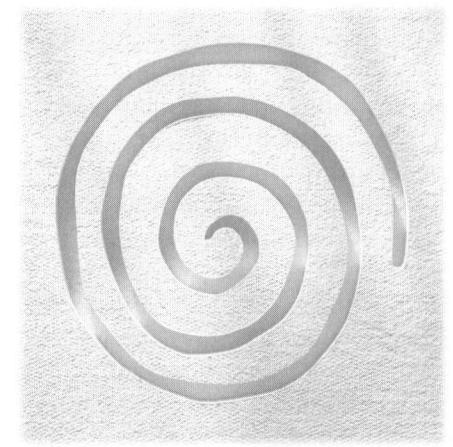

Barry S. Levy, MD, MPH

Barry S. Levy is Director of Barry S. Levy Associates, Sherborn, Mass; Adjunct Professor of Community Health at Tufts University, School of Medicine, Boston; and Immediate Past President of the American Public Health Association.

In 1872, Dr. Steven Smith and 9 colleagues founded the American Public Health Association (APHA), and we are very grateful to all of them today. In 1921, at the 50th annual meeting of the Association, Dr. Smith returned, at the age of 99, to give the principal address. He was very pleased that APHA had been contributing, and was continuing to contribute, in many ways to public health. If Dr. Smith and the other co-founders were with us today, they would be astounded at the many contributions APHA has made, and continues to make, to improving the public's health, not only here in the United States, but also throughout the world, by advancing public health policy, by stimulating public support for public health, and by improving public health practice.

But Dr. Smith and the other cofounders would probably be dismayed that the question asked most frequently of many of us is "What is public health?" How many of you have been asked that question at least once? How many of you have been asked it 10 or more times? How many of you have been asked it 100 or more times? I am among you, for I have had to answer that question hundreds of times.

What Public Health Is

In response to those who ask this question, I say that public health is a whole series of activities that are designed to promote health, to prevent disease and injury, to prevent premature death—to assure conditions in which we all can be safe and healthy. And I tell them that many public health activities are invisible—you do not see them, but you see their results throughout the day.

I tell them that all of us use the public health system daily, whether we know it or not. We get up in the morning, turn on

the faucet, and know that our water is safe. That is public health—that is the result of public health. And, if we are fortunate, that water is also fluoridated—that, too, is public health. We sit down at the breakfast table and eat a more nutritious breakfast, and there are even "Nutrition Facts" on the cereal box. That, too, is public health. We get into our cars (or, better yet, onto our bicycles) to go to work or school or elsewhere, and those cars are less polluting and safer, with air bags, seat belts, child restraints. Not only are these features present, but we and people across the country are more likely to use them. All of that is public health. And when we get to work, even though our workplaces still have many hazards, they are much safer today than ever before and much safer than those in many other countries. That, too, is public health.

Many other parts of our daily lives, such as our healthier exercise patterns, are the results of public health. Our access to comprehensive quality health care

From *American Journal of Public Health,* February 1998 (Vol. 88, No. 2), pp. 188–192. Reprinted with permission from The American Public Health Association.

that provides not only diagnosis, treatment, and rehabilitation but also preventive services—that, too, is public health. All of the community-based preventive services that prevent disease and injury and promote and protect health are critical parts of public health. So are education, research policy analysis and development, and the organizational infrastructure that supports it all.

All of this is public health, and most of it is invisible. We don't see it unless there is a crisis—an outbreak of foodborne disease (*E. coli* in the meat or hepatitis A virus in the school-lunch dessert), an increase in diabetes, a flood, an episode of community violence, or a war.

When I tell people what public health is, I sometimes add the Institute of Medicine's definition from *The Future of Public Heath* report published approximately 10 years ago: "Public health is what we, as a society, do collectively to assure the conditions in which people can be healthy." It takes a society to practice public health.

The Harris Poll

A Harris Poll performed in December 1996 reinforced my experience that few people know what public health is. Louis Harris Associates asked a random sample of approximately 1000 people across the country several questions about public health. In fact, they asked, "What is public health?" Only 3% of those questioned, perhaps representing those of us who work in public health, responded correctly with answers like "health education," "health promotion," and "immunization." Ninety-seven percent of those questioned did not know what public health is.

Many respondents said that public health is health care for the indigent. It should therefore not surprise us that many of our elected officials believe that when you move so-called indigent people into private-sector managed care programs, there is no need for public health anymore. Some of these officials believe that we have wiped out all the serious health problems of the earlier part of the century. "Who needs public health?" And, indeed, in several communities in Texas and Colorado and elsewhere across the country, health departments have even been closed until the public has cried out, "We need public health!"

The Harris Poll also provides some good news: More than 90% of the same people, when asked, "Do you support communicable disease control? Do you support immunization?" answered, "Yes." When asked about clean air, clean water, control of toxic waste, more than 80% said they support efforts to achieve these goals. When asked about safer lifestyles (and, in other surveys, when asked about controlling youth access to tobacco), more than 70% said, "Yes, we support that." So there is a paradox, or a huge disconnect, here: Only 3% of the American people know what public health is, but the vast majority support the goals, the values, and even the principles of public health. Clearly, we need to give much more attention to putting the public back into public health. It takes a society to practice public health.

For the rest of my presentation, I will focus on creating the future of public health. The future of public health is not in a crystal ball somewhere; it is not some predetermined fate that we live out. Instead, as APHA Past President Dr. Bill Foege often

says, we create the future of public health together. We have the capabilities to create the future we want in our society—and, indeed, throughout the world. To accomplish this, we must engage the public in public health. At the same time, we also need to understand some major trends that are occurring and will continue to occur which will have a profound impact on the future of public health as we create it with all of society.

Ten Trends: Dangers and Opportunities

Each of the following trends holds dangers and opportunities—serious dangers for the health of the public as well as serious opportunities for us to improve the health of the public.

I. Changes in the Financing and Organization of Health Care and Other Health and Human Services

Many changes are occurring, from so-called "welfare reform" (or "welfare repeal," as some of you call it), to for-profit conversions of community hospitals, to the growth of managed care. Clearly, managed care is neither an evil nor a panacea. It does provide, however, many opportunities for public health agencies and managed care organizations—and all the health professionals within them—to work together much more closely on improving not only the care of the "covered," or enrolled, populations, but also the health of all society.

At the same time, many of us are very concerned that, increasingly, we have a system of market-driven health care. "Products" are replacing "services," cost containment is replacing compassion, stockholders are replacing stakeholders. We should be concerned about all of this. And we should be concerned that there are more than 40 million Americans—an additional 100,000 more each month—who are uninsured. Look at your own health care delivery plan—your own health insurance policy if you have one—and see what it says. For those of us who are insured, health insurance is very expensive and not at all comprehensive. It usually does not cover mental health, dental health, podiatric health, vision care, and other important services. We do not have a holistic health care system in this country. And we in public health should be very concerned about this.

2. The Increasing Recognition of Alternative and Complementary Health Care

More than one third of the U.S. population uses products such as minerals and vitamins and services such as chiropractic and acupuncture on an annual basis. How many of you or your family members use these products and services regularly? We in public health should be concerned that these products and services are evaluated for efficacy and safety, just like products and services in mainstream health care. At the same time, we should be building bridges to alternative and complementary health care providers; many people get their health care only from these providers. We should also have sensitivity to traditional healers and traditional health care, from which we in public health and in mainstream health care can learn much.

3. The Information and Communication Revolution

Breakthroughs in information and communications technologies present many dangers and opportunities. There are potential dangers, such as breaches in confidentiality of data and depersonalization of services. But there are enormous opportunities to gather, analyze, and use data better, to communicate better with other public health professionals, even those halfway around the world, and to engage the public in public health.

4. The Biotechnology and Genetics Revolution

Biotechnology offers great opportunities to improve the efficacy and safety of many of the things we do. For example, within a year or 2, biotechnology will enable us to administer 8 childhood vaccines in 1 dose. The human genetics revolution is moving forward very quickly as well. By the year 2005, the Human Genome Project will have determined the chromosomal location for all 75,000 to 100,000 human genes and we will be well on our way to knowing what each of them does. Ultimately, it is estimated that every human being will be determined to have, on average, 20 to 25 high-risk genetic traits.

There are important legal and ethical issues here. For example, do you want your government, your insurance company, even your family members to know your genetic code? Do you want your employer to have that information? We in public health need to get ahead of the wave, we need to be addressing the legal and ethical issues that are being raised by the genetics revolution, and we need to start doing this now.

5. Changes in Our Population

The United States has an increasingly diverse population.

Diversity is, indeed, the strength of our nation and the strength of our Association. We need to celebrate that diversity, and we also need to make sure that all types of health services are available to all people—no matter what their language, no matter what their culture, no matter what their immigration status.

At the same time, we need to prepare for the aging of the population. The fastest growing segment of the U.S. population is 85 years of age and older; by the middle of the next century, there will be 1 million people over the age of 100 in the United States. Aging presents important challenges and opportunities for public health professionals. We need to make sure that more attention is paid not only to preventing chronic diseases and injuries, but also to preventing the complications of these diseases and injuries once they occur. And we need to make sure that we work toward improving not only the length of life, but also the quality of life.

6. Changes in the Economy, Both in the United States and Abroad

Many economic indicators in our nation look wonderful: Wall Street is booming, our unemployment rate is low. However, most people are working longer hours—the average work week is now 47 hours; it was 41 hours a decade ago. Americans are certainly not living in the era of leisure that was anticipated at that time. Indeed, many parents are working 2 or more jobs, a fact that has profound impacts on the care of children and results in more and more "latchkey children" and more and more childhood public health problems because parents are working so much of the time.

We should also be concerned with the globalization of the economy. Yes, the gross national product is growing quickly in some "newly industrializing countries," but in many of them—Mexico, for example—the government is so desperate for economic development and people are so desperate for employment that they are willing to take jobs subject to unfair labor practices or health and safety problems, in companies that are polluting the environment. We should be concerned about all of this—sweat shops, child labor, contaminated air and water, the export of hazard. Not very long ago, 2 American companies exported a pesticide known to cause sterility in men, though it had been banned in the United States; they exported it to many less-developed, or "developing," countries. More than 25,000 men in those countries are now either sterile or have reduced fertility as a result of exposure to that pesticide. The export of hazard continues—tobacco, unsafe drugs, dangerous pesticides, toxic and radioactive wastes, hazardous industries. We in the United States need to do something about this.

7. The Changing Role of Government

Although there seems to be much government-bashing in the United States, in the Harris Poll that I previously mentioned approximately 3 out of every 5 people questioned supported government's taking the lead in public health. If we apply the political definition of a landslide vote, there is a "landslide" of people who want government to take the lead in public health by working closely with educational institutions, nongovernmental organizations, private-sector organizations, and other groups in society. Sometimes those people who complain the loudest about government's being too big or too costly are among the first people asking for government services. Ask public health professionals from Minnesota and North Dakota, who provided many necessary services during the flood crisis there last spring.

8. Unraveling of the Fabric of Our Society

Most of our civic and other nongovernmental organizations are in serious decline. On average, there is one third less participation in these organizations than there was 3 decades ago. These are the organizations where we communicate our public health message. These are the organizations where we engage the public in the work of public health, where we engage people in the public health issues that affect, or may affect, them or their families or their communities. We should be concerned about what is happening in these organizations, and we should work to strengthen them. One of the positive developments in recent years has been the establishment of the APHA Caucus on Public Health and the Faith Community, with the leadership of Dr. Caswell Evans. This is an important step in rallying behind these organizations and building bridges with them for better public health.

9. Deterioration of Our Sociocultural Environments

Throughout the world, sociocultural environments are being weakened. When I was growing up in Bayonne, New Jersey, I had 20 first-degree relatives living within 6 blocks of my home. How many of you grew up in a similar situation? Today, my parents are the only family members who live there; everyone else has died or is scattered across the country. Although we send e-mail messages, write letters, and see each other from time to time, it's not quite the same. Our sociocultural environments—our families, our neighborhoods, our communities—support the healthy attitudes and behaviors that we in public health most want to promote.

We need to be concerned about this trend, not only in this country but throughout the world. In many less-developed countries, it is typical for young men to go to the cities in search of jobs, leaving their families behind in the countryside. Their wives must cope with the physical, social, and psychological burdens of raising the family, and they must also provide some economic support. Meanwhile, the men face uncertainty of finding jobs and serious public health risks, from unsafe working conditions, to substance abuse, to sexually transmitted diseases, including HIV/AIDS. We need to help strengthen sociocultural environments, not only here in the United States but throughout the world.

10. A Crisis of Values

There is increasingly more apathy in our population about issues of social justice. The federal government spends a relatively trivial amount of resources for the poor, both at home and abroad. Author Marianne Williamson, in her book *The Healing of America*, says that the United States has created a system that "comforts the comfortable and afflicts the afflicted." Instead of waging a war on poverty, we seem to be waging a war against the poor. The gap between the rich and the poor in the

United States is the largest that it has been in 70 years; the gap between the rich and the poor globally has doubled in the past 30 years. There are many other gaps in social justice. Hubert Humphrey, former U.S. Senator from Minnesota, said that the moral test of government is how it treats people who are young, old, needy, sick, or physically or mentally disabled. We should use this measure to help determine public health needs and our responses to them.

All of us should be concerned about and understand these trends. We need to get ahead of the wave, so that we can not only react to these trends but also proactively create opportunities to improve the public's health.

What We Need to Do

The theme of our 1997 annual meeting, "Communicating Public Health," gives us 4 clues about what we need to do.

1. Listen

The first aspect of communication is listening. We need to listen to people in the communities we serve; we need to listen to what they believe is needed and wanted. We need to understand their perceptions of health and public health and what they see as their roles in public health.

2. Educate and Inform

It takes a society to practice public health, and I believe that an educated society will ultimately make the right decisions. We need to educate and inform the public in many different ways. We need to educate and inform people directly, where they work, where they live, where they play—in their communities and

in their homes. We also need to work more effectively with the media and to take advantage of "teachable moments." When parents have a newborn infant, there is a teachable moment when we can educate them about a whole range of preventive measures for good child care, such as immunization, good nutrition, and use of car seats and seat belts.

There are also teachable moments for society. When I was at the Hawaii Public Health Association (HPHA) meeting last year, for example, I learned that public health professionals in Hawaii took advantage of such an opportunity. At the time, "mad cow disease" was on the front pages of newspapers. When the reporters telephoned the HPHA, the Association said, "No, we don't have 'mad cow disease' here in Hawaii. But, before you hang up, you may be interested to know that multiply-resistant tuberculosis—also an infectious disease—is increasing in the state and so are HIV/AIDS and several other infectious diseases. And you should also know that the state legislature is about to 'reinvent' and downsize disease-control activities of the state health department, privatize the state laboratory, and close the University of Hawaii School of Public Health." Now, that is what I call taking good advantage of a teachable moment.

3. Advocate

We need to advocate for strong public health policies and programs and to teach ourselves and others how to advocate more effectively. Ms Byllye Avery, recipient of the 1995 APHA Presidential Citation, has said that we in public health are much too shy. We need to assert ourselves much more at the federal, state, and local levels.

We need to advocate not only for specific public health policies and programs, but also for support of the overall infrastructure of public health—the research institutions, the educational institutions, and the public health agencies, particularly at the state and local levels. We need to support the entire infrastructure and ensure that it is responsive to community needs. And our advocacy needs to be based on sound public health science.

4. Develop Partnerships

We need to develop partnerships, which are so critical in the work that we do—not only partnerships made with like-minded public health and health-related organizations, but also partnerships established by reaching out to all groups in society. I can give many examples of wonderful partnerships that I have see this past year while visiting many public health organizations, agencies, and institutions across the country. One example is in the state of Washington, where, when public health leaders develop the statewide public health plan, they have more than 500 community groups and other organizations and agencies not only give input into the development of the plan but also participate in its implementation. These groups have essentially "bought into" the plan. Public health professionals there and elsewhere really believe that it takes a society to practice public health, and they are indeed putting the public into public health.

A different kind of example comes from New Mexico, where public health professionals have even found common ground with the National Rifle Association on issues of educating parents and children about gun safety. I maintain that whatever are our differences with other groups, we can always find some common ground for the good of society. It takes a society to practice public health, and we cannot write off any person or any group.

Who We Need to Be

In addition to thinking about what we need to do, we should answer a question we usually do not consider "Who do we need to be?"

In answering this question, we should think about values, vision, and leadership.

Values

Values define us as a group of public health professionals; values draw many of us into public health in the first place. Ultimately, we often feel most passionate about values. General values include respect for human dignity, health and well-being, and quality of life. They include social justice and community responsibility—we are indeed our sisters' and brothers' keepers. We need to support these general values and also specific values, such as environmental justice and a woman's right to choose.

Dr. John Hurty, Indiana Secretary for Health and APHA President 85 years ago, said in his presidential address at our 1912 Annual Meeting that prevention was under-valued. Dr. Hurty became a champion for prevention, and today there are many champions for prevention in our Association. Like John Hurty, we must be champions for prevention. And we must be champions for social justice. We need to make sure not only that everyone has a slice of the pie; we need to make sure that everyone has access to the kitchen.

Vision

We need to have visions, visions of healthy and safe lives in healthy and safe communities— even visions that seem impossible. Robert Kennedy used to say often, "Some people see things as they are and ask, 'Why?' I dream things that never were and ask, 'Why not?' " We need to dream things that never were and ask "Why not?"

If it were not for the impossible-seeming visions of people 25 years ago, we would not have the progressive smoking policies that we have today—we would probably not be meeting in a smoke-free facility. If it were not for the visions, the seemingly impossible visions, of people 50 years ago, we would not be on the brink of worldwide polio eradication today. And if it were not for visions of people many years before, visions that appeared to be impossible, the American Public Health Association and many other health-related organizations, including our state and local public health associations, might not exist today. The philosopher Sören Kierkegaard once said, "Life can only be understood backwards, but it must be lived forwards." To do so effectively, we must have visions —even seemingly impossible visions—and the courage and persistence to see those visions come to reality.

Leadership

Finally, we need to have leadership—leadership that translates these values and visions into actual policies and programs. We need to call forth leadership, not only in ourselves, but also in others. We need to be leaders who not only do things right but also choose to do the right things. We

need to demonstrate what public health is all about—not only by what we say, but also by what we do. As Mahatma Gandhi said, "Be the change you want to see in the world."

About a year ago, a visiting professor from England visited Tufts University School of Medicine, where I have an adjunct faculty appointment. I told him, "We in public health are fighting to get a seat at the managed care table," and he responded, "We in England consider ourselves the table." At first, I thought his remark was arrogant, but I now see the wisdom in it. We in public health should, figuratively, be the table—for managed care and many other issues. Indeed, society gives us the mandate to be the table. We need to go out and listen to people, gather the relevant data, frame the issues, pose the questions, and bring everyone, or at least their representatives, to the table—our table.

We also need to have leaders who are not seeking credit for what they have accomplished but know that their acknowledgment is in seeing the fruition of their values, their visions, their leadership.

A wonderful poem from the Chinese tradition addresses these qualities of leadership:

Go to the people,
Learn from them,
Love them,
Start with what they know,
Build on what they have;
But of the best leaders,
When their task is accomplished,
Their work is done,
The people will remark,
"We have done it ourselves."

That's the kind of leadership we need to call forth.

Now, you may ask, "Where are the people who have these values, generate these visions, and provide this kind of leadership?" Of course, they are the people sitting in your chairs and your colleagues across the country. If not you, who? If not now, when?

Creating the Future of Public Health

So, as we move forward and create the future of public health together, let us remember the values that brought us into public health in the first place and not be afraid to articulate them, even in unfavorable political climates—to articulate them with passion, with courage, and with persistence.

Let us remember our visions—even seemingly impossible visions—for healthy and safe lives in healthy and safe communities.

Let us be the leaders of public health, leaders to shape the future of public health.

And let us not forget that it takes a society to practice public health, a society in which the public is in public health.

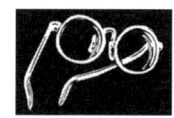 **Article Review Form at end of book.**

Meeting the challenge of cultural sensitivity will require what? Define and describe *cultural relativity*.

Becoming Culturally Sensitive:

Preparing for Service As a Health Educator in a Multicultural World

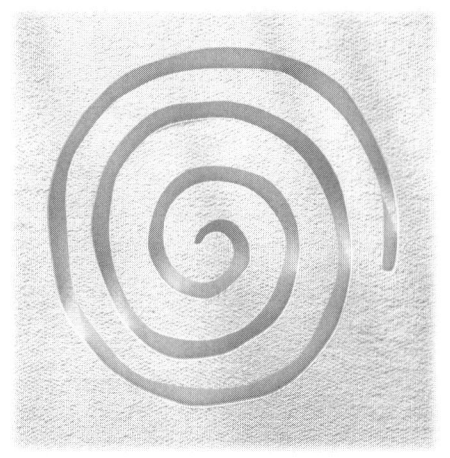

Martha O. Loustaunau, PhD, CHES

Martha O. Loustaunau is an Associate Professor of Sociology, Department of Sociology/Anthropology, New Mexico State University, Las Cruces., NM.

Abstract

In the field of education, it is well known that learning takes place at a more accelerated pace and at a higher level when there is empathy and communication between teacher and learner. In health education, this is especially vital, since information given may affect the learner's general state of health and well-being. In a world of cultural diversity and mobile populations, there will be an increasing cultural mix of teachers and learners that will challenge the skills of educators to bridge the culture gap and convey a culturally sensitive, caring, meaningful, and effective message. But what does it really mean to be culturally sensitive? Does it mean we accept everything and that everything is relative? What are the culturally relevant re-sponsibilities of the educator toward those being educated and how do we become sensitive to culture? In working with diverse populations, in communication and education, related problems arise concerning personal bias, cultural interpretation, and respect. This paper explores a few of the pressing issues involving cultural sensitivity and health education that an entry-level health educator may confront.

Culturally Insensitive Education

Many health educators may have heard the story about the attempt of health workers in a tropical village to create an awareness of the dangerous malaria mosquito. They set a large screen in the village square, and projected upon it a large photograph of the malaria-carrying insect while describing the dangers and means of eradication to the villagers. When the presentation was over, one villager remarked that he was certainly glad they didn't have anything to worry about. The health worker was shocked, and asked, "Why, whatever do you mean?" "We don't have any mosquitoes that large around here!", answered the villager.

This snippet indicates that health educators must be aware of cultural diversity and differences in perceptions of the population they serve. In the process of education, whether of patients, providers, or community, health educators will be dealing more and more with culturally diverse groups, and will encounter a corresponding diversity of beliefs, attitudes, and behaviors, including their own, which will present challenges to their efforts and educational (as well as medical) outcomes (Loustaunau & Sobo 1997; Matiella 1994). Meeting this challenge will require skills in acquiring cultural knowledge and sensitivity, in communication and mediation, and in many cases, in compromise. If the goal of health education is, indeed, the best possible level of health and well-being for an individual, a family, or an entire population, such skills will be mandatory. Health educators without a solid appreciation and understanding of the cultural context, may not only be ineffective, but may backfire.

Population and Cultural Diversity

We are truly a "multicultural" or pluralist nation, maintaining a multitude of culturally diverse identities and not the "melting pot" that was at one time predicted (Gordon, 1964). And the problem promises to become even more pressing. Day's (1997) report predicts that from 1990 to 2050, as a percentage of the racial and ethnic composition, the White Anglo population will drop from 75.8% to 52.5%. African Americans will increase from 11.7% to 14.4%, Asians and Pacific Islanders from 2.8% to 9.7%, Native Americans from 0.7% to 0.9%, and the Latino population will increase from 9.0% to 22.5%.

Not only will those who receive education and care become more diverse, but so will those who provide them. Due to demographic trends, for example, "older adults, including the baby boomers, will be cared for by large numbers of health care professionals who are people of color. . . ." (Feagin, Vera, & Zsembik, 1996).

It also is also important to remember that even were we to "melt down" racially and ethnically, which we have not done, culture also is defined by age, gender, social class, religion, and occupational group, all of which affect how we perceive and define health and illness, as well as what we do about them. Being "culturally sensitive," then, also

must involve how well we can, in a sense, put ourselves in the shoes of others outside our own frame of reference.

Problems of Multiculturalism

The arguments against multicultural education, as well as multicultural health care, depict recognition of cultural diversity as divisive and dangerous (Bennett, 1992; Bloom, 1987). Feagin et al. (1996), however, point out that "if they are well implemented, programs of multiculturalism represent a way to bring diverse peoples together in mutual respect for one another and for the equal rights and privileges promised by the Declaration of Independence" (p. 18).

The challenge to health educators is even more pressing, not only in the schools (Matiella 1994), but in communities. And that means understanding how a culture affects values, beliefs, and behavior. But there is an additional problem. The biomedical model, although highly successful, frames illness and health care in a purely scientific and mechanistic way. Scientific medicine, a culture in itself (Loustaunau & Sobo, 1997), has left little or no room for taking account of the tremendous cultural diversity in our population or for the recognition of how this cultural diversity may directly affect the health, illness, beliefs, and practices of people. There also is little or no consideration of the possibility that many tested "folk" practices can work, and may offer viable alternatives and a way for client and practitioner to learn from each other (Micozzi, 1996).

However, gaining an understanding, and particularly an ap-

preciation of other cultural beliefs, attitudes, and practices, is not always easy. Time constraints, lack of knowledge sources, energy, motivation, and personal biases get in the way. It may seem much easier to try to bring people to "our own way of thinking."

In some cases involving medical practice, there is obviously little room for cultural considerations as in emergency situations or when resources are simply not available. Often, however, such sensitivity is possible. In a case that relates directly to the educative function, a nurse caring for a rural Hispanic agricultural worker recommended that the client drink orange juice, high in vitamin C, for a respiratory ailment. Hispanic folk tradition, however, considers the ailment as a "cold," to be treated with a "hot" remedy. Orange juice was considered "cold" and, therefore, inappropriate. If the nurse had understood the concept of hot and cold illnesses and remedies, she could have recommended an appropriate "hot" remedy high in vitamin C, such as red chile (Rose, 1978).

Ethnocentric Bias

The disciplines of sociology and anthropology have a great deal to teach us about cultural sensitivity. The concept of "ethnocentrism," for example, refers to the judgment of other cultures, customs, and beliefs as false, or inferior to one's own. Modern medicine, based upon scientific principles and investigation, ethnocentrically views cultural interpretations and perceptions of illness and treatment which do not fit within the scientific medical framework as "illegitimate" (Loustaunau & Sobo, 1997). People who see the world in a different way from one's own cultural world view are, thus, considered to be misinformed, ignorant, or even dangerous (Kreps & Kunimoto, 1994).

Cultural Relativity

Cultural relativity, the opposite of ethnocentrism, implies respect and understanding within the specific context. When customs, beliefs, and practices are examined and viewed in this way, the reasons for them may become clear or understandable (Loustaunau & Sobo, 1997). For example, we may "know" that a virus causes certain symptoms and not the evil eye of a malevolent neighbor. However, an objective study of the values and norms of the culture allows us to evaluate the belief within the context of that culture. The culturally relative view makes no judgmental conclusions about what is "culturally good" or "culturally bad."

Limitations of Cultural Relativity

But how does one deal with those practices and beliefs that one finds in extreme cases, that may actually be harmful to health? Personal attitudes and biases may be dealt with through experience and education. Harmful beliefs and practices, however, may require a deeper understanding and highly sensitive educational efforts. The interpretation of what is "harmful," may be, to a degree, subjective. Other cases, however, may be more obvious.

In some Hispanic communities, for example, it is believed that a depression at the top of a baby's skull, known as the "mollera caida," or fallen fontanelle, must be pushed back into place by pressing on the baby's soft palate, by holding the baby upside down over a pan of water, or by using herbs and raw eggs to "draw" the depression out (Rose, 1978).

Such depressions are now known to be primarily caused by dehydration and must be treated by giving the baby adequate fluids. The problem here is not to denigrate or portray the belief as "ignorance" or "superstition," but to find the way to modify such long-held beliefs and offer alternatives with proven results.

At a community educational meeting, while discussing the topic of "mollera caida," one "curandero" or local healer, remarked that with his treatment, many babies recovered, while with biomedical treatment, some babies did not recover. If efforts at education were to be successful, recognizing that he had considerable status in the community, it was important to create a link with him and to gain his friendship, allowing him to become part of the process of reeducation, showing him how the odds of recovery may be affected by treatment and how dehydration can be extremely dangerous to the baby's health.

Another case of a harmful belief and practice is more extreme. The practice of female circumcision, also known as female genital mutilation, or FGM, is common in various Arab and African countries and has accompanied immigrants to the U.S. as well as to other countries. It is based on the belief that females are not "clean" or "marriageable" until they are ritually circumcised by cutting away the clitoris and sometimes the inner and outer labia, and then sewing the wound shut with only a tiny opening remaining. The procedure is often performed on very young girls and causes incredible pain and suffering, often infection, and sometimes death. Even so, the belief is sometimes very strongly ingrained and difficult to counter (Toubia, 1994). One American physician talked to me of delivering a baby from a woman who demanded that afterward she be sewed up exactly as before.

Such customs and practices found to be physically and mentally harmful can be considered a violation of human rights, as stated in the United Nations' International Bill of Human Rights (1978). Education here is vital, but must still be approached with caution and with recognition of the strong cultural values and attachments certain practices may retain, even for those who suffer from them.

Becoming Culturally Sensitive

Health educators, perhaps more than anyone, must, therefore work to develop broad cultural understanding and familiarity with other frames of reference. And as sociologist, C. Wright Mills contended, in order to become more open minded, we must first admit and examine our own biases (Mills, 1959). Self analysis is crucial.

The literature on becoming more culturally sensitive does not imply that we must know everything about everyone. Nor does it suggest a simple acceptance or even simple tolerance for the attitudes, beliefs, and behaviors of others. Cultural sensitivity is described as a skill that must be consciously developed, comprised of a willingness to read, listen, ask, learn, and appreciate the fact that there may be many paths to the same goal (Kavanagh & Kennedy 1992; Locke 1992; Majumdar 1995).

This is illustrated by a situation described in recent letters to the *Journal of the American Medical Association* (Blackhall, Murphy, Frank, Michel, & Azen, 1996; Carrese & Rhodes, 1996; Fenyvesi, 1996; Fitzgibbons, 1996; Gostin, 1996; Kazal, 1996; Pantilat, 1996; Pastorek, 1996). The need to inform people as to their diagnosis and prognosis is being strongly stressed as a "right to know" (as far as it can be known) in order to make informed decisions about one's options and outcomes, and as a personal right. Among the Navajo, however, speaking of such things is not done, since it is believed that to speak of them makes them likely to happen. While one doctor insisted that such a belief was ridiculous and that the Navajo patients should be informed in any case, other health workers found that the problem could be easily solved by discussing the case in the third person plural. This was perfectly acceptable and also increased the cooperation and trust of patients for practitioners.

In a multidisciplinary examination of the relationships of culture to health, illness, and medicine, Loustaunau and Sobo (1997) discussed the unique role of health care providers and educators in "caring" for others. Achieving the goals of cultural sensitivity, they point out, must include understanding the influence of a broad range of cultural elements which include age, gender, race/ethnicity, and socio-economic status, in health, illness, and care, and developing the skills to use that understanding in a productive way. Scientific knowledge and critical thinking must be accompanied by tact and facility for transmitting, accumulating, and adapting knowledge. Without these skills, education, and even treatment may be thwarted, with unsatisfactory outcomes.

As an example, an African American woman from a poverty background who becomes pregnant, may encounter the biases of her health care provider, who strongly disapproves of women on welfare becoming pregnant. The physician's "signals" of disapproval may be obvious. The possibility of sterilization may even be mentioned. Prescriptions of medications, rest, mild exercise, vitamins, diet, and follow-up visits may not take into consideration the lack of economic means, other children at home, a job with no sick leave or maternity leave, distance between home and clinic, lack of transportation or time off, and many other considerations that will prevent good prenatal care and a positive outcome (Loustaunau & Sobo, 1997).

The cultural experiences of being Black, poor, and a southern or Caribbean Black woman, all have an impact on this woman's perceptions and behavior. In addition, a background of well-founded lack of trust in a white male medical physician, lack of health insurance, the irrationality and, indeed, impossibility of compliance, and possible fear of ridicule of folk practices and customs may all conspire against her and result in a poor pregnancy outcome ultimately costing her and society a great deal more than culturally relative care (Snow, 1993). This woman has taken a first step by making clinical contact, but cooperation and education can only take place within the realm of possibilities as she perceives them.

So what is cultural sensitivity? "The multicultural person," says Hoopes (1981), "is the person who has learned how to learn culture—rapidly and effectively" (p. 10). Majumdar (1995) referred to such persons as "individuals who have mastered the knowledge and skills necessary to feel comfortable and communicate effectively with people of similar and dissimilar backgrounds by any situation involving a group of people of diverse ethnocultural backgrounds" (p. 2). Loustaunau and Sobo (1997) suggested that it goes even further, in translating knowledge into effective holistic caring not only for the individual, but for the whole family or household unit, within the cultural context.

There is much debate and controversy in the field of medicine as to the place of cultural considerations in training of physicians and in medical practice (Loustaunau & Sobo, 1997). For health educators whose role is to educate individuals, groups, or communities, cultural sensitivity becomes an integral part of their role. There are increasing resources available for becoming more culturally sensitive (Kavanagh & Kennedy, 1992; Kreps & Kunimoto, 1994; Locke, 1992; Majumdar, 1995). Cultural sensitivity, however, is not learned only from a book, but is a skill that must be developed and cultivated in an increasingly globally-connected, yet culturally diverse world.

References

Bennett, W. (1992). *The de-valuing of America: The fight for our culture and our children.* New York: Summit Books.

Blood, A. (1987). *The closing of the American mind.* New York: Simon and Schuster.

Blackhall, L. J., Murphy, S. T., Frank, G., Michel, V., & Azen, S., (1996). Patient-physician communication: Respect for culture, religion, and autonomy [Letter to the editor]. *Journal of the American Medical Association, 275,* p. 109.

Carrese, J. A., & Rhodes, L. A. (1996). Patient-physician communication: Respect for culture, religion, and autonomy [Letter to the editor]. *Journal of the American Medical Association, 275,* p. 109.

Day, J. (1997). *Population projections of the United States, by age, sex, race, and Hispanic origin: 1995 to 2050; U.S. Bureau of the Census, Current Population Report* (pp. 25–1104). Washington, DC: U.S. Government Printing Office.

Feagin, J., Vera, H., & Zsembik, B. (1996). Multiculturalism: A democratic basis for U.S. society. In B. C. Calhoun & G. Ritzer (Eds.), *Perspectives on sociology,* (pp. 1–22). New York: McGraw-Hill.

Fenyvesi, T. (1996). Patient-physician communication: Respect for culture, religion, and autonomy [Letter to the editor]. *Journal of the American Medical Association, 275,* p. 107.

Fitzgibbons, S. (1996). Patient-physician communication: Respect for culture, religion, and autonomy [Letter to the editor]. *Journal of the American Medical Association, 275,* p. 108.

Gay, G. (1994). *At the essence of learning: multicultural education.* West Lafayette, IN: Kappa Delta Pi.

Gordon, M. (1964). *Assimilation in American life.* New York: Oxford University Press.

Gostin, L. O. (1996). Patient-physician communication: Respect for culture, religion, and autonomy [Letter to the editor]. *Journal of the American Medical Association, 275,* p. 110.

Hoopes, D. (1981). International communication concepts and the psychology of intercultural experience. In M. Pusch (Ed.), *Multicultural education* (pp. 10–38). New York: Intercultural Press.

Kazal, L. A. (1996). Patient-physician communication: Respect for culture, religion, and autonomy [Letter to the editor]. *Journal of the American Medical Association, 275,* p. 108.

Kavanagh, K., & Kennedy, P. (1992). *Promoting cultural diversity strategies for health care professionals.* Newbury Park, CA: Sage.

Kreps, G., & Kunimoto, E. (1994). *Effective communication in multicultural health care settings.* Thousand Oaks, CA: Sage.

Locke, D. (1992). *Increasing multicultural understanding: A comprehensive model.* Newbury Park, CA: Sage.

Loustaunau, M., & Sobo, E. (1997). *The cultural context of health, illness, and medicine.* Westport, CT: Bergin and Garvey.

Majumdar, B. (1995). *Culture and health: Culture-sensitive training manual for the health care provider* (4th ed.). Hamilton, Ontario: McMaster University.

Matiella, A. (Ed.). (1994). *The multicultural challenge in health education.* Santa Cruz, CA: ETR Associates.

Micozzi, M. (Ed.). (1996). *Fundamentals of complementary and alternative medicine.* New York: Churchill Livingston.

Mills, C. (1959). *The sociological imagination.* London: Oxford University Press.

Pantilat, S. Z. (1996). Patient-physician communication: Respect for culture, religion, and autonomy [Letter to the editor]. *Journal of the American Medical Association, 275,* p. 107.

Pastorek, J. (1996). Patient-physician communication: Respect for culture, religion, and autonomy [Letter to the editor]. *Journal of the American Medical Association, 275,* p. 108.

Rose, L. (1978). *Disease beliefs in Mexican-American communities.* San Francisco: R & E Research Associates.

Snow, L. (1993). *Walkin' over medicine.* Boulder, CO: Westview Press.

Toubia, N. (1994). Female circumcision as a public health issue. *New England Journal of Medicine, 331,* 712–716.

United Nations. (1978). *International bill of human rights.* New York: United Nations Office of Public Information.

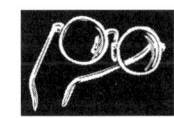 **Article Review Form at end of book.**

WiseGuide Wrap-Up

- The top ten self-reported health problems are arthritis, high blood pressure, depression, asthma, cancer, heart disease, diabetes, anxiety disorder, skin cancer, and alcoholism.

- The future of health education includes program advocacy, community empowerment, and credentialing.

- Surveys conducted in California and nationwide show widespread support for community-oriented disease-prevention and health-promotion activities.

- *Globalization* is defined as the process of increasing economic, political, and social interdependence and global integration that takes place as capital, traded goods, persons, concepts, images, ideas, and values diffuse across state boundaries.

- Global public health in the twenty-first century requires thinking globally and acting globally and locally.

- All of the community-based preventive services that prevent disease and injury and promote and protect health are critical parts of public health.

- For health educators, whose role is to educate individuals, groups, and communities, cultural sensitivity is an integral part of their role.

R.E.A.L. Sites

This list provides a print preview of typical **Coursewise** R.E.A.L. sites. (There are over 100 such sites at the **Courselinks**™ site.) The danger in printing URLs is that web sites can change overnight. As we went to press, these sites were functional using the URLs provided. If you come across one that isn't, please let us know via email to: webmaster@coursewise.com. Use your Passport to access the most current list of R.E.A.L. sites at the **Courselinks** site.

Site name: Health Resource Links

URL: http://www.whitehouse.gov/WH/pointers/html/health.html

Why is it R.E.A.L.? This page is an introduction to online health-related resources from the U.S. government and is comprised of the following major sections:

Leading Causes of Death; Health Care; Health and Environment; and Alcohol, Smoking, and Drug Information

Key topics: leading causes of death; health care; health and environment; alcohol, smoking, and drug information

Try this: Select Leading Causes of Death. How do the top four causes of death compare with the top reported concerns from the Clements and Hales article (Reading 1)?

Site name: The Michigan Electronic Library: Health Information Resources

URL: http://mel.lib.mi.us/health/health-statistics.html

Why is it R.E.A.L.? This site provides health information resources. This project is sponsored by The Library of Michigan and the University of Michigan, University Library. It is funded, in part, with Library Services and Technology Act (LSTA) funds administered by The Library of Michigan.

Key topics: health statistics, data, Healthy People 2000, health care financing

section 2

School-Based Programming

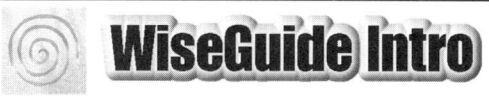 **WiseGuide Intro** All states have mandated some form of health-education programming designed to help students develop and maintain behaviors conducive to good health. Historically speaking, this programming has taken the shape of health education or personal health in the classroom environment. Beyond the academic setting of the traditional classroom, many innovative approaches are being taken to improve the health of our youth.

In this section, we will examine several school-based programs, including peer-led programs, a worksite health-promotion model adapted to school health promotion, the collaboration of school health and managed care, a school-based nutrition improvement program, and preservice training for early childhood and elementary teachers.

David Black (Purdue University), Nancy Tobler (State University of New York at Albany), and John Sciacca (Northern Arizona University) present "Peer Helping/Involvement: An Efficacious Way to Meet the Challenge of Reducing Alcohol, Tobacco, and Other Drug Use among Youth?" Peer-led drug-prevention programs for middle school youth are reviewed as to whether or not they are a vital resource in an overall effort to minimize the use of alcohol, tobacco, and other drugs (ATOD).

James Eddy (University of Alabama), Eugene Fitzhugh, (University of Tennessee), Robert Gold (Macro International Inc.), and G. Greg Wojtowicz (University of North Carolina) collaborate on "A Worksite Health Promotion Model for Public Schools." The purpose of this article is to propose a different approach to school health education, one that implements the key features of the worksite health-promotion model to improve student health.

Howard Taras, M.D., Philip Nader (University of California at San Diego), Holly Swiger (San Diego School Health Innovations Project), and John Fontanesi (Kaiser-Permanente) present "The *School Health Innovative Programs:* Integrating School Health and Managed Care in San Diego." This article describes the first two years of a San Diego–based collaborative program consisting of managed care organizations, school districts, and other health care agencies. Various challenges, such as data collection, parental consent, and new forms of communication among health professionals, are also addressed.

Kari Jo Harris (University of Kansas Medical Center), Kimber Richter and Jerry Schultz (University of Kansas), and Judy Johnston (Kansas LEAN) present "Formative, Process, and Intermediate Outcome Evaluation of a Pilot School-Based 5 a Day for Better Health Project." This paper reports the formative, process, and intermediate outcome results of a five-month school-based project that was linked to the National 5 a Day for Better Health campaign to increase young children's consumption of fruits and vegetables.

William English (Clarion University of Pennsylvania) and Charles Duke (Appalachian State University) present "Dealing with the Health Crisis in Our Schools: Clarion University's Health Education Model for Elementary and Early Childhood Education Majors." To address the

Learning Objectives

- To examine the use of peer-led programs in school-based health promotion

- To review the application of a worksite model for pubic school health promotion

- To study the collaboration of school health and managed care as it relates to school health services

- To examine the outcomes of a school-based nutrition program

- To review a preservice training model for elementary and early childhood education majors

problem of lack of professional preparation, with regard to knowledge and skills for health-education issues, for elementary and early childhood education teachers, the Health and Physical Education Department at Clarion University of Pennsylvania has developed and implemented a model health-education emphasis for preservice teachers in the university's College of Education and Human Services.

? Questions ?

Reading 8. An interactive (peer-led or peer involvement) program involves _____; a noninteractive (teacher-led) program involves _____. What are the two main criteria for the development and use of screening tests?

Reading 9. The school-based health promotion model is founded on which two notions? Describe social marketing as it relates to school health.

Reading 10. List the three common elements of each collaborative agreement between the schools and managed care organizations. Discuss the principles developed by the *SHIP* collaborative partners.

Reading 11. Describe the focus of Phases I and II of the pilot project. Differentiate between formative and process evaluation.

Reading 12. The key to meeting the health education crisis in this country continues to lie with _____. Although most of the health education within the elementary school is carried out by the classroom teacher, most elementary teachers are ill-equipped to teach health education effectively. How has this problem been perpetuated?

An interactive (peer-led or peer involvement) program involves
_____; a noninteractive (teacher-led) program involves
_____. What are the two main criteria for the development
and use of screening tests?

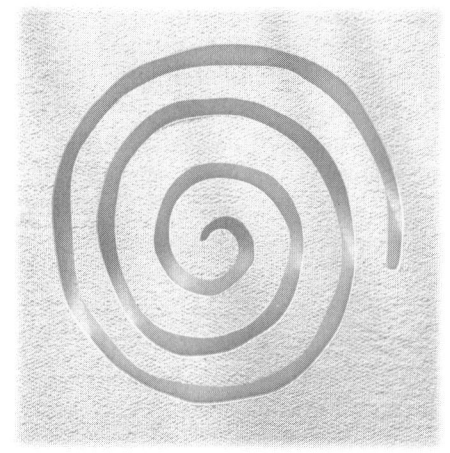

Peer Helping/ Involvement:

An Efficacious Way to Meet the Challenge of Reducing Alcohol, Tobacco, and Other Drug Use among Youth?

David R. Black, Nancy S. Tobler, and John P. Sciacca

David R. Black, PhD, MPH, CHES, FASHA, Professor, Health Promotion; Health Sciences; Foods and Nutrition; and Nursing, Division of Health Promotion/HKLS, Purdue University, Nancy S. Tobler, PhD, Research Associate Professor, State University of New York at Albany, and John P. Sciacca, MPH, PhD, CHES, Professor, Health Education and Promotion, Dept. of Health, Physical Education, Exercise Science, and Nutrition, College of Health Professions, Northern Arizona University.

Abstract

Peer-led drug prevention programs for middle school youth are reviewed as to whether or not they are a vital resource in an overall effort to minimize the use of alcohol, tobacco, and other drugs (ATOD). The paper focuses on the following: a) results of a 120-study meta-analysis of school-based drug prevention programs and positive program features; b) considerations for falsely concluding that peer programs are ineffective; c) features of two model or stellar programs that compared interactive (peer leadership) to teacher/researcher-led (non-interactive) programs that followed National Peer Helpers Association (NPHA) Programmatic Standards; and d) suggestions for designing and implementing high-quality, peer-led programs. The authors conclude that interactive peer interventions for middle school students are statistically superior to non-interactive didactic, lecture programs led by teachers/researchers. Programs implemented according to NPHA Programmatic Standards may eliminate Type II (false negative) and III ("implementation failure" or ineffec- tively designed and implemented program) errors. Opportunities for prudent application of well-designed peer programs appropriately implemented and evaluated must remain a salient priority. (J Sch Health. 1998;68(3):87–93)

This paper explores peer helping programs for youth as a vital resource in an overall effort to minimize the use of substances that are undermining the vitality of society. Evaluation of peer programs is particularly timely because there is increased interest in prudent fiscal accounting and deciding which programs should receive funding to curb the menacing drug problems confronting today's youth. Accordingly, this paper focuses on the following: a) the efficacy of adolescent alcohol, tobacco, and other drug (ATOD) prevention programs

David R. Black, Nancy S. Tobler, and John P. Sciacca, "Peer Helping/Involvement: An Efficacious Way to Meet the Challenge of Reducing Alcohol, Tobacco, and Other Drug Use among Youth?" *Journal of School Health,* (Vol. 68, No. 3), pp. 87–93, March 1998. Reprinted with permission from the American School Health Association.

based on a meta-analysis of 120 studies; b) reasons why conclusions might be mistakenly drawn that characterized results of peer programs as equivocal, contradictory, or inconclusive; c) the outcomes of two stellar programs that adhere to the Programmatic Standards National Peer Helpers Association (NPHA) *Checklist for a Peer Helper Program;* and d) recommendations for designing and implementing high-quality, peer-led programs.

Meta-Analysis Results

Results of 120 adolescent drug prevention programs conducted in North America were reviewed that concurrently addressed the use of alcohol, cigarettes, cannabis, and other illicit drugs. None of the 120 programs focused on illicit drugs only. Most studies focusing on drug use were conducted with children in grades six to eight, where drug use is low; generalizations to older age groups should be made with caution. The programs were universal interventions targeted at the general student population rather than selective or indicated interventions. Selected interventions target individuals or subgroups at risk and indicated intervention focus on those who are users but do not meet diagnostic criteria for a drug disorder.

The findings presented are based on a recent meta-analysis funded by the National Institute on Drug Abuse and conducted by Tobler and Stratton.[1] Their findings are in agreement with those presented in other review articles.[2-6] What is presented are general lessons learned from the entire meta-analysis on school-based drug prevention programs, but have application to peer-led programs as well as those conducted by teachers. Table 1 contains the characteristics of programs that were statistically superior, and results are presented in Figure 1.

A summary of the data in Table 1 indicates interactive programs are statistically superior to non-interactive programs in preventing drug use among adolescents. An interactive (peer-led or peer involvement) program involves communications based on face-to-face *peer* interactions. Planned activities are used to stimulate active participation. Students may generate role plays, which provide a real world, age-appropriate experience. Inter-personal skills also may be modeled and rehearsed, and feedback may be received from peers. A non-interactive (teacher-led) program involves a passive approach, where content is introduced by teachers in a didactic, instructive manner in a lecture format and also may include experiential activities that are mainly between teacher and student, not student to student.

An important factor to note in Table 1 is that results are significant in comparison to other programs in which subjects received a bona fide, full-fledged treatment as opposed to a no-treatment or control group. This suggests that interactive programs are effective, the degree to which is discussed in a practical context below. Figure 1 graphically depicts the efficacy of these results. What is quickly observed is that, regardless of whether only high quality experimental studies [56 (46.6%) out of 120 studies] or all studies are included in the analyses, interactive programs are statistically superior to non-interactive programs across different drugs to include tobacco, alcohol, cannabis, and other illicit drugs.

Although not graphically displayed, interactive programs also are statistically superior to DARE, a well-known, national program. Tobler and Stratton[1] noted that the interactive programs had higher weighted effect sizes (WES, proportional to the sample size) in comparison to the four project DARE programs and another group of non-interactive programs. Their WESs were .19, .07, and .08, respectively.

The efficacy of four leader categories were assessed to include teachers, peers, clinicians, and others. Figure 2 shows that effect sizes for teacher, peer, and other leaders are statistically equivalent when results are reviewed for interactive programs, independent of whether the study was high-quality or included in the total set. Effect sizes for the mental health clinicians were exceptionally high. However, when clinicians were compared to the combination of all other leaders and sample size was a covariate, no statistically significant differences were observed across different types of leaders. It appears that the same benefits can be achieved with peer helpers as with more educated and experienced adults; but all leaders, regardless of educational level, need to be trained to be effective facilitators and peer helpers. They need to understand and endorse the value of an interactive versus a non-interactive approach.

Table 1 further shows that the most effective programs dispel the myth that everyone is using drugs by including components that acquaint participants with local statistics; teach drug refusal skills under conditions that can be transferred and used in real life situations; and present the negative consequences (e.g., physical, social, emotional, and

Table I Characteristics of Superior Adolescent Drug Prevention Programs

	Description	Outcome
Program		
Interactive (I) (Social Influence, Comprehensive life Skills, and Others)	Focused on: • Interpersonal competence • Knowledge about short- and long-term consequences of drug and prodrug influences • Drug refusal skills taught under realistic conditions to build confidence • Challenged amount of drug use via local statistics	$I > NI, p = .05$
	or combined with • Strengthening of personal competence and intrapersonal functioning • Self-esteem building, decision making, coping skills, public commitment activities	$I > NI, p = .05$
Non-Interactive (NI) (Knowledge-only, Affective-only, Knowledge and Affective)	Focused on: • Intrapersonal factors • Examination of personal beliefs, values, and decision-making • Decision to abstain based on ethics and morals • Content directed at person and internal perceptions and not those of peers	Very Ineffective
Delivery		
Interactive	Teaching method: • Contact, intercommunication, and exchange of ideas • Interactions included everyone and the activities were participatory and between peers • Structured small group activities used to introduce program and promote acquisition of drug-refusal skills • Corrective feedback in order to use skills in situations of higher stress	
Non-Interactive	Teaching style: • Lecture/didactic with discussion and experiential activities • Communication mostly between teacher and student, not student-to-student	
Size		
Small (S)	≤ 400 students	$S > L, p = .05$
Large (L)	> 400–4,000	
Large Interactive (LI)	> 400–4,000	$LI > LNI, p = .05$
Large Non-Interactive (LNI)	> 400–4,000	
Attitude and Use		
Drug Pathway	Increased perceived risk of using cannabis associated with decreased use of marijuana Converse also true	
Interactive (I)	Significant changes in knowledge, attitudes, and decrease in drug use	
Non-Interactive (NI)	Significant change in knowledge only	
Length of Program		
Intensity	68% only six hours Longer programs of 18 hours did only slightly better	
Statistical Differences		
Interactive (I)	Effect size	$I = 0.02$ vs $NI = 0.20$
Clinical Success		
Interactive (I) Non-Interactive (NI)	Clinically important differences	$I = 9.5\%$ vs $NI = 1.0\%$

economical problems) of using drugs. The drug pathway for cannabis that was identified was that if students perceive drug taking as risky, then drug use declines. If drug use is not perceived as risky, then the converse is true.

The delivery method that was most effective emphasized sharing, cooperating, and contributing. The style was not di-

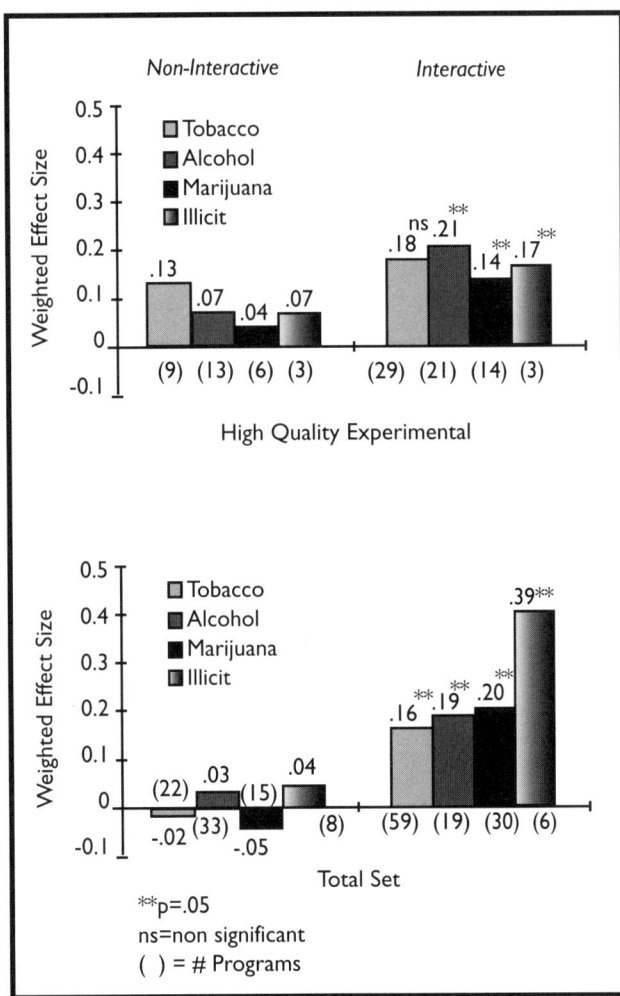

Figure 1 Different types of drugs by type of program.

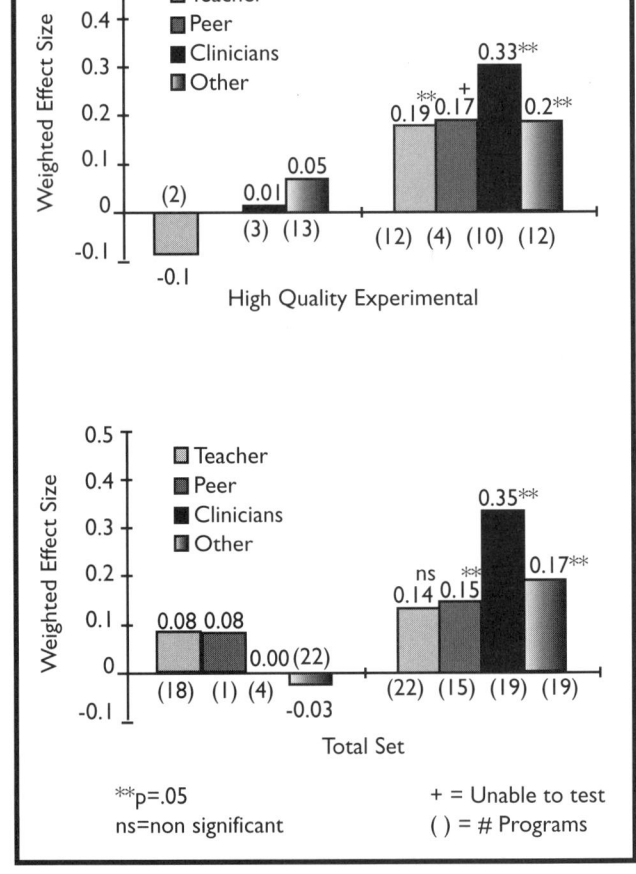

Figure 2 Leaders by type of program.

dactic, but highly interactive and participatory. The ethnographic results reported by three Dundee High School peer leaders and their peer trainer at one of the workshops at The Scottish Conference on Drug Education, held in Edinburgh in 1997, helps exemplify and clarify what is meant by interactive and participatory, and why students seem to value a peer approach.[7] Students reported the following about their peer leaders: "They're not teachers, they were very up to date on drugs and understood our views"; "I feel more comfortable talking to seniors than adults"; "We felt we could tell them more than we could tell a teacher, and we were more likely to listen to them"; "Peers are more like a friend"; "[They are] nearer our age"; "They knew what we were thinking, and we also had a bit of a laugh"; "It was more fun"; and "They knew quite a lot about drugs."

Small group instruction also was prized, along with constructive peer feedback to hone and sharpen refusal skills. Programs that were best included no more than 400 participants. The length of 68% of the interactive programs was only 6 hours and produced clinically important changes; it is yet to be determined, however, whether there is a "dose-response" relationship because programs of 18 hours did only marginally better. The difference of 8.5% change between the interactive and non-interactive programs is important, especially when compared to the use of medicine such as aspirin to treat coronary heart disease. As Tobler[8] noted in a perusal of a double-blind study on the effects of aspirin and heart disease, the success rate among the 22,000 physicians who had participated in the study was only 3.5%. This percentage is less than half of the change produced by peer drug prevention programs. Yet, authors of the medical study on aspirin and heart disease concluded that it was unethical not to offer aspirin to the control group because of the reduction in heart attacks. If similar logic were applied to drug use, it seems it would be unconscionable not to advocate a peer-led program as a viable option for drug reduction or prevention.

Tobler[8] also indicated that several program and research policy recommendations be considered. She suggested the following actions: a) implement interactive programs and shift focus from instructing classes to facilitating groups; b) initiate training in conducting interactive groups for current teachers and new teachers; c) develop appropriate interactive programs for high school youth, since developmentally appropriate programs are available for junior high youth; d) establish as a funding priority initiatives to develop and test innovative high school programs that acknowledge that these adolescents use drugs; e) fund programs so long-term objectives can be met, such as coordination of programs throughout high school and addressing certain subjects and populations; f) modify expectations that low-intensity programs of 10 hours will produce long-term results; and g) fund programs that include yearly booster sessions or increase program intensity in other ways.

Mistaken Conclusions

Professionals may hear that peer programs are ineffective or results are equivocal, contradictory, or inconclusive.[9] Based on results of the meta-analysis, this is untrue. The reason for the erroneous

conclusion seems to relate to a Type III or "implementation" error.[10] A Type III error indicates the program was poorly designed, the program protocol was not adhered to, or the program received little administrative support. In other words, the program was doomed from the outset and had little chance of succeeding.

Type III errors also increase the probability of a Type II error, falsely concluding that the intervention is ineffective when it may actually have potential if it had been properly designed and implemented. As far as can be detected by reading summaries of methods of various studies, a common problem was that program supervisors had not followed or had incompletely implemented the intervention according to tenets listed in *Programmatic Standards* published by the National Peer Helpers Association (NPHA).[11] The idea about incompletely or partially adhering to the program also is supported by Botvin et al[12] who reported that some teachers did not include all parts of the program because they seemed to have been uncomfortable with certain components, such as role plays. Teachers may need to be trained and convinced of the value of the techniques they will be implementing. Programs must be planned that provide an adequate "dose" of intervention, and then the program must be implemented as designed.

Another way to evaluate adherence to protocol, especially if it is for an interactive program, is to observe the amount of student involvement. Wilhelmsen et al[13] found students in the interactive as compared to non-interactive condition reported more involvement; more group work satisfac-

tion and benefits; and active participation and satisfaction with program participation. To determine if the program is being implemented as designed, process evaluation or a quality assurance review must be a mainstay of the evaluation to be certain that a program works or not. It may ultimately be found that peer programs simply do not work for certain problems or populations, but are effective with others as demonstrated in this instance by the meta-analysis conducted by Tobler and Stratton.[1] The time may also come when effective components from otherwise ineffective programs can be identified and incorporated into efficacious packages.

Model Programs

It is a formidable challenge and perhaps unwise to select a single study, or even a few, as exemplars of how programs might be designed and implemented. Nevertheless, the studies selected were chosen because of their superior effect sizes and their commendable methods. The results of two studies are presented: one a clinical trial and the other a large scale study conducted in four different countries. Admittedly, the studies had some design limitations. However, the studies were conducted according to the NPHA *Programmatic Standards*,[11] and their results were exceptional.

Botvin and colleagues[12] conducted a 20-session cognitive-behavioral program for substance abuse prevention with 1,311 7th grade students from 10 suburban New York junior high schools. The program was designed to reduce interpersonal pressure to smoke, drink excessively, or use cannabis. Tables 2 and 3 contain the results of these studies. The values in the tables are adjusted based on pretest scores; therefore, the meaning of the numbers in absolute terms is difficult to interpret. However, the fact that the magnitude of the values is different is the critical issue. Table 2 shows that peer-led programs were statistically superior to teacher-led and control groups on monthly measures of cigarette smoking and cannabis use as well as weekly measures of cannabis use. Table 3 again depicts that peer-led programs were superior to teacher-led and control groups on smoking, drinking, and cannabis knowledge and attitude measures as well as on locus of control and ability to influence smoking. Another finding not given in the tables, but of importance, is that significantly less drunkenness occurred among students in the peer-led group than both the teacher-led and control groups.

In summary, the peer-led prevention programs were superior to teacher-led programs and the control condition in their effect on cigarette smoking, excessive drinking, and cannabis use. Significant changes were noted in select cognitive, attitudinal, and personality predisposing variables. The lack of significant teacher results may be because teachers received no monitoring or assistance. Conversely, peers were trained in that they were provided a series of presession briefings and their programs were monitored by the research staff. A lesson learned is that everyone needs training regardless of educational level and amount of professional experience.

The second study selected to demonstrate the efficacy of peer programs was conducted by

Table 2	Adjusted Posttest Response Proportions for Cigarette Smoking and Marijuana Use among Treatment and Control Groups		
Measure	**Peer**	**Teacher**	**Control**
Cigarette smoking			
Monthly measure	.15[a]	.22	.21
Weekly measure	.07	.11	.12
Daily measure	.03	.06	.08
Marijuana Use			
Monthly measure	.02[b]	.07	.07
Weekly measure	.01[c]	.04	.06

[a] $p < .05$; [b] $p < .01$; [c] $p < .005$

Reprinted with permission: Elsevier Science Ltd., Oxford, England.

Table 3	Covariate Adjusted Posttest Means for the Cognitive, Attitudinal, and Personality Variables: Comparison of the Experimental and Control Conditions		
Variable	**Peer**	**Teacher**	**Control**
Smoking knowledge	6.80[d]	6.74[d]	5.53
Drinking knowledge	7.61[d]	7.16	7.04
Marijuana knowledge	7.16[d]	6.78[a]	6.06
Smoking attitudes	47.04[b]	45.42	45.48
Drinking attitudes	41.60[d]	39.90	39.80
Marijuana attitudes	48.51[d]	45.54	45.87
Assertiveness	69.20	68.40	68.60
Locus of control	7.56[a]	8.16	7.92
Social anxiety	26.64	26.73[a]	25.92
Self-esteem	37.90	37.50	37.50
Smoking influenceability	7.47[c]	7.68	7.83
General influenceability	13.10	13.05	13.30

[a] $p < .05$; [b] $p < .01$; [c] $p < .001$; [d] $p < .0001$

Reprinted with permission: Elsevier Science Ltd., Oxford, England.

Perry and Grant.[14] Like the first study, there were two intervention groups, teacher-led and peer-led. This study was selected because it focused on four different countries. Depending on priorities and perspective, its primary limitation is that the intervention was designed only to reduce alcohol consumption.

The primary results of the Perry and Grant[14] study indicate that peer-led programs overall demonstrated significantly lower alcohol use scores than the teacher-led and control conditions for both nondrinkers ($p < .0003$) and drinkers ($p < .04$). Students in the peer-led program also had significantly higher knowledge scores than students in the control group for nondrinkers ($p < .01$), but the peer-led and teacher-led programs did not significantly differ. Students in both the peer-led and teacher-led programs demonstrated significantly higher attitude scores than controls whether they were nondrinkers ($p < .01$) or drinkers ($p < .03$), but no significant differences existed between the two experimental conditions. Students in the peer-led program who were non-drinkers and drinkers reported significantly fewer friends were drinking than students in the teacher-led programs ($p < .0003, .0003$; respectively) or in the control groups ($p < .005, .005$; respectively).

Several conclusions can be drawn from the study. First, the peer-led approach was superior to the teacher-led and control conditions among drinkers and nondrinkers. Second, students in the peer-led groups reported significantly less alcohol use than other students. Last, students in peer-led programs acquired more knowledge of drinking, improved their attitudes about drinking, and had fewer drinking friends than those in the other two conditions. An interesting addendum is that Perry and Grant[14] noted: "Within some countries, the teacher-led program actually had more negative outcomes than the control group; thus the teacher-led program is not recommended" (p. 1167).

The Botvin et al[12] and Perry and Grant[14] studies complied with NPHA standards in a number of significant ways. Both concentrated on peer training. Training was *comprehensive* and involved a workshop, experiential activities, and training manuals. In essence, peer leaders were provided with both accurate information and behavioral skills to resist pressure to engage in harmful behaviors. Specifically, training focused on the consequences of drug use; the role of the peer helper; listening and

communication skills; problem solving and decision making strategies; provision of local drug use norms; classroom management skills; and on-going regular supervision. The second major way in which the studies complied with NPHA *Programmatic Standards*[11] was that prior to program implementation careful planning occurred that took into account rationale, purpose, goals, and objectives of the program. The last area was screening and selecting peers. The objective in both studies was to identify prospective students who were helpful, trustworthy, concerned for others, good listeners, and positive role models. In the Botvin et al[12] study selection occurred via an interview with a project staff member and a teacher; in the Perry and Grant[14] study, this was accomplished by teachers very familiar with the student population.

Recommendations
Target Behaviors and Activities and Target Drugs

Do priorities need to be reviewed as to which drugs to concentrate on in terms of drug prevention? Data from Johnston, O'Malley, and Bachman's[15] national study on drug use shows that the most preferred drugs by far among 8th, 10th, and 12th grade students "using daily" are tobacco products, such as cigarettes and smokeless tobacco, and alcohol. Their study found that the percentage using daily for these products increased with grade level and varied between 9.3% to 21.6% for cigarettes, 1.2% to 3.6% for smokeless tobacco, and .7% to 3.5% for alcohol. The percentage using cannabis daily was similar to those using smokeless tobacco

and varied between .8% to 4.6% as the grade levels increased. For stimulants, steroids, cocaine, inhalants, crack, sedatives, other opiates, LSD, hallucinogens other than LSD, heroin, and tranquilizers, the percentage of daily use was no greater than .3% for each of the three grade levels. More typically, for all of these illicit drugs daily use hovered around zero. Though any number is of concern, especially because of the devastating effects of these drugs on people's lives, all drugs cannot be given the same priority unless resources are unlimited. It seems that greatest benefits would occur by focusing on alcohol and tobacco products.

A host of serious medical and economic sequela relate to the consumption of these products. For example, the cost of alcohol problems in America is estimated to exceed $70 billion per year.[16] Tobacco is responsible for more than one of every six deaths in America and is the most important single preventable cause of death and disease.[17,18] Cigarette smoking accounts for 390,000 deaths yearly, including 21% of all coronary heart disease deaths, 87% of lung cancer deaths, and 30% of all cancer deaths.[16] Fortunately, school-based programs target drugs that have substantial negative influences on health and well-being of the largest percentage of the population and not a small proportion of students. Continuation of this focus should be reinforced through grant awards for such programs.

Efficient Ways to Target At-Risk Populations

Few, if any, school-based programs focus on select, identified at-risk youth. Use of behavioral epidemiologic surveillance procedures from the field of public health may be a prudent method for identifying such populations. Various types of screening tests have been applied to large groups or populations to include vision, blood pressure, pap smear, blood, chest x-ray, and breast and testicular self-examination tests. Several behavioral epidemiologic paper-and-pencil screening tests also exist, such as marital adjustment scales, eating disorder surveys and a forthcoming test specifically developed for athletes with eating disorders/disordered eating.[19] Why not develop or utilize a paper-and-pencil screening test appropriate for at-risk youth who are potential alcohol and tobacco users?

Two main criteria for development and use of screening tests are that the condition being screened should be relatively prevalent and an important health problem. Alcohol and cigarettes meet these criteria. The real advantage would be to focus on and involve those students in interventions who most need the services. This is especially important in an era of economical constraints and limited resources. Perhaps it is time to rethink the use of resources, which is so difficult when problems are so apparent and social, economic, health, and personal consequences so evident. Discussions about priorities are often controversial and painful once the realization comes that all needs cannot be met. Current methods of drug prevention education do not emphasize individual differences. Instead, they seem to treat all subjects the same. Development or utilization of paper-and-pencil screening tests which focus on increased specificity for identifying at-risk youth should be considered a funding priority.

New Peer Helping Service Delivery Model

Besides developing screening tests, there may be other ways to prudently use resources. A new peer-helping service-delivery model may have merit. The framework is an extension of the Stepped Approach Model of Service Delivery,[20-24] which has shown to be reasonably efficacious with problems such as alcohol use and problem drinking, tobacco, obesity, hypertension, and increasing physical activity.[16] The framework developed by Black and Scott[23] is called Lay Opportunities-Collaborative Outreach Screening Team (LO-COST): A Model for Peer Health Education. It is a combination of recruitment strategies, systematic use of interventions beginning with those that are simplest and least costly, and collaboration between professionals as peer trainers and volunteers or peers.

The model capitalizes on incorporating and using peers or volunteers as primary service providers who are trained and supervised by subject matter experts skilled in the problem area of focus, such as STDs/HIV and alcohol. The services provided are delivery of programs which range from those that are predominantly self-administered by the participant to those that are time intensive and depend on a higher level of professional training, such as group and individual counseling. The model is proposed to stimulate research, to ultimately decide which peer "delivery system" is most efficacious and cost-effective, and to encourage the incorporation of "volunteers" who often remain a viable untapped "national" resource.

Conclusions

Interactive school prevention programs for middle school students seem effective in reducing drug use. However, it is important not to over-represent or under-represent the efficacy of these programs because there are a few qualifiers. First, most studies have been conducted with middle school children where drug use is lower. The focus has been on a combination of drugs and not on illicit drugs only. Failures of programs may be due to Type III errors or poorly designed interventions that have little chance of producing an effect from the outset. Use of the NPHA *Programmatic Standards* is highly recommended to reduce the possibility of Type III errors and the occurrence of Type II errors. Programs that follow NPHA *Programmatic Standards* seem to be efficacious. It also is important not to misconstrue the results presented as a condemnation of teachers or that teacher/researcher programs are of no value. Instead, an interactive peer program represents an important potential resource or method for reducing ATOD use in youth and should be considered as a welcome adjunct to existing school ATOD reduction programs.

If priorities must be set due to limited resources, it is advocated, because of greater public health benefits, that legal drugs receive primary attention. However, this statement should not be misconstrued to mean that illicit drugs are unimportant and should be overlooked. Perhaps, a more prudent way to maintain a comprehensive drug use program is to utilize surveillance procedures to identify at-risk youth and those with a drug problem rather than to treat everyone and proceed as if "One size fits all." If screening measures are developed, then using a service delivery procedure that incorporates recruitment as a primary objective and delivery of services in an incremental, sequential manner may be promising alternatives.

References

1. Tobler N, Stratton H. Effectiveness of school-based drug prevention programs: a meta-analysis of the research. *J Primary Prev.* 1997;18:71–128.
2. Bangert-Drowns R. The effects of school-based substance abuse education: a meta-analysis. *J Drug Educ.* 1988;18:243–264.
3. Bosworth K. Sailes J. Content and teaching strategies in 10 selected drug abuse prevention curricula. J Sch Health. 1993;63:247–253.
4. Botvin G. Substance abuse prevention: theory, practice and effectiveness. In Tonry M, Wilson J, eds. *Drugs and Crime (Crime and Justice).* 1990;11:461–520). Chicago, Ill: University of Chicago Press.
5. Brown J, D'Emidio Caston M. On becoming at-risk through drug education: how symbolic policies and their practices affect students. *Eval Review.* 1995;19:451–492.
6. Hansen W. School-based substance abuse prevention: a review of the state of the art in curriculum, 1980–1990. *Health Educ Res.* 1992;7:403–430.
7. Storier F. *Scottish peer-led programme.* Workshop conducted at the meeting of The Scottish Conference on Drugs Education: meeting the Front Line Challenge, Edinburgh, Scotland, February 1997.
8. Tobler N. Adolescent drug programs. Congressional Forum on Drug Education sponsored by the Drug Policy Foundation, Washington, DC, May 1996.
9. Milburn K. A critical review of peer education with young people with special preference to sexual health. *Peer Facil Q.* 1996;14:6–17.
10. Windsor R. Baranowski T, Clark N, Cutter G. *Evaluation of Health Promotion, Health Education, and Disease Prevention Programs* (2nd ed.). Mountain View, Calif. Mayfield; 1994.
11. National Peer Helpers Association. Programmatic Standards. *Peer Facil Q.* 1990;4(7):8–12.
12. Botvin GJ, Baker E, Renick NL, Filazzola AD, Botvin EM. A cognitive-behavioral approach to substance abuse prevention. *Addic Behav.* 1984;9:137–147.
13. Wilhelmsen BU, Laberg, JC, Klepp, K. Evaluation of two student and teacher involved alcohol prevention programmes. *Addictions.* 1994;89:1157–1165.
14. Perry CL, Grant M. Comparing peer-led to teacher-led youth alcohol education in four countries. *Alcoh Health Res World* 1988;12:322–326.
15. Johnston LD, O'Malley PM, Bachman J. *National Survey Results on Drug Use from the Monitoring the Future Study,* 1975–1994: College Students and Young Adults. Washington, DC: US Government Printing Office publication 96-4020;1996:Vol 1.
16. U.S. Dept of Health and Human Services. *Healthy People 2000: National Health Promotion and Disease Prevention Objectives.* Washington, DC: US Government Printing Office publication 91-50212; 1992.
17. Harwood HJ, Napolitana DM, Kristiansen PL, Collins JJ. *Economic Costs to Society of Alcohol and Drug Abuse and Mental Illness: 1980.* Research Triangle Park, NC. Research Triangle Institute; 1984.
18. Rice DP, Kelman LS, Dunmeyer S. *The Economic Costs of Alcohol and Drug Abuse and Mental Illness.* San Francisco, Calif: Institute for Health and Aging, University of California–San Francisco; 1990.
19. Black DR, Leverenz L, Coster DC, Nagel D, Larkin LS. Evaluation of a screening test for female college athletes with disordered eating. *Suppl. J Athletic Train.* 1997;32:S-23.
20. Black DR, Cameron R. Self-administered interventions: A health education strategy for improving population health. *Health Educ Res.* in press.
21. Black DR, Hultsman JT. The Purdue stepped approach model: a heuristic application to health counseling. *Counsel Psychol.* 1988;16:647–667.
22. Black DR, Hultsman JT. The Purdue stepped approach model: sequencing community and clinical interventions to reduce cardiovascular risk factors. *Int Q Comm Health Educ.* 1988/1989;10:19–37.
23. Black DR, Scott LA. Lay opportunities-collaborative outreach screening team (LO-COST): a model for peer health education. *Peer Facil Q.* 1996;13(2):29–38.
24. Black DR, Scott LA. Self-administered interventions: an alternative to service delivery. In Blechman EA, Brownell KD, eds. *Behavioral Medicine for Women: A Comprehensive Handbook.* New York, NY: Guilford; in press.

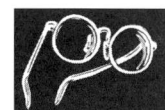 **Article Review Form at end of book.**

The school-based health promotion model is founded on which two notions? Describe social marketing as it relates to school health.

A Worksite Health Promotion Model for Public Schools

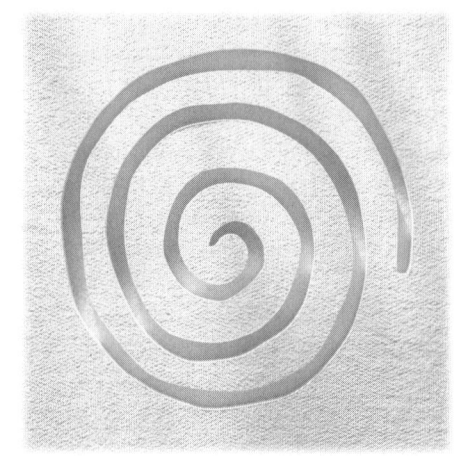

James M. Eddy, Eugene Fitzhugh, Robert S. Gold, and G. Greg Wojtowicz

James M. Eddy is Professor of Health Studies, Health and Human Performance Studies, University of Alabama, Tuscaloosa, Eugene Fitzhugh is an Assistant Professor, Department of Health, Leisure, and Safety Sciences, University of Tennessee, Knoxville, Robert S. Gold is Vice President of Macro International Inc., Calverton, MD, G. Greg Wojtowicz is Professor of Health Education, Department of Health and Kinesiology, University of North Carolina at Charleston.

Over the past several decades worksite-based health promotion efforts have slowly evolved. Although there are no standard program components common to all corporate programs, it is generally accepted that comprehensive, effective health promotion programs include corporate culture modification, social marketing efforts, and health promotion programming activities. These programs are designed to help employees develop positive health behaviors to achieve corporate goals such as improving morale and productivity, and reducing health care cost and rates of absenteeism.

Similarly, all states have mandated some form of health education programming also designed to help students develop and maintain behaviors conducive to health. Although the ultimate goals of these programs are similar (to encourage the adoption or maintenance of healthy lifestyle behaviors), the methods used to achieve these goals are often quite disparate. The purpose of this article is to propose a different approach to school health education, one that implements the key features of the worksite health promotion model to improve student health.

A synopsis of general program characteristics for school health education and worksite health promotion programs is provided in Table 1. These generalities explain differences in health promotion programs designed for these two settings. The School Based Health Promotion Model (SBHPM), outlined in Table 1, reflects the notion that the outcomes of improving health of students should be viewed differently. Instead of improved knowledge, attitudes, and behavior as outcomes of the health education program, the school based health promotion program would address goals such as improved student morale, increased productivity (in this case, learning as measured by grades), and reduced absenteeism. In essence, the SBHPM encourages health education and health promotion to be viewed from the micro and macro perspectives. Traditional school health education programs tend to view outcomes from a micro perspective, or knowledge gained by the student. The SBHPM encourages us to view health education and promotion from a macro perspective which mandate a careful examination of the social, organizational, and political factors that impact the health of children. Viewing school health from a macro perspective also encourages us to examine ways to include faculty and staff in health promotion programs and to develop programs

This article is reprinted with permission from the *JOURNAL OF HEALTH EDUCATION*, January/February, 1996, pages 48–50. The *JOURNAL OF HEALTH EDUCATION* is a publication of the American Alliance for Health, Physical Education, Recreation and Dance, 1900 Association Drive, Reston, Virginia 20191.

Table 1 General Program Characteristics for School Health Education, Worksite Health Promotion, and a Model School Health Promotion Program

	School Health	Worksite Health Promotion	School-Based Health Promotion Model

Proposed Outcomes	• Increased knowledge
	• Improved attitude
	• Maintenance and/or adoption of healthy behaviors
		• Improved productivity
		• Reduced health care cost
		• Decreased absentee rate
		• Improved morale
			• Increased average daily attendance
			• Improved student productivity
			   1. Academic performance
			   2. Extracurricular involvement
			• Decreased student health services utilization and need
			• Improved health knowledge
			• Improved health attitudes
			• Maintenance and/or adoption of healthy behaviors
			• Decreased incidence of accidents

Planning Process	• Minimum curriculum scope and sequence established by State Department of • Local curriculum designed and implemented by school district	• Needs assessment usually conducted at local level	• Student needs assessment administered regularly • Coordination by a Comprehensive School Health Education Education
Mode of Implementation	• Classroom instruction	• Personal assessment & prescription • Incentives • Classroom instruction • Use of on-site and off-site facilities	• Classroom instruction • Multimedia messages • Health screenings • Incentives • Improvement of healthy school environment • Utilization of on and off-site facilities
Levels of Evaluation	• *Outcome Evaluation—*the majority of school districts evaluate through student knowledge evaluation, while a small percentage of schools use student attitude and behavior as evaluation criteria.	• Formative evaluation (Needs Assessment) • Process evaluation • Outcome evaluation • Cost benefit evaluation	• Formative evaluation • Process evaluation • Outcome evaluation • Cost benefit evaluation

that don't "blame the victim" for health problems of society.

Schools are uniquely suited to approaching health promotion in this manner. Four student related factors contribute to the potential validity of the school based health promotion model. First, most children and adolescents are enrolled in school so potential access to the group is a given. Second, the potential for successful implementation of a health promotion program exists simply because the participants tend to stay in school for a long period of time. Third, data collection, especially longitudinal data, is relatively easy and schoolsites provide opportunities to study specific problems of interest, track specific subgroups, and evaluate the effect of the entire program. Finally, students tend to be enthusiastic, willing participants in innovative, action oriented programming. Programs which deviate from the normal school routine are usually accepted by students.

The School-Based Health Promotion Model

The School-Based Health Promotion model is founded on two notions: (1) students will voluntarily choose to participate and complete program activities, and (2) behavioral outcomes found in successful worksite programs will also occur in schoolsite interventions. The SBHPM is based on voluntary participation with students electing to become involved in various health promotion activities. The voluntary nature of such a program would put the onus on the administrator of the health promotion program to insure that the program meets the needs and interests of students.

The nature and scope of Comprehensive School Health Education programs is established by teachers, parents, local administrators, or state agencies. In the SBHPM, the needs and interests of the consumer (students) would set the agenda. (It should be noted that state mandated health instruction would continue and serve as a social marketing effort.) (See discussion below.) Pre-assessment of student needs allows for participant ownership in the program and would serve to enhance student involvement. In addition, student needs assessments provide direction and emphasis for program activities and the foundation upon which post participation evaluations can be measured to determine program success and efficacy.

For many school districts, state and district guidelines mandate the scope and sequence of an instructional program. In the school based health promotion model each school district would determine their program by student need and would be subject to modification on a regular basis. In essence, while it is a laborious process to modify a statewide health education instructional mandate, in this model program, change at the local school district level would be encouraged and mandated.

In order to achieve the desired benefits from implementation of a school-based worksite health promotion program, a meaningful intervention program should be designed and implemented. Ideally, a school-based health promotion program would include social marketing, education and program activities, and environmental/corporate cultural support.

Social Marketing

Social marketing is the marketing of ideas. Social marketing includes design, implementation, and control of programs seeking to increase the acceptability of a social idea or practice in a target audience. In the context of the public schools, social marketing activities contained within the SBHPM would include activities designed to provide students with health information and to change attitudes in regard to the acceptability of a health behavior or concept. In a public school setting, social marketing activities would include, but not be limited to:

1. Health education instructional courses required by state mandate

2. Health newsletters

3. Pamphlets, brochures, fact sheets

4. Video spots on closed circuit TV

5. Bulletin boards, posters

6. Existing community-based health screening, health fairs, and related activities.

It is important to note that in this paradigm the traditional health education class would support the interventions included within the school-based health promotion model. For example, information disseminated in a mandated health education class on stress would provide background information that may encourage students to participate in targeted stress management programs offered in the school-based health promotion model.

Program and Educational Activities

Program and educational activities refer to structured interventions designed to maintain and improve health or decrease health risks. These interventions can take a variety of forms: screening activities (BMI, blood pressure, percent body fat), incentive programs (safety belt use, healthy weight loss, fitness competition), and educational programs targeted at specific health risk behaviors (physical fitness to reduce percent body fat, weight reduction through diet management, medical self-care procedures). Again, it should be noted that these program and educational activities should be based on the needs and interests of the target population. The SBHPM requires that specific programs be developed for segments of the target audience. For example, physical activity programs would vary based on the desired benefits of the target audience. The programs for students who want to engage in various forms of physical activity for social reasons would differ from those designed for students seeking competition.

Environmental/ Cultural Factors

Environmental and cultural factors refer to a composite of all factors which influence the school-based health promotion programs. The key component is the development of an expanded "healthy school" environment. The school environment and culture are shaped by policies, procedures, and attitudes, both written and unwritten, that are established at the building and district level. Development of an environment of this type is clearly tied to:

- Study/learning conditions (class size, lighting);

- Opportunities for student participation in decision making and problem solving situations;

- Student/Teacher/ Administrator/Parent relations;

- Opportunities for students to succeed in health promotion activities of their choice; and,

- Well-managed change with appropriate opportunities for feedback. In essence, a student-based health promotion program would influence and be influenced by the school environment. These factors cannot be isolated from the success or failure of the program.

Summary

The purpose of this article was to outline a different approach to improving the health of school age children. The basic premise of the School Based Health Promotion Model is that a program designed to meet the problems, needs, and interests of the target audience and one that includes social marketing, program and educational activities, and environmental/cultural support would be an effective way to enhance the health of students and improve educational outcomes. This notion is similar to procedures and outcomes proposed for worksite health promotion programs. We believe that if this model were used in public schools, it would enhance the feeling of local ownership and reduce the level of controversy that often surrounds school health education. Clearly, a carefully constructed ongoing assessment process which includes input from students, teachers, staff, and parents should ameliorate much of the controversy that surrounds some school health programs. In addition, this model would strive for goals that are perceived as a common good by most people; improved attendance, improved grades, and enhanced health behaviors. We hope that this Personal Perspective initiates a dialogue that will advance the notion of implementing the worksite health promotion model in schools.

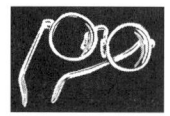 **Article Review Form at end of book.**

List the three common elements of each collaborative agreement between the schools and managed care organizations. Discuss the principles developed by the *SHIP* collaborative partners.

The *School Health Innovative Programs:*

Integrating School Health and Managed Care in San Diego

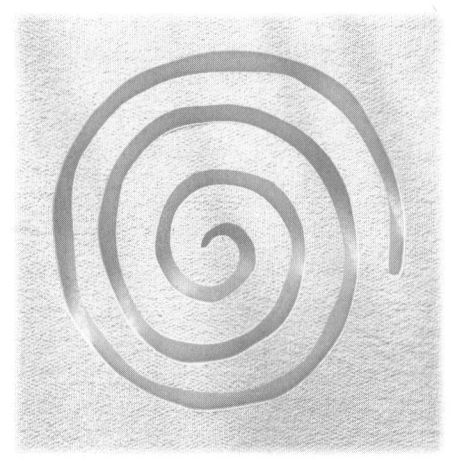

Howard Taras, Philip Nader, Holly Swiger, John Fontanesi

Howard Taras, MD, Associate Professor; and Philip Nader, Chief; Division of Community Pediatrics, University California, San Diego, 9500 Gilman Drive, Dept. 0927, La Jolla, CA 92093-0927; Holly Swiger, Project Coordinator, San Diego School Health Innovations Project, 3913 Summer Way, Escondido, CA 92025-7942; and John Fontanesi, PhD, Clinical Neuropsychologist, Pediatrics Center for School Problems, Kaiser-Permanente, 7060 Clairemont Mesa Blvd., 3rd Floor, San Diego, CA 92111. This article was submitted July 18, 1997, and accepted for publication October 5, 1997.

Abstract

Managed care organizations (MCOs) are being recruited to support school health services delivered in school clinics. Schools without clinics already provide numerous health services and could provide more if they had support from managed care organizations. This article describes the first two years of a San Diego-based collaborative consisting of MCOs, school districts, and other health care agencies. By establishing trust, developing overriding principles, and creating an interagency communication infrastructure, this collaborative has encouraged shared management of many student health issues. Because the agreements apply to all schools, programs can reduce high rates of absenteeism district-wide and avoid unnecessary doctor appointments for common health problems. These collaborative agreements are designed to be financially self-sustaining. However, data collection, the logistics of obtaining parental consent, and getting health professionals to communicate with each other in new ways remain to be significant challenges. (J Sch Health. 1998; 68(1):22–25)

A national trend has developed for both privately insured and Medicaid-insured populations to receive health services through managed care organizations (MCOs). Concomitantly, an unre-lated trend to develop school-linked and school-based health services has emerged, which can improve access to medically under-served populations.[1,2] Much of the work to bridge these trends has focused on how MCOs can support services at school clinics and how school clinics can improve access to care for MCO clients.[3–6]

About 600 school-based health centers operate in the United States at this time. This statistic represents an enormous increase from the number of school clinics that existed a decade ago, but it is an insignificant proportion of the schools whose student populations could benefit from such services. School health centers struggle financially to remain open after start-up funds expire. Various experimental agreements among school districts, health departments, and MCOs have helped many school clinics stay open.[3–6] Yet, no mas-

Howard Taras, Philip Nader, Holly Swiger, and John Fontanesi, "The *School Health Innovative Programs:* Integrating School Health and Managed Care in San Diego." *Journal of School Health,* (Vol. 68, No. 1), pp. 22–25, January 1998. Reprinted with permission from the American School Health Association.

ter plan addresses the feasibility for MCOs to support school clinics if clinics were to operate in each school that needs one but does not yet have one.

The *School Health Innovative Programs (SHIP)*, developed in San Diego, explored how MCOs and schools can work together to improve the health of students who attend all schools, whether or not a school-based or school-linked clinic exists. This article summarizes the first two and a half years of the project's accomplishments.

Background

California's San Diego County enrolls families with Medicaid into MCOs, accounting for a large number of students with MCO-Medicaid insurance in schools. A project was initiated in a cluster of 12 schools (two secondary and 10 elementary) in a region with a high Medicaid-MCO penetration. A school nurse is assigned to each school in this district for at least one day per week. Although other school districts have joined *SHIP* more recently, this report addresses the initial two years.

SHIP participants met monthly. Schools were represented by district-level staff from three departments: health; billing and contracts; and management information services. School health staff from pilot sites also attended meetings. Three MCOs (Kaiser Permanente, Great American, and Community Health Group) have participated in *SHIP* since its inception. Others have joined as Medicaid contracts with more MCOs. Each MCO representative has access to the local chief executive officer of his or her organization. To implement pilot collaborative arrangements

between MCOs and schools, primary care doctors and school health staff receive in-service training from project representatives at intervals during the course of the project.

The Division of Community Pediatrics at the University of California at San Diego, the local public health department, local community clinics, the local children's hospital, and the local chapter of the American Academy of Pediatrics each send representatives to *SHIP*'s monthly meetings. The initial year's efforts were supported by a grant from the Foundation Consortium of California. The group has since been self-supported.

Project Development
Establishing Trust: The Initial Six Months

Initially, MCOs and school staff were suspicious of each other's intentions to collaborate. School personnel suspected health plans did not want to encourage service utilization for populations that did not normally seek services. MCO administrators and health providers suspected school health staff were competing with traditional health care providers for the health care dollar.

MCO representatives learned that most school health services— such as vision screenings, administering medication, and special health care procedures for students with special health care needs—are mandated by law. By visiting school sites and speaking to school nurses, MCO representatives began to appreciate the utility of school health services. Medicaid populations are more likely to over-utilize emergency services,[7] and it became more apparent to MCOs that school

health staff can identify and assist families that do not know how to optimally utilize preventive and acute care health services. Without case management, immunizations, and physical health examinations available at schools, these students are either absent from school or not well enough to learn optimally and may eventually incur higher health care costs to MCOs and their providers.

Also during the initial six-month period, school district representatives learned that MCOs operate under constraints of limited Medicaid capitation rates. MCOs rely on control of health resource utilization to provide quality care at low Medicaid reimbursement rates. Over time school staff came to understand the MCOs' hesitation to tacitly support any school clinic that already existed or would exist in the future. The complexity for MCOs to form individual agreements with numerous schools in numerous districts was appreciated. Staff decided that each collaborative agreement would be piloted and evaluated before making large-scale commitments. Because of this doctrine, *SHIP* participants worked on numerous issue-based arrangements in a step-wise manner.

Development of Overriding Principles

SHIP collaborative partners developed and adhered to the following principles:

- Each partner would recognize and respect the institutional goals of others, how they differ from their own, and where they overlap. Health goals for schools are to keep students healthy so they are available to learn optimally and attend school. For health plans and primary care providers, members need to be kept healthy by delivering care in a cost-effective, coordinated, and accessible manner.

- Collaborative activities would maintain principles of confidentiality,[8] parent involvement, preventive care, and continuity of care.

- The project endorsed the "medical home" principle as defined by the American Academy of Pediatrics.[9] A student's health plan, or more appropriately the student's designated health provider, is regarded by *SHIP* participants to be the optimal medical home, not the school.

- Collaborative agreements have to be replicable to student populations with varying demographic characteristics and applicable to each school in any one district.

- To be financially sustainable without grant or governmental funding, aside from Medicaid, each agreement needs to make business sense for MCOs, their health providers, and schools.

Coordination of Collaborative Activities

Most project funds were spent on a project coordinator, a nurse with extensive experience in project management and group facilitation, who acted as a moderator of meetings. Once collaborative pilot projects between schools and MCOs were planned, the coordinator was responsible for assuring that information was disseminated to staff at participating schools and to health providers of participating MCOs.

Creation of a Communication Infrastructure

Schools asked parents for consent when their children registered for school. This allowed schools and MCOs to exchange pertinent information. Each MCO assigned a contact person and phone number to *SHIP* participating schools so school staff could quickly elicit student enrollment status information and exchange health information. A participating MCO donated a fax machine to each pilot school's health office, so confidential health information would not be sent to nonhealth areas of the school.

Project Protocols

Several protocols were developed by the third year of the project.

Utilization of Health Services

Anonymous data on students in pilot schools enrolled in MCOs were shared to measure utilization of services, duplication of services, and service gaps such as students with incomplete immunizations or required health screenings. Some 238 students simultaneously enrolled in an MCO-Medicaid plan and a pilot school in 1995–96. Of these, 206 students received Medicaid billable services at school. These services were mostly mandated vision and hearing screenings, immunizations, learning problem assessments, and some counseling for behavioral problems. These activities totaled 534 services. Many more students received medical services not accounted for in these

numbers because they were not recorded, or the service did not meet the 15-minute minimum billing criterion. Of the 238 students, 63 received 210 health services through their MCOs. Surprisingly, there were no service duplications. To improve the value of this data, *SHIP* participants are working on standardized nomenclature and descriptions for health services and on better documentation of the services.

Vision, Hearing, and Other Health Screening Referrals

If a student fails his or her school vision or hearing screening, this information is recorded on a computerized form and on the school health record. Aside from notifying parents to seek medical follow-up, the computerized system also indicates which designated MCO representative to notify. Parental permission to release information is necessary for computerized notification of the MCO.

Tuberculin Skin Testing

Most Mantoux Skin Tests placed on children in their health providers' offices often fail to be read two to three days later.[10] For reasons of transportation, parent employment, and missed classroom time, it is inconvenient for families to keep these follow-up visits. The *SHIP* collaborative arranged for school nurses to verify skin test results placed by MCO health providers. MCO reimbursement to schools for the service is currently pending and depends on program utilization and its evaluation.

Mental Health Referrals

This first phase of collaboration concentrated on attention- and learning-related problems. Health providers have complained that students are needlessly referred to them for suspected attention deficit disorder, and referrals are often based on the opinion of only one school staff member. Pertinent information on students' school behavior often do not accompany referrals, which necessitates an additional appointment and wasted time. This situation also leads physicians to over-refer students for special education evaluations. As such, this situation has been costly to school districts and MCOs, and it delays diagnosis and management.

The collaborative agreement required that a multidisciplinary review team at school ("student study team") address student's learning, attention, or behavioral issues before recommending that parents seek a pediatric or mental health appointment. The written report of this multidisciplinary discussion and any other pertinent materials, including the most appropriate contact person at the school, were sent with the parent to the first appointment. The index of suspicion for a learning disorder was addressed by the school's resource specialist, who was part of the team, in this report. This information was expected to reduce the number of students unnecessarily referred by physicians for comprehensive psychological testing.

Head Lice

An inordinate number of student attendance days are lost to head lice infestation. Because most plans require a physician's prescription if treatment is to be covered by insurance, this procedure delays treatment and wastes physician time. New arrangements between schools and MCOs allow school nurses to make the diagnosis. Depending on the MCO, school nurses can either call the student's primary care provider to arrange for a prescription at a local pharmacy, call the pharmacy themselves on behalf of the health provider, or dispense treatment that is supplied at the school by one MCO.

First Grade Physical Examinations

The largest school district in San Diego performs EPSDT examinations on first graders who do not receive them elsewhere. Without an agreement, this program would not continue, and students would be temporarily suspended from school until these examinations were done. With the agreement, school nurse practitioners can continue to conduct these examinations and be reimbursed by the MCO. The exam occurs only after MCOs are notified in advance and still fail to perform examinations through their traditional providers.

Several *SHIP* collaborative arrangements currently are under discussion: 1) to jointly monitor, educate, and manage asthmatic students since chronic diseases,[11] and asthma in particular,[12] cause considerable and preventable expenses to schools and MCOs; 2) to systematically share school-derived speech, occupational, and physical therapy reports with health providers; 3) to jointly address preadolescent risk-taking behaviors; 4) to coordinate identification and treatment of sexually transmitted diseases; 5) to address health management of students at schools with onsite clinics. Aside from expanding the number of schools, MCOs, and students served, the next phase of *SHIP* will concentrate on ways to collect better data and evaluate the utilization and cost-effectiveness of each interagency agreement.

Project Implications

Three common elements were part of each collaborative agreement between schools and MCOs. First, regular systems of communication between health plans and schools were developed. Second, joint management was developed to benefit students, parents, schools, health providers, and/or MCOs. Third, inexpensive and simple ways were found to improve access to health care.

Two major time and funding costs affected implementing San Diego's *SHIP* model for MCO and school collaboration. First, attaining parent permission to exchange basic information is a time-consuming and inefficient hurdle. Second, changing the practices of physicians[13–15] and their office staff is time consuming. Yet both of these factors are necessary to the success of San Diego's model because school health office staff and primary-care provider offices are not yet accustomed to coordinating or communicating directly on matters like TB skin tests and head lice management. Collaborative agreements with schools will be more commonly utilized in primary care physician offices when *SHIP* agreements expand to larger numbers of schools and all MCOs so that the protocols can apply to all school-aged patients of a physician's practice.

As *SHIP* agreements are adapted to school districts with fewer school nurses, MCOs are recognizing the value of the medical expertise that school nurses bring to school sites, their ready access to students and families, and their case-management skills. School nurses have found an ally for school nursing services through this process.

In this pilot program, MCO reimbursement for school health services does not lower the capitation rates that MCOs negotiate with health providers. However, because more school health services may be used in larger numbers of schools instead of physician offices, it is possible that reimbursement can come from capitation rates as the program expands beyond the pilot phase. Involvement and endorsement of health providers is essential to the process of negotiation between MCOs and schools. *SHIP*'s overriding principal that each negotiated agreement make business sense for all needs to include health providers. Staff must demonstrate that primary care providers benefit from this as well.

The prevalence of managed health care for children with private and publicly funded health insurance is not unique to San Diego. Opportunities for school districts to reach large numbers of health providers through MCOs are opening up in other communities across the nation. School health staff must recognize this opportunity and initiate dialogue with these systems when they are still new and malleable enough to accommodate school health principles. Many states have instituted or are considering legislation that mandates a defined relationship with schools. The collaborative work begun in San Diego may influence the nature of such legislation.

Conclusion

The San Diego *SHIP* experience may be instructive for other parts of the nation going through similar transitions in health care delivery. The time is favorable for MCOs and school districts to work together toward their separate and common missions. This process should include the participation of all health entities with a stake in the relationship between school districts and health plans. The development of a trusting relationship between negotiating parties should not be overlooked nor regarded as misspent time. Effecting institutional change, even if done incrementally, seems to be a good recipe for initial success. School agreements with MCOs can be inexpensive, reach large numbers of students, and address the most prevalent health problems when they are not limited to the school clinic as the sole model of school health service delivery.

References

1. *Linking local health centers with schools serving low income children. An idea book.* Washington, DC: U.S. Dept of Health and Human Services, Bureau of Primary Health Care, Health Resources and Services Administration; 1996.
2. *Making the Grade. Medicaid, Managed Care, and School-Based Health Center.* Proceedings of a meeting with policy makers and providers. Washington, DC; 1995.
3. Hacker K. Integrating school-based health centers into managed care in Massachusetts. *J Sch Health.* 1996;66(9):317–321.
4. *School-based health centers and managed care.* Washington. DC: U.S. Dept of Health and Human Services, Office of Inspector General; 1993.
5. *A Partnership for Quality and Access: School-based Health Centers and Health Plans.* New York. NY: School Health Policy Initiative, Montefiore Medical Center; 1996.
6. Grant R, Maggio L. Import of Medicaid managed care on school-based clinics. *Res Soc Health Care.* 1997;14:289–303.
7. Davidson AEF, Klein DE, Settipane GA, Alario AJ. Access to care among children visiting the emergency room with acute exacerbations of asthma. *Ann Allergy.* 1994;72:469–473.
8. American Academy of Pediatrics. Task force on Medical Informatics, Committee on Practice and Ambulatory Medicine. *Pediatrics.* 1996;98(5):984–986.
9. American Academy of Pediatrics. Ad hoc task force on definition of the medical home: The medical home. *Pediatrics.* 1992 Nov;90(S):774.
10. Sewint, JR, Hall BS, Baldwin RM, Virden JM. Outcomes of annual Tuberculosis screening by Mantoux Test in children considered to be at high risk: results from one urban clinic. *Pediatrics.* 1997;99:529–533.
11. Newacheck PW, Stein REK, Walker DK, Gortmaker SL, Kuhlthau K, Perrin JM. Monitoring and evaluation managed care for children with chronic illnesses and disabilities. *Pediatrics.* 1996;98(5):952–958.
12. Lozano P, Fishman P, VonKorff M, Hecht J. Health care utilization and cost among children with asthma who were enrolled in a health maintenance organization. *Pediatrics.* 1997;99:757–764.
13. Davis DA, Thomson MA, Oxman AD, Haynes B. Changing physician performance—a systematic review of the effect of continuing medical education strategies. *JAMA.* 1995;274:700–705.
14. Greco PJ, Eisenberg JM. Changing physicians' practices. *N Engl J Med.* 1993;329:1271–1273.
15. Weiss R, Charney E, Baumgardner RA, et al. Changing patient management: what influences the practicing pediatrician. *Pediatrics.* 1990:85:791–795.

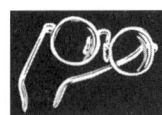 **Article Review Form at end of book.**

Describe the focus of Phases I and II of the pilot project. Differentiate between formative and process evaluation.

Formative, Process, and Intermediate Outcome Evaluation of a Pilot School-Based 5 a Day for Better Health Project

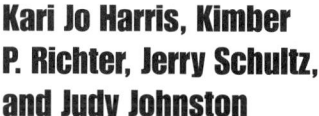

Kari Jo Harris, Kimber P. Richter, Jerry Schultz, and Judy Johnston

Kari Jo Harris, MPH, is at the Department of Preventive Medicine, University of Kansas Medical Center. Kimber P. Richter, MPH, and Jerry Schultz, PhD, are at the University of Kansas, Lawrence, Kansas. Judy Johnston, MS, RD, LD, is at Kansas LEAN, Wichita, Kansas.

Purpose

Low consumption of fruits and vegetables is associated with higher rates of chronic diseases.[1] Children consume less than the optimal number of fruits and vegetables.[2] Several school-based health initiatives have successfully influenced children's diets,[3] few of which targeted children's consumption of fruits and vegetables.[4,5] This paper reports the formative, process, and intermediate outcome results of a 5-month school-based project that was linked to the National 5 A Day for Better Health campaign[6] to increase young children's consumption of fruits and vegetables. This project, The Kansas LEAN School Health Project, PHASE II: 5 A Day for Better Health, was implemented in three elementary schools. Two years prior to the start of this project, these schools completed PHASE I of the Kansas LEAN School Health Project, a more extensive intervention targeting nutrition education, physical activity, and dietary fat.[7,8] While PHASE I focused on reducing children's consumption of dietary fat and increasing exercise, PHASE II focused on increasing children's consumption of fruits and vegetables.

Methods

Design

The project team, consisting of dietitians and evaluators, used two designs to address the formative, process, and intermediate outcome level questions outlined in Table 1. A formative case study design was used to develop the intervention and collect information about the implementation of the project. The team also explored one intermediate outcome of the project (tasting new foods) using a one-group pretest-posttest design.

Sample

Three elementary schools in the Kansas communities of Salina (population 42,300) and Dighton (population 1400) participated.

Reprinted by permission from *American Journal of Health Promotion,* July/August 1998 (Vol. 12, No. 12), pp. 378–381.

Table 1 Evaluation Questions and Assessment Tools

Evaluation Questions	Assessment Tools
Formative	
What barriers to consuming fruits and vegetables exist at home?	Preliminary focus groups
What barriers to consuming fruits and vegetables exist at school?	Preliminary focus groups
What incentives would facilitate the consumption of fruits and vegetables at school?	Preliminary focus groups
How acceptable were candidate recipes to students and food service employees?	Sensory evaluation
Process	
Was the project implemented as planned?	Teachers' activity logs
	Food service activity logs
	Coupons redeemed
	Follow-up focus groups
How satisfied were participants?	Follow-up focus groups
How might the project be improved?	Follow-up focus groups
Intermediate outcome	
Did students taste fruits and vegetables prepared in new ways?	Taste testing data sheets
What were the effects of the project on students' tasting of new fruits and vegetables?	Follow-up focus groups tasting
	Written survey
What were the effects of the project on the cost and participation in the school food service program?	Food service records

These schools were selected because they had track records for addressing childhood risk factors for cardiovascular diseases through their participation in PHASE I of the project. The Salina intervention school housed 488 students, and an offsite kitchen served lunch. The two Dighton intervention schools housed 284 students, and lunches were provided by an onsite kitchen in one of the elementary schools. All students (n = 772), teachers (n = 28), and food service programs (n = 2) were invited to participate. Both food service programs participated. Five teachers in one school declined to participate in the project because of other demands on their time; students (n = 126) in these teachers' classes were unable to participate in the classroom-based components.

Measures

Eight assessment tools listed in Table 1 provided information to address the evaluation questions. Team members conducted preliminary focus groups with homogeneous groups of parents, children, and food service staff and sensory evaluations with food service staff and children to design the intervention. Teacher and food service activity logs, coupons redeemed, and tasting data sheets provided information about project implementation. Follow-up focus groups with homogeneous groups of parents, children, and food service staff at both schools provided information on how satisfied participants were and suggestions for improvements. The project team used three dependent measures to explore one intermediate outcome of the project. Students' tasting of the recipes introduced by the intervention was assessed using tasting data sheets, which consisted of tally sheets for marking new recipes tasted by students. Younger (grades K–3) students' tasting new foods was assessed by a written survey, the "Foods I have tried" section of the Changing the Course assessment.[9] A formative evaluation of this assessment established high content validity and calculated Cronbach's alpha reliability coefficient of .92 for the entire questionnaire.[10] Archival food service records tracked the intervention's effect on the cost and participation in the school lunch program.

Intervention

The intervention, based on the 5 A Day model, was facilitated by Kansas LEAN (Leadership to Encourage Activity and Nutrition)[11] and promoted five fruits and vegetables: apple, zucchini, pear, tomato, and broccoli. Table 2 summarizes the setting and components of the intervention, which occurred in school classrooms (e.g., 21 potential classroom activities, recording of tasting 25 new recipes and incentives for tasting), school cafeterias (e.g., 25 new recipes, 38 cafeteria activities), supermarkets (e.g., five coupons, supermarket tours), homes (promotional items sent home at the discretion of teachers), and the community (one community-wide event). Teachers and food service programs were encouraged to use as many of the activities as they wished.

Table 2	Setting and Components of the LEAN 5 a Day Project

Setting	Components
Classroom	Information and posters
	Tasting raw foods
	Activity sheets and group projects
	Cooking activities
	Recording of taste testing and incentives
	Mini grants for teachers
Cafeteria	New recipes served
	Posters
	Games and activities
Supermarket	Tours
	Coupons
Home	Brochures
	Menus
	Promotional items (e.g., magnets)
Community	Your Produce Man community event

Analysis

The project team analyzed comments made during focus groups by identifying patterns and themes in participants' responses and drew conclusions about program implementation and functioning based on themes that emerged from the verbal data. Activity logs and taste testing data sheets were tallied, coupons redeemed were counted, and data from food service records were averaged. To determine statistical significance of changes in new foods tried from before and after the intervention, researchers calculated one-tailed z-scores[12] based on the proportion of students who tried the foods at posttest compared to an estimate (5%) of the proportion of students expected to try new foods in a 6-month period.

Results

Formative Evaluation

The project team used preliminary focus groups to select the intervention foods. These were foods that (1) were not eaten frequently, and (2) students reported neither a strong dislike nor a strong like for. Focus group data also aided in the selection of classroom materials (e.g., hands-on activities and games), incentives for children (e.g., T-shirts, pogs, stickers), and food preparation procedures that fit in with current food service practices (e.g., holding times for foods). Results from the sensory evaluations were used to correct recipes before dissemination.

Process Evaluation

There was a consensus among those participating in focus groups that the project was successful in increasing the students' ability to recognize new foods, their willingness to try them, and their awareness of their nutritional value. Some teachers chose not to participate because of the regular demands placed on them by the school. However, most teachers and all food service workers, parents, and students would recommend the project to other teachers and schools, especially if slight modifications were made. Overall, the project was implemented as planned in each setting.

Classroom. The project was implemented by most (82%) teachers in the participating schools, and teachers used many (41%) of the classroom materials. In addition, most (80%) of the teachers facilitated students' tasting of the new recipes by completing data sheets and providing incentives to students.

Cafeteria. Food service staff prepared and served samples of nearly all (96%) of the new recipes and used many (55%) of the promotional materials, including posters, buttons, and T-shirts.

Supermarket. The project was not completely implemented as planned in the supermarket. Only one teacher reported taking a class on a supermarket tour and, during focus groups, teachers reported distributing only some of the food coupons. Only 80 coupons were redeemed in Dighton, which, if all teachers distributed all five coupons to every student, is a 9% return rate. Similar data are not available in Salina since the coupons redeemed were inadvertently destroyed at the supermarket.

Home. Focus group results indicated that parents received promotional materials from their children, including flyers, coupons, and recipes. Parents appreciated the materials and felt they prompted them to provide more fruits and vegetables to their children. Overall, however, parents were unaware of the specific foods promoted.

Community. Both communities held a community event featuring a nationally recognized newscaster who provided fun facts about fruits and vegetables. Participants in focus groups reported that the community events were a strength of the project and served to kick off the promotion.

Intermediate Outcome Evaluation

Tasting New Recipes. On average, most (96%) students in Dighton and half (50%) of the students in Salina tasted new recipes on days when sampling data were collected.

Tasting New Fruits and Vegetables. Most (80%) of students had, at pretest, tasted three of the featured foods (apples, pears, and broccoli) and a number of other foods. For the other foods, a significant ($p > .01$) percent of students who had not tried the foods at pretest had tried the foods at posttest.

Lunch Cost and Participation. The project did not appear to affect cost or participation in the school food service program. Food service records were available only for Dighton, where the per student cost of lunch for months that the project was implemented ($1.29) was nearly identical to the months when the project was not implemented ($1.27). Participation in the school lunch program remained at nearly 100% throughout the school year.

Discussion
Summary and Interpretation of Results

Overall, this process and intermediate outcome evaluation showed that the project was implemented as planned and increased students' tasting of fruits and vegetables. The project team used data from preliminary focus groups and sensory evaluations to choose the intervention foods, select materials, determine incentives, and develop new recipes. Data from activity logs, redeemed coupons, and follow-up focus groups indicated that the project was implemented throughout the target schools in all intended settings. In general, participants were satisfied with all components of the project. Teachers, food service employees, students, and parents provided a number of suggestions to improve the project. The project team reviewed data from follow-up focus groups, taste testing data sheets, surveys, and food service records to explore the intermediate outcomes of the project. Many students tasted food prepared using the new recipes, younger students tasted a variety of new foods, and the project did not seem to affect the cost of the school meal programs or students' participation in school lunch.

Significance

The project team used a combination of qualitative and quantitative research methods to obtain formative, process, and intermediate evaluation data for an intervention that was designed to be short term, implemented by community members, low cost, flexible, and easy to adopt by schools. The evaluation provides a model of how to conduct formative research for program improvement while at the same time collecting data on the intermediate outcomes of the project. Kansas LEAN will use data from this evaluation to modify the intervention for dissemination across the state. Broad-scale dissemination of such an intervention may likely reduce risks for cardiovascular diseases among large groups of young people.

Limitations

There are a number of limitations associated with evaluating a relatively brief intervention implemented by community members in real settings. First, the level of implementation varied across settings (e.g., high implementation of new recipes, low implementation in supermarkets) and communities (e.g., more students tasted new recipes in Dighton). The evaluation tracked level of implementation rather than controlling it. Second, since the intervention was very brief, the project team did not continually feed process or intermediate outcome data back to community members so they could improve the project. Third, no control sites were used to compare intervention students' increase in tasting new foods. The increase might have been a result of maturation, which the project team attempted to control for in their statistical analysis. Fourth, data on students' consumption of fruits and vegetables are not available. Students may have tried new foods and new recipes, but may not have consumed quantities necessary to affect their risks for chronic diseases. Finally, the intervention occurred in only two communities, which may limit the generality of these findings.

References

1. Block G, Patterson B, Subar A. Fruit, vegetables, and cancer prevention: a review of the epidemiological evidence. *Nutr Cancer* 1992:18:1–29.
2. McPherson RS, Montgomery DH, Nichaman MZ. Nutritional status of children: what do we know? *J Nutr Educ* 1995;27:225–34.
3. Contento C, Balch GI, Bronner YL, et al. The effectiveness of nutrition education and implications for nutrition education policy, programs, and research: a review of research. *J Nutr Educ* 1995;27:275–418.
4. Havas S, Heimendinger J, Damron D, et al. 5 a day for better health—nine community research projects to increase fruit and vegetable consumption. *Public Health Rep* 1995:110:68–80.

5. Domel SB, Baranowski T, Davis H. Development and evaluation of a school intervention to increase fruit and vegetable consumption among 4th and 5th grade students. *J Nutr Educ* 1993;25:345–349.

6. Heimendinger J, Van Duyn MA, Chapelsky D, et al. The national 5 A Day for Better Health Program: a large-scale nutrition intervention. *J Public Health Manage Pract* 1996;2:27–35.

7. Harris KJ, Richter KP, Paine-Andrews A, et al. Community partnerships: review of selected models and evaluation of two case studies. *J Nutr Educ* 1997;29:189–95.

8. Harris KJ, Paine-Andrews A, Richter KP, et al. Reducing elementary school children's risks for chronic diseases through school lunch modifications, nutrition education, and physical activity interventions. *J Nutr Educ* 1997;29:196–202.

9. American Cancer Society. *Changing the Course (Lower Elementary Curriculum)*. Atlanta, Georgia: American Cancer Society, 1993.

10. Contento IR, Kell DG, Keiley MK, et al. A formative evaluation of the American Cancer Society Changing the Course nutrition education curriculum. *J Sch Health* 1992;62:411–6.

11. Johnston JA, Marmet PF, Coen S, et al. Kansas LEAN: an effective coalition for nutrition education and dietary change. *J Nutr Educ* 1996;62:115–8.

12. Glass GV, Hopkins KD. *Statistical Methods in Education and Psychology*. 2nd ed. Englewood Cliffs, New Jersey: Prentice-Hall, 1984.

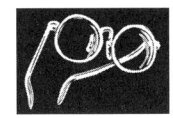 **Article Review Form at end of book.**

The key to meeting the health education crisis in this country continues to lie with _____. Although most of the health education within the elementary school is carried out by the classroom teacher, most elementary teachers are ill-equipped to teach health education effectively. How has this problem been perpetuated?

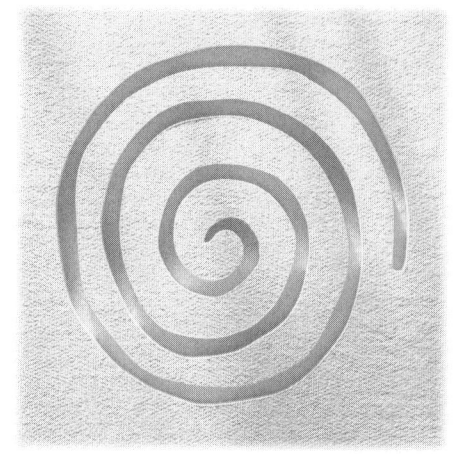

Dealing with the Health Crisis in Our Schools:

Clarion University's Health Education Model for Elementary and Early Childhood Education Majors

William English and Charles R. Duke

William English is with the Department of Health and Physical Education, Clarion University of Pennsylvania 16214. Charles R. Duke is with Appalachian State University, Boone, NC and was formerly Dean of the College of Education and Human Services at Clarion University of Pennsylvania.

Abstract

The training of elementary and early childhood education teachers often does not involve professional preparation to develop knowledge and skills for introducing effective health education into the classroom. To address this problem, the Health and Physical Education Department at

Clarion University of Pennsylvania has developed and implemented a model health education emphasis for preservice teachers in the university's College of Education and Human Services. The program addresses key issues in health education and offers professional preparation for providing health education as a part of an overall comprehensive health program for schools.

Much of the hope for prevention and the implementation of health promotion programs has been placed in the hands of educators because many of the significant health related problems facing our nation can be traced to inappropriate behaviors, habits, and attitudes developed during the

early school years. School health programs also have been given increased attention because what traditionally have been considered adult health issues (drug and alcohol abuse, weight problems, sexuality, abuse, AIDS, and pregnancy, to name just a few) now appear on a daily basis in our elementary and secondary schools.

Pennsylvania can serve as an example of a state with problems in health education similar to those in many other states. For example, among the findings from a 1988–89 drug and alcohol survey of 38,757 Pennsylvania school students, and the 1989 Youth Risk Behavior Survey of 4,548 Pennsylvania public school

This article is reprinted with permission from the JOURNAL OF HEALTH EDUCATION, March/April 1995, pages 78–80. The JOURNAL OF HEALTH EDUCATION is a publication of the American Alliance for Health, Physical Education, Recreation and Dance, 1900 Association Drive, Reston, Virginia 20191.

students (Cinelli, B. A. et al., 1992) were the following:

- Almost 50 percent of seniors drink once a month, and 24 percent drink weekly or more often.

- Thirty percent of ninth graders, 13 percent of seventh graders, and eight percent of sixth graders have a drink at least once a month.

- Twenty-one percent of seniors and seven percent of ninth graders smoke cigarettes daily.

- Fourteen percent of seniors and seven percent of ninth graders smoke marijuana at least once a month.

- Fifty-six percent of Pennsylvania high school students engage in sexual intercourse and nearly 21 percent have multiple sex partners.

The picture concerning nutrition and exercise is no less alarming. For example, in a survey of 2,495 students in grades nine through 12, the Pennsylvania Department of Health (Cinelli, B. A. et al., 1992) determined that 18 percent had not taken part in at least 20 minutes of strenuous physical exercise during the two weeks prior to the survey and 10 percent had not attended a physical education class during the same period.

The initial response to these data might well be that more emphasis needs to be placed on health education at the high school level. Although there is no denying the need for education at that level, to have any great impact, effective health education must begin during the early formative years (K–6) when a child's attitudes and priorities relating to many health concepts are established. Elementary school health education, therefore, has always had long standing support as an important component of the curriculum. In 1984 an article appeared in the *Journal of School Health* in which many national professional school health education organizations re-affirmed their positions that a comprehensive school health education program should be in place from pre K–12. State legislatures at various times also have enacted legislation holding schools responsible for teaching drug and alcohol education at every grade level K–12; in Pennsylvania, for example, HIV/AIDS education and education about steroids have been mandated recently.

But position statements and practice do not always match. Unfortunately for Pennsylvania's students as well as students around the country, emphasis upon health education and health related issues at the elementary school level appears to be minimal. For example, the percentage of Pennsylvania elementary classroom teachers who spent less than two hours per year on various health topics (Cinelli, B. A. et al., 1992) is indicated below:

- 30 percent taught community health for less than two hours.

- 67 percent taught consumer health for less than two hours.

- 51 percent taught disease prevention and control for less than two hours.

- 76 percent taught family health for less than two hours.

- 32 percent taught safety and first aid for less than two hours.

- 37 percent taught fitness for less than two hours.

- 37 percent taught growth and development for less than two hours.

- 20 percent taught nutrition for less than two hours.

- 51 percent taught personal health for less than two hours.

- 21 percent taught tobacco, alcohol, and drugs for less than two hours.

Currently at the elementary level, the regular classroom teacher or other personnel such as a school nurse, counselor, or special education teacher can teach health. However, only one percent of the curriculum supervisors who are responsible for health education programs possess an undergraduate degree in health education, although 39 percent do hold a dual degree in health and physical education (Cinelli, B. A. et al., 1992). An examination of the dual degree, however, reveals severe inadequacies related to the health education component of the dual degree.

Although most of the health education within the elementary school is carried out by the classroom teacher, most elementary teachers are ill-equipped to teach health education effectively. In fact, the completion of courses in health education is not a requirement for elementary teacher certification in Pennsylvania and many other states. A Pennsylvania School Health Education Study found that 54 percent of elementary school teachers have not attended a health education in-service program in the past two years and 83 percent of elementary classroom teachers have six or fewer credits in health education as undergraduates. Fifty-four percent of the teachers surveyed believed that improved undergraduate preparation in this area was needed if instruction in health education is to improve (Cinelli, B. A. et al., 1992).

Because of these deficiencies, efforts should be initiated to improve the preparation of undergraduate elementary education candidates in health education. In addition to calling for the strengthening of preparation programs for health educators, the Pennsylvania Department of Health's report, "Healthy Children: The Key to Our Future" (Cinelli, B. A. et al., 1992) recommends that institutions of higher education develop a concentration or minor in health education to meet the professional preparation needs of early childhood and/or elementary education majors.

Clarion's Elementary Health Emphasis Program

At Clarion University of Pennsylvania, the Department of Health and Physical Education initiated a study of health curriculum in 1991 that anticipated the state's call for reform. As a result of its investigation into health issues related to teaching in the elementary school, the department was able to capitalize on the expertise of its faculty and developed a model program designed for elementary and early childhood majors. The Elementary Health Emphasis program requires 16 credits of professional preparation coursework as follows:

Introduction to Elementary Health Concepts and Promotion	3 credits
CPR	1 credit
First Aid and Safety	2 credits
HIV/AIDS Education	1 credit
Fitness for Wellness	3 credits
Food, Diet, and Weight Management	3 credits
The Elementary Health Curriculum	3 credits

Clarion University's Elementary Health Emphasis is not a minor but does require 16 credits of coursework in health education. Currently all elementary education majors in the College of Education and Human Services at Clarion are required to declare an area of emphasis of at least 15 credits; traditionally these areas have included mathematics, science, English, art, or music. The Department of Health and Physical Education at Clarion, recognizing the need for training elementary educators in health, went to the Department of Education, which houses Elementary Education, and worked collaboratively with the faculty to develop the present Elementary Health Emphasis. The College's administration also enthusiastically endorsed the program. During its initial year, the HPE department enrolled 30 students in its new emphasis.

Central to the program are "Introduction to Elementary Health Concepts and Promotion" and "The Elementary Health Curriculum." The two courses are designed to assist students in synthesizing content knowledge related to health and help prepare them for teaching effective health education programs in the schools. "Introduction to Elementary Health Concepts and Promotion" is an introductory level course designed to introduce students to selected health concepts and issues faced by the elementary teacher and the young child. A significant part of the course is designed to develop within students an appropriate understanding and appreciation for health education as an important component within any early childhood or elementary school curriculum. This is accomplished through an in-depth investigation of current health issues that can be addressed through quality health education in the schools. Among the issues explored are child abuse, alcohol and drug use, nutrition, childhood stress, and sexuality. Also addressed in the course are the development of a sound background of entry level health information necessary for the understanding and eventual teaching of health education programs to elementary students. The preservice teachers also are expected to be familiar with the national and state health promotion and disease prevention goals and objectives for both individuals and communities, particularly as they impact upon the elementary school population.

The second key course, "Elementary Health Curriculum," is designed specifically for the elementary education major who may eventually teach health in a classroom setting. The course provides an in-depth study of the development and structure of contemporary health education as well as the specific teaching methods needed for effective health education instruction. Students in the course also examine the evolution of health education and health promotion to increase their appreciation and understanding of health education as an important discipline within the elementary school. The full course is designed to match the overall goals of a comprehensive health education program in the schools (see Cornacchia et al., 1991, for further information about these goals.)

Within Pennsylvania, the primary responsibility for teaching health education at the elementary level usually lies with the regular classroom teacher. "Elementary Health Curriculum" assesses the present status of Health Education within Pennsylvania and leads students to develop their knowledge and teaching skills needed to implement effective health education programs in elementary schools. Particular emphasis is placed on making comprehensive health education an integral part of an overall comprehensive school health program.

Complementing the two keystone courses in the health education emphasis are two other courses—"CPR" and "First Aid and Safety." In addition, students also explore the issues related to HIV/AIDS. In "HIV/AIDS Education," students are introduced to the facts relating to AIDS and the emotional issues involved in teaching about HIV infection. Psychosocial issues covered in the course include values, attitudes, and beliefs, and their effects on teaching and learning about HIV, drugs and drug use, and sex and sexuality. Emphasis also is placed on helping students develop the skills needed to make effective AIDS presentations with a nonjudgmental perspective and with sensitivity to the cultural diversity within their communities.

Nutrition and healthy lifestyles also form a part of the program. In "Fitness for Wellness," for example, students develop strategies for attaining appropriate health status through fitness and stress management. A practical experience in developing one's own exercise prescription, for instance, is one of the main focuses for the course along with understanding the common pitfalls to exercise adherence. In general, the core of the course provides the message that exercise, stress management, and time management skills can provide a buffer against illness and disease as well as enhancing an individual's quality of life.

"Food, Diet, and Weight Management" provides students with an opportunity to study in depth the subject of nutrition and its application in weight management. As an extension of weight management, students in the class also are exposed to critical issues about eating disorders and their effect on "wellness" and the "quality of life" for the individual.

The main objective behind Clarion University's Elementary Health Emphasis is to prepare the elementary school teacher to implement effective health education and health promotion programs within the school system. Currently many elementary school teachers who are responsible for teaching health education are ill-prepared for carrying out such an important responsibility because they do not understand the philosophy or the need for comprehensive health education programs. In addition, many of them do not have appropriate training or an adequate knowledge of health related issues to present health information effectively in classroom settings. Some teachers also avoid the whole topic of health education because of what they perceive to be controversial and sensitive issues.

The Elementary Health Emphasis program at Clarion University is an initial attempt to address these deficits in the preparation of elementary school teachers. Never before in our history has the need for effective health education been so important. Our society is bursting with escalating health concerns and costs. The key to meeting the health education crisis in this country continues to lie with prevention efforts that begin at the earliest ages of our children and continue throughout their schooling. Clarion's program is designed to equip prospective elementary school teachers with the leadership and teaching skills necessary to improve the quality of health instruction in elementary schools and serve as health promoters and wellness models for all students and staff.

Cinelli, B. A., Rose-Colley, M., & Bechtel, L. (1992). *Healthy children: The key to our future.* Harrisburg, PA: Pennsylvania Department of Health.

Cornacchia, H. J., Olsen, L. K., & Nickerson, C. J. (1991). *Health in elementary schools.* 8th ed. St. Louis: Mosby-Year Book, Inc.

National professional school health education organizations: Comprehensive school health education. (1984). *Journal of Health, 54*(8), 312–315.

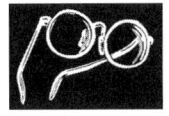 **Article Review Form at end of book.**

WiseGuide Wrap-Up

- Peer-led prevention programs were superior to teacher-led programs with regard to smoking, excessive drinking, and cannabis use.

- The basic premise of the school-based health promotion model is that a program designed to meet the problems, needs, and interests of the target audience and one that includes social marketing, program and educational activities, and environmental/cultural support would be an effective way to enhance the health of students and to improve educational outcomes.

- School agreements with managed care organizations (MCOs) can be inexpensive, can reach large numbers of students, and can address the most prevalent health problems when they are not limited to the school clinic as the sole model of school health service delivery.

- Broad-scale dissemination of such interventions as the school-based 5 a Day for Better Health may reduce risks for cardiovascular disease among large numbers of young people.

- The key to meeting the health-education crisis in this country continues to lie with prevention efforts that begin at the earliest ages of our children and continue throughout their schooling. In order to meet this educational need, early childhood and elementary teachers must receive appropriate training in health education.

R.E.A.L. Sites

This list provides a print preview of typical **Coursewise** R.E.A.L. sites. (There are over 100 such sites at the **Courselinks**™ site.) The danger in printing URLs is that web sites can change overnight. As we went to press, these sites were functional using the URLs provided. If you come across one that isn't, please let us know via email to: webmaster@coursewise.com. Use your Passport to access the most current list of R.E.A.L. sites at the **Courselinks** site.

Site name: Youth Risk Behavior Surveillance System (YRBSS)

URL: http://www.cdc.gov/nccdphp/dash/yrbs/ov.htm

Why is it R.E.A.L.? The purposes of YRBSS are to determine the prevalence and age of initiation of health-risk behaviors; to focus the nation and relevant agencies on specific health-risk behaviors of young people; to assess whether health-risk behaviors increase, decrease, or remain the same over time; to provide comparable national, state, and local data; and to monitor progress toward achieving the Healthy People 2000 and Healthy People 2010 objectives and the National Education Goals.

Key topics: youth risk behavior, adolescent health

Try this: Select At-a-Glance. Review the CDC leadership role and the uses for YRBSS data.

Site name: ERIC Clearinghouse on Teaching and Teacher Education

URL: http://www.ericsp.org/schooled.html

Why is it R.E.A.L.? This provides comprehensive school health education resources, organizations, and associations.

Key topics: school health, health education

Try this: Select National Health Information Center. Preview the available links to various federal resources.

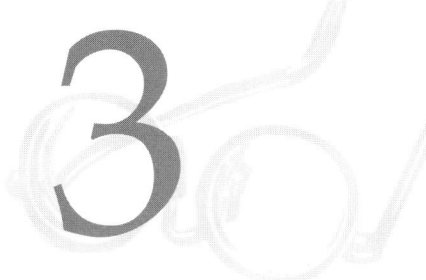

section 3

Learning Objectives

- To examine the association of trade unions to workplace health-promotion programs

- To review the factors associated with availability and participation in worksite health-promotion programs

- To analyze the health- and cost-effective outcomes of worksite health-promotion programs

- To examine the cost of employee assistance programs

- To review the relationship among health, unemployment, and underemployment

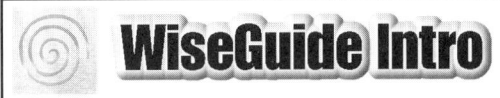

WiseGuide Intro

"An ounce of prevention is worth a pound of cure." This may well be the motto for worksite health promotion. In the past two decades, efforts have increased to promote healthier behaviors among the workforce.

This section will address the association of unionism with worksite health promotion abroad, worksite health promotion in the U.S., the cost-effectiveness of worksite health promotion, employee assistance programs (EAPs), and the relationship between unemployment and health.

C. D'Arcy Holman, Billie Corti, Robert Donovan, and Geoffrey Jalleh, all at the University of Western Australia, present "Association of the Health-Promoting Workplace with Trade Unionism and Other Industrial Factors." This study raises the hypothesis, but cannot confirm, that trade unions could provide a means for employees to pursue the creation of a health-promoting workplace. The study examines associations of five healthy workplace attributes with trade unionism and nine other industrial and sociodemographic factors.

James Grosch, Toni Alterman, Martin Petersen, and Lawrence Murphy, all at the National Institute for Occupational Safety and Health, present "Worksite Health Promotion Programs in the U.S.: Factors Associated with Availability and Participation." This study concludes that, although availability of worksite health-promotion programs remains high, participation by employees in specific types of programs can vary widely. Attempts to increase participation should look beyond individual, health, and organizational variables to specific features of the work environment that encourage involvement in health-promotion activities.

Kenneth Pelletier (Stanford University School of Medicine) presents "A Review and Analysis of the Health and Cost-Effective Outcome Studies of Comprehensive Health Promotion and Disease Prevention Programs at the Worksite: 1993–1995 Update." This article represents the updated summaries of the impact of comprehensive health-promotion programs on health and financial outcome measures. It also recognizes that not all health-promotion and disease-prevention programs at the worksite are health- and/or cost-effective.

Michael French (University of Miami) and Gary Zarkin, Jeremy Bray, and Tyler Hartwell (all at the Research Triangle Institute) present "Costs of Employee Assistance Programs: Findings from a National Survey." This study represents the first attempt to generate national estimates of EAP costs. The findings have at least two important uses: (1) EAP coverage is growing rapidly and (2) considerable attention is currently focused on state and federal health care reform, and especially on the role of employers.

David Dooley and Jonathan Fielding (both at the University of California) and Lennart Levi (Karolinska Institute) present "Health and Unemployment." This paper reviews the relationship between health and inadequate employment, especially unemployment. Few studies have evaluated interventions to prevent or reduce the adverse health effects of job loss. There have been even fewer studies of the health effects of other types of inadequate employment, such as the increasingly prevalent forms of underemployment.

? Questions ?

Reading 13. _____ was consistently associated with a higher level of healthy workplace attributes. Discuss the implications of this research for health-promotion practitioners.

Reading 14. The results of this study indicate that, from an employee's perspective, worksite health promotion programs are _____. What are the recommendations for increasing participation in worksite health promotion programs?

Reading 15. Is the renewed interest in health promotion and disease prevention really buoyed up by better health and cost outcomes data and research? How has managed care impacted worksite health promotion?

Reading 16. What are the two primary types of employee assistance programs (EAPs)? What are the benefits of each type of EAP?

Reading 17. Studies have found links between unemployment and such behaviors as _____. Describe underemployment.

_____ was consistently associated with a higher level of healthy workplace attributes. Discuss the implications of this research for health-promotion practitioners.

Association of the Health-Promoting Workplace with Trade Unionism and Other Industrial Factors

C. D'Arcy J. Holman, Billie Corti, Robert J. Donovan, and Geoffrey Jalleh

C. D'Arcy J. Holman, PhD, is a Professor of Public Health; Robert J. Donovan, PhD, is an Associate Professor of Management; Billie Corti, M. App. Sc, is a Lecturer in Health Promotion; and Geoffrey Jalleh is a Research Assistant, all at the Health Promotion Development and Evaluation Program, Department of Public Health and Graduate School of Management, The University of Western Australia.

Abstract

Purpose

The study examines associations of five healthy workplace attributes with trade unionism and nine other industrial and sociodemographic factors. The aims were to illustrate the measurement of workplace health promotion indicators in Western Australia and to identify associations leading to a better understanding of determinants of the healthy workplace.

Introduction

The complex dynamic between behavior and environment in the workplace has led several authors to propose ecological models of workplace health promotion.[1-4] At first, programs evolved from those targeting single health habit interventions to those embodying many single health habit interventions into a general risk reduction strategy.[5] In line with the comprehensive approach to health promotion adopted in other settings, much contemporary health promotion practice in the workplace now combines individualistic strategies with actions tackling structural barriers to health at the levels of work organization and environment that lie outside the control of individual workers.[1-6]

The ecological paradigm has implications for the measurement of health promotion outcomes. Motivated originally by a framework that emphasized the measurement of behavior change and, ultimately, reductions in morbidity and mortality, evaluators of workplace health promotion now face the challenge of devising indicators to assess the extent to which a workplace is supportive of good health, i.e., the health-promoting workplace. These developments are evolving along two somewhat orthogonal paths: measures that provide a broad "horizontal" indication of organizational climate and aspects of workplace design such as task demand and worker control[7,8] and measures that provide a more fractional and "vertical" indication of workplace attributes concerned with specific occupational health issues such as smoking restrictions or adaptation of worksites for disabled people.[9-11] Other options in the design of indicators of a health promoting workplace include, for example, that the object of measurement

Reprinted by permission from *American Journal of Health Promotion*, May/June 1998 (Vol. 12, No. 5), pp. 325–334.

may be a policy, practice, or physical feature. The term "attribute" covers all of these possibilities. The unit of observation may be set at levels ranging from a discrete organization or worksite to the environment experienced by the individual worker. Data obtained directly from organizations have the advantage of immediacy to the level where policy decisions are made. Community survey data collected from individuals have the advantages of improved representation of working conditions in small, unregistered, or diffuse settings, which may be undernumerated in worksite sampling frames; reduction of misclassification error due to within-site variation in attributes; and fewer "false positives" due to health-promoting policies that are endorsed officially, but not put into practice.

Health promotion activities in the workplace are increasing in the United States, but trend data are not available in Australia.[4,5,12] A U.S. national survey of 1507 worksites in 1992 found that 81% offered at least one health promotion activity, compared with two-thirds of those surveyed 7 years earlier.[12] Smoking cessation, health risk appraisal, back care, injury control, stress management, and physical fitness programs were the most frequently cited health promotion activities at these worksites.[12] Two recent reviews of 48 studies evaluating the effectiveness of workplace health promotion programs found convergent evidence of improved health outcomes in the areas of smoking cessation, weight loss, and reduction of other coronary heart disease risk factors.[13,14] Similarly, a review of 22 workplace intervention studies undertaken on behalf of the International Union for Health

Promotion and Education found evidence of effectiveness of programs targeting smoking, nutrition, and other risk factors for cardiovascular disease, but less conclusive evidence with respect to several other interventions.[15]

The interventions evaluated to date have varied enormously in their mix of individual and environmental strategies, and it has been impossible to assess the independent contributions of environmental modifications of worksites to improved health outcomes. The one exception is that the effects of restrictive smoking policies in the workplace have been extensively researched.[10,16–22] The results indicate that restrictive smoking policies are highly effective in the control of passive smoking at work and are associated with an overall reduction in tobacco exposure among smokers in the order of 15%.[10,16–22] The independent effectiveness of other "vertical" healthy workplace attributes, such as healthy catering and sun protection practices, remains uncertain. A successful program of research into the effectiveness of environmental strategies to promote health in the workplace will depend, in part, on the development of appropriate systems of measurement.

This report represents the combined results of two cross-sectional surveys in Western Australia, undertaken in 1992 and 1994, and covering 2423 household respondents in paid employment and working mainly at locations other than home. We use the data to examine the associations of five healthy workplace attributes, specifically, a restrictive smoking policy, healthy catering practices, sun protection practices, disability access features, and the presence of a formal workplace health promotion

program, with 10 sociodemographic and industrial factors. The purpose is to illustrate a system for the measurement of "vertical" workplace health promotion indicators in a defined population and to apply the system to identify associations that might lead to a greater understanding of the determinants of healthy workplaces. A unique feature of the study was to examine the relationships of healthy workplace attributes to the prevalence of trade unionism and to separate any observed effect of unionism from those of potential confounders such as workplace location, size, sector, and industrial classification. Finally, we draw on the results to discuss improvements in targeting future efforts at workplace health promotion.

Methods
Design

Two cross-sectional household surveys of the general population aged 16 to 69 years were conducted from August to September 1992 and from May to July 1994. The numbers of respondents in paid employment and not working mainly at home were 1310 and 1113, respectively. The surveys were undertaken as part of a 3-year evaluation of the Western Australian Health Promotion Foundation, a statutory agency that provides grants and sponsorship to promote health in community settings such as sports and arts venues, schools, and workplaces.[23–27] The variables of interest in this study were gender, age, social disadvantage, and occupation; location, size, sector, industrial classification, and degree of unionization of the respondent's workplace; and presence of the five healthy workplace attributes described below.

Sample

The surveys used a hybrid of personal and telephone interview methods, the latter being required in rural areas. Apart from differences in sample size, the methods used in 1992 and 1994 were identical. Respondents interviewed in person were drawn from a two-stage cluster sample based on private dwellings within the Perth metropolitan area. Clusters were derived from random start points using Australian Bureau of Statistics collectors' districts as the sampling frame. A collector's district consists of 200 to 300 households. Two start points were randomly generated within each selected collector's district, and five interviews were obtained from each start point, after applying a skip interval of two dwellings.

For telephone interviews, the sample was based on randomly selected listed and unlisted private numbers. It was important to ensure that unlisted numbers were included, as they comprised 15% of all private telephone numbers. A sampling frame of unlisted numbers was generated by drawing on a database of listed private numbers, duplicating the database with a constant of 9 added to each telephone number, and matching the preconstant and postconstant databases to remove listed numbers.

A single respondent was interviewed in each selected household. He or she was selected as the household member with his or her birth date nearest to the date of first contact. A quota was applied to ensure equal numbers of male and female respondents in the personal and telephone interview strata. The aim of the quota was to avoid the oversampling of female respondents due to their greater time spent in the home.

All interviews took place on weekends and after 4:00 P.M. on weekdays. The study was offered to potential participants as a voluntary "survey of recreation and health," performed by The University of Western Australia. There were up to three attempts at contact to an empty house/unanswered number, at least one of which was made on a separate day. Once contact was made, there were up two additional callbacks, at different times of the day and/or on different days, to obtain the desired respondent. Subjects who would have been otherwise eligible for interview were excluded if they did not speak English with sufficient fluency or if their mental faculties were not sufficiently sound to provide for a reliable interview. A response rate of 72% was achieved based on the 6408 households contacted, with at least one potential respondent known to be in scope and in quota. The 4620 respondents to the survey were asked their present occupation, the industry in which they worked, and if they worked mainly at home. On this basis, 1809 people who were unemployed, retired, students, or homemakers and 388 others who worked mainly at home were excluded. A total of 2423 subjects remained, who were included in the study.

Measurement

Occupations and industries were coded using the Australian Standard Classification of Occupations and the Australian Standard Industrial Classification published by the Australian Bureau of Statistics. In the results, "white-collar" workers include para-professional, clerical, and sales occupations and "blue-collar" workers include tradespeople, machinery operators, and labor-

ers. "Heavy industries" were the mining, construction, forestry, agriculture, and energy resource industries; "light industries" were manufacturing, transport, storage, wholesale, and retail; and "service industries" were those involved in communications; finance; property; public administration; and community, recreational, and personal services.

Respondents were asked where their workplace was located, to estimate how many people worked in the same location as themselves, whether they worked mainly in the public or private sectors, and if the majority of the employees at their place of work were members of a union. The age and gender of the respondent were recorded, and their postcode of residence was used to assign them to one of five levels of social disadvantage falling between the 0th, 25th, 50th, 75th, 90th and 100th percentiles of the distribution of a census-derived index, incorporating measures of household income, educational attainment, and home and motor vehicle ownership.[28]

The five healthy workplace attributes assessed in the surveys were those most frequently promoted by the Western Australian Health Promotion Foundation. They were defined as follows:

1. Restrictive smoking policy: No smoking allowed anywhere. This measure was restricted to respondents who worked mainly at one location and mainly indoors.

2. Healthy catering practices: The canteen or snack bar provided either a lot of fresh fruit or a lot of fresh salad rolls. This measure was restricted to respondents who worked mainly at one location with an onsite canteen or snack bar.

3. Sun protection practices: Provision by the employer of any type of protection from the sun such as a sunshade, a hat or sunscreen, or avoidance of working outside during the middle of the day. This measure was restricted to respondents working mainly outdoors.

4. Disability access features: Provision of two or more of the following: special parking places for disabled people, ramps or lifts in place of stairs, and special toilet facilities. This measure was restricted to respondents who worked mainly at one location.

5. Worksite health promotion program: Provision of any type of health promotion program such as keep-fit groups or health check-ups available at the place of work or provided by the employer.

The presence of a healthy workplace attribute was assessed using the combination of yes/no responses to two or more questions pertaining to each separate element of the definition. Thus, for example, respondents were asked three separate questions about the provision of special parking places for disabled workers, ramps or lifts in place of stairs, and special toilet facilities. If they answered yes to at least two questions, then their workplace met the criteria, as defined above, for disability access features. Variations in restriction that logically applied to each healthy workplace attribute caused the numbers of respondents available for analysis to differ between attributes. The reliability and validity of measures of healthy workplace attributes were not assessed.

Analysis

The survey data were used to estimate the prevalence of exposure to healthy workplace attributes in different sections of the working population of Western Australia, according to sociodemographic and industrial factors. The prevalence figures were obtained by weighting the survey samples to the actual distribution of the Western Australian population aged 16 to 69 years according to health administration region in the 1991 Australian Census. The system of balanced weights was designed to adjust for the higher sampling fractions of rural residents.

A multivariate analysis was also performed. The four sociodemographic factors (gender, age group, social disadvantage, and occupational group), five industrial factors (location, sector, number of workers at site, trade unionism, and industrial classification), and the calendar year of survey (grouped with the industrial factors) were included as covariates in an unconditional logistic regression model, along with binary indicators of each healthy workplace attribute in turn as the outcome variable.[29] Logistic regression was performed on unweighted data, as there was no prior justification to believe that the relative effects of sociodemographic or industrial factors were modified by the survey stratification.[30]

A system of progressive adjustment of potential confounding was implemented in three phases. It was considered essential to adjust for confounding due to strong associations between the determinant variables. Trade unionism, for example, was correlated with the public sector, large worksites, service industries, and earlier calendar time; male gender was correlated with blue-collar occupations, private sector employment, large worksites, and nonservice industries; and so on. First, a "crude" analysis was performed relating each outcome variable to each separate sociodemographic and industrial factor in a bivariate model. In the second phase, the effect of each sociodemographic factor was adjusted for potential confounding by the combination of all industrial factors and *vice versa*. In the final phase of adjustment, all sociodemographic and industrial factors were included as covariates in the model. Indicator coefficients and standard errors obtained from the Statistical Package for the Social Sciences were used to calculate adjusted prevalence odds ratios and associated confidence intervals.[31]

Results

There were 2423 respondents who were in paid employment and who did not work mainly at home. The average respondent was aged 36.8 years and was more likely to be male (61%) than female (39%). Thirty-eight percent were blue-collar workers, 31% white-collar workers, and the remaining 31% were professionals or managers. Aboriginal people comprised 2.4% of the sample compared with 2.5% of the general population, and thus appeared to be adequately represented. Between one-third and two-thirds of respondents were exposed to healthy workplace attributes: 52.3% worked in a smoke-free environment, 67.6% had healthy catering available, 67.7% had working conditions that protected them from excessive sunlight exposure, 38.7% worked at a location with disability access features, and 33.4% had

Table I Prevalence of Healthy Workplace Attributes According to Sociodemographic Factors in Respondents Aged 16–69 Years in Western Australia in 1992/1994

	Prevalence of Healthy Workplace Attribute* (%)				
Sociodemographic Factor	Restrictive Smoking Policy (n = 1583)	Healthy Catering Practices (n = 535)	Sun Protection Practices (n = 520)	Disability Access Features (n = 1388)	Worksite Health Promotion Program (n = 2175)
Gender					
Female	61.7%	73.4%	63.5%	46.3%	31.7%
Male	43.9%	62.3%	68.2%	31.8%	34.4%
Age group					
16–24 yr	46.6%	58.1%	61.0%	38.4%	25.8%
25–39 yr	49.6%	69.4%	68.0%	38.6%	34.0%
40 + yr	57.3%	68.7%	53.4%	38.9%	35.7%
Social disadvantage					
Least disadvantage	58.8%	69.5%	64.3%	41.3%	32.9%
Low disadvantage	53.4%	65.7%	65.7%	35.7%	31.9%
Medium disadvantage	51.1%	70.4%	64.0%	37.0%	29.8%
High disadvantage	48.6%	60.7%	79.7%	37.2%	40.0%
Most disadvantage	49.8%	69.7%	68.8%	44.0%	37.0%
Occupational group					
Professionals and managers	60.8%	75.7%	70.8%	38.7%	36.8%
White collar	60.5%	67.7%	72.2%	49.9%	37.7%
Blue collar	30.4%	55.2%	65.7%	21.8%	26.1%

*Weighted to the Western Australian Census Population 1991.

access to a worksite health promotion program.

Sociodemographic Factors Associated with Healthy Workplace Attributes

Table 1 shows the prevalence of healthy workplace attributes according to gender, age group, social disadvantage, and occupational group, weighted to the census population of Western Australia in 1991. Crude prevalence odds ratios and those adjusted for confounding effects are shown in Table 2. Categories not reported in Table 2 were used as baselines for calculation of prevalence odds ratios.

A lower prevalence of restrictive smoking policies was reported by male than female workers and by respondents in blue-collar occupations compared with professionals, managers,

and white-collar occupations (see Table 1). Respondents aged 40+ years were more likely to report a restrictive smoking policy at work than younger people. Table 2 shows that these crude associations were attenuated by adjustment for other factors, but even after full adjustment, a smoke-free workplace was inversely associated with male gender and blue-collar occupations. The association of restrictive smoking policies with social disadvantage was inconsistent and weak.

Healthy food catering was reported less often by males than females and less often by blue-collar workers and by those aged 16 to 24 years compared with other workers (Table 1). These results were explained by chance, albeit after adjustment in the case of blue-collar occupations (Table 2). There was no consistent pattern of association of sun

protection with sociodemographic factors.

Disability access was reported more often by female than male workers and by those in the most socially disadvantaged group. Wide variations were found in the prevalence of disability access features reported by different occupational groups (Table 1). The effects of gender and blue-collar occupation were largely removed by progressive adjustment in Table 2, whereas positive associations with social disadvantage and with white-collar work were strengthened.

The provision of worksite health promotion programs was associated with male gender and social disadvantage, but was inversely associated with blue-collar occupation. The positive association with social disadvantage increased after adjustment for industrial

Table 2

Relationship of Healthy Workplace Attributes to Sociodemographic Factors in Respondents Aged 16–69 Years in Western Australia in 1992/1994

Healthy Workplace Attribute/Sociodemographic Factor	Prevalence Odds Ratios for Healthy Workplace Attribute			
	Crude*	Adjusted (1)*†	Adjusted (2)*‡	95% CI for (2)
Restrictive smoking policy				
Male gender	0.49***	0.66***	0.76*	0.60–0.98
Ages 25–39 yr	1.16	1.02	1.03	0.75–1.42
Ages 40 + yr	1.46*	1.26	1.21	0.87–1.68
Most disadvantaged	0.90	0.69*	1.20	0.92–1.56
White-collar occupation	1.05	0.96	0.92	0.70–1.20
Blue-collar occupation	0.30***	0.42***	0.45***	0.33–0.61
Healthy catering practices				
Male gender	0.71	0.70	0.71	0.44–1.12
Ages 25–39 yr	1.55	1.01	0.98	0.52–1.84
Ages 40 + yr	1.46	0.89	0.87	0.46–1.66
Most disadvantaged	1.32	1.25	1.27	0.76–2.12
White-collar occupation	0.89	0.92	0.82	0.50–1.37
Blue-collar occupation	0.61*	0.70	0.73	0.42–1.28
Sun protection practices				
Male gender	1.15	1.14	1.11	0.59–2.08
Ages 25–39 yr	1.47	1.09	1.09	0.63–1.89
Ages 40 + yr	1.56	1.19	1.20	0.67–2.14
Most disadvantaged	0.96	1.25	1.75	0.62–4.96
White-collar occupation	1.18	0.93	0.94	0.47–1.90
Blue-collar occupation	1.11	0.97	0.98	0.58–1.64
Disability access features				
Male gender	0.55***	0.72*	0.84	0.63–1.12
Ages 25–39 yr	0.92	0.67*	0.69	0.48–1.00
Ages 40 + yr	1.03	0.71	0.75	0.51–1.09
Most disadvantaged	1.33	1.11	1.42*	1.05–191
White-collar occupation	1.41**	1.73***	1.62**	1.19–2.21
Blue-collar occupation	0.47***	0.97	0.97	0.66–1.41
Worksite health promotion program				
Male gender	1.30**	1.25	1.33*	1.05–1.69
Ages 25–39 yr	1.48**	1.01	1.01	0.74–1.38
Ages 40 + yr	1.58**	1.05	1.06	0.78–1.46
Most disadvantaged	1.15	1.24	1.52**	1.14–2.03
White-collar occupation	0.89	0.95	1.00	0.78–1.30
Blue-collar occupation	0.73**	0.78	0.76*	0.58–1.00

*$0.05 > p \geq 0.01$, **$0.01 > p \geq 0.001$, ***$p < 0.001$.

†Adjusted for industrial factors: location, sector, no. of workers at site, unionism, and industrial classification.

‡Adjusted for industrial factors and all other sociodemographic factors.

and other sociodemographic factors (Table 2).

Industrial Factors Associated with Healthy Workplace Attributes

Healthy workplace attributes were strongly associated with several industrial factors. Table 3 shows the weighted proportions of respondents reporting attributes according to workplace location, sector, number of workers, trade unionism, industrial classification, and calendar year. Corresponding crude and adjusted prevalence odds ratios are given in Table 4. There was little evidence of a change in the prevalence of attributes between 1992 and 1994.

Workplaces in rural locations were less likely than those in metropolitan Perth to have a restrictive smoking policy, healthy catering, and disability access features and were less likely to offer worksite health promotion programs. Results in

Table 4 show that none of these results was explained by confounding or by chance variation. Sun protection was more prevalent in rural locations than in the capital city. This was explained, in part, by confounding with other industrial factors, although the adjusted prevalence odds ratio remained at 1.47.

Workers in the public sector experienced a higher weighted prevalence of healthy workplace attributes (range 52.6 to 80.2% in Table 3) than their private sector counterparts (21.4 to 61.1%). These results were explained entirely by confounding with sociodemographic and other industrial factors in the case of restrictive smoking policies and healthy catering (Table 4). However, sun protection, disability access, and worksite health promotion programs remained more prevalent in the public sector after adjustment.

The differences in health-promoting attributes between medium-sized and small worksites were inconsistent, but large worksites, with 50 or more workers, had several distinctive characteristics (see Table 3). After adjustment, respondents from large worksites were more likely to have access to a health promotion program and to report disability access features and sun protection practices (Table 4). However, large worksites were less likely to have a restrictive smoking policy.

Respondents in unionized workplaces reported a higher weighted prevalence of all five health-promoting attributes (range 49.1 to 80.3% in Table 3) than those in situations where the majority of workers were not members of a trade union (19.9 to 58.5%). The corresponding adjusted prevalence odds ratios in

Table 4 for healthy catering (2.05; 95% CI 1.30 to 3.23), sun protection (2.66; 1.69 to 4.17), disability access (1.47; 1.10 to 1.95), and worksite health promotion programs (2.56; 2.07 to 3.17) remained high, even after adjustment for sociodemographic and other industrial factors. A lower adjusted prevalence odds ratio of 1.21 was found to compare restrictive smoking policies in trade unionized and non-unionized workplaces (95% CI .95 to 1.55).

Compared with workers in the services sector, those in light industries had a consistently reduced prevalence of exposure to healthy workplace attributes (Table 4). Taking a five-attribute average of the weighted prevalence measures in Table 3, the wholesale and retail industries (36.4%) had the least healthy work environment of any of the 12 industry classifications. The second lowest five-attribute average was observed in the manufacturing industry (38.0%). Energy resources had the highest five-attribute average (73.8% from Table 3). The pattern of results in heavy industries varied across attributes (Table 4): restrictive smoking policies and disability access features were uncommon, whereas healthy catering, sun protection practices, and worksite health promotion programs were associated with heavy industry, albeit at a statistically significant level only in the latter instance.

Discussion
Occurrence of Healthy Workplace Attributes

In this study, between one-third and two-thirds of the labor force in Western Australia had the purported benefits of each of five healthy workplace attributes. Healthy catering and sun protec-

tion practices were the most frequently reported attributes, whereas an organized health promotion program at the worksite was the least common attribute. Healthy workplace attributes were reported less often by respondents from rural areas and by those working in the private sector and at small worksites. Although there was no consistent relationship with sociodemographic factors, including social disadvantage, blue-collar workers reported a low prevalence of restrictive smoking policies compared with other occupational groups. The most striking results were those pertaining to trade unionism. This factor was strongly associated with sun protection practices, organized health promotion programs, and healthy catering practices. There was a moderate and statistically significant association of trade unionism with disability access features, but only a weak and statistically nonsignificant association with restrictive smoking policies.

Several limitations should be taken into account in the interpretation of these results. Although the response fraction of 72% was adequate, it may have led to a potential for selection bias. Whether nonrespondents would have been less likely to work in a health-promoting workplace is unknown, and caution should be exercised in generalization of levels of attributes reported by respondents to the general population. All information collected was based on self-reports and was not validated from any other source, nor was the instrument tested for reliability. A further limitation, which other investigators should consider in future research, was that respondents were asked only about the observable presence of attributes. They were not asked

Table 3	Prevalence of Healthy Workplace Attributes According to Industrial Factors Reported by Respondents Aged 16–69 Years in Western Australia in 1992/1994				
	Prevalence of Health Workplace Attribute* (%)				
Industrial Factor	**Restrictive Smoking Policy (n = 1583)**	**Healthy Catering Practices (n = 535)**	**Sun Protection Practices (n = 520)**	**Disability Access Features (n = 1388)**	**Worksite Health Promotion Program (n = 2175)**
Location					
Metropolitan	54.2%	70.5%	63.7%	41.7%	34.5%
Rural	46.5%	57.6%	73.5%	29.0%	30.2%
Sector					
Private	46.6%	61.0%	61.1%	26.3%	21.4%
Public	61.5%	72.8%	80.2%	57.4%	52.6%
No. of workers at site					
1–4	54.6%	51.6%	76.0%	27.1%	14.6%
5–9	52.0%	63.1%	53.0%	28.9%	24.3%
10–49	53.2%	62.4%	79.0%	35.8%	33.7%
50–199	48.3%	70.1%	87.7%	48.9%	48.8%
200+	51.4%	78.6%	85.8%	61.9%	66.9%
Unionized					
No	50.2%	58.5%	55.0%	28.2%	19.9%
Yes	54.6%	72.0%	80.3%	50.5%	49.1%
Industrial classification					
Agriculture and forestry	7.2%	57.3%	68.9%	24.6%	25.4%
Mining	25.3%	73.1%	91.4%	20.9%	50.9%
Manufacturing	33.0%	46.9%	66.8%	10.2%	33.3%
Energy	51.1%	87.3%	100.0%	57.6%	72.8%
Construction	31.8%	100.0%	51.2%	12.3%	13.7%
Wholesale and retail	45.4%	51.7%	46.9%	28.3%	9.9%
Transport and storage	45.3%	44.2%	63.4%	27.1%	35.0%
Communication	84.1%	73.1%	90.4%	49.6%	58.5%
Finance and property	67.7%	71.1%	52.9%	30.7%	26.0%
Public administration	68.8%	78.2%	84.0%	62.7%	61.8%
Community services	68.0%	75.5%	84.2%	60.7%	45.3%
Recreational and personal services	32.3%	46.0%	59.5%	40.2%	19.5%
Calendar year					
1992	52.4%	68.7%	68.6%	38.0%	34.5%
1994	52.3%	66.2%	66.4%	39.7%	32.1%

*Weighted to the Western Australian Census Population 1991.

how they were affected personally, if at all, by the health-promoting attribute. Although we adjusted for gender, age, social disadvantage, occupation, and the location, size, sector, and industrial factors of the workplace in the analysis, residual confounding may have occurred due to other extraneous determinants of healthy workplace attributes that were unevenly distributed between unionized and nonunionized worksites.

International comparisons of the occurrence of healthy workplace attributes are possible only for smoking restrictions, reported by 52.3% of respondents in Western Australia. This figure is comparable to that of a household survey in Maryland, U.S., in 1992–1993, which found that of 1018 workers, 51.6% were covered by a comprehensive smoking ban.[32] Although based on recent surveys of organizations rather than individuals, smoking restrictions have been implemented at 66% of workplaces in the Western Cape Region of South Africa and in 59% of those in Singapore.[33,34] These data,

| Table 4 | Relationship of Healthy Workplace Attributes to Industrial Factors Reported by Respondents Aged 16–69 Years in Western Australia in 1992/1994 |

Healthy Workplace Attribute/Industrial Factor	Prevalence Odds Ratios for Healthy Workplace Attribute			
	Crude*	Adjusted (1)*†	Adjusted (2)*‡	955 CI for (2)
Restrictive smoking policy				
Rural location	0.70***	0.71**	0.77*	0.60–0.98
Public sector	1.86***	1.44**	0.83	0.62–1.11
Medium worksite (10–49)	0.98	1.00	0.86	0.66–1.11
Large worksite (50+)	0.68**	0.76*	0.60**	0.44–0.81
Unionized	1.15	1.26*	1.21	0.95–1.55
Light industries	0.46***	0.62***	0.62***	0.48–0.80
Heavy industries	0.22***	0.31***	0.35***	0.25–0.50
1994	0.98	0.97	0.98	0.78–1.22
Healthy catering practices				
Rural location	0.55**	0.58**	0.42***	0.26–0.65
Public sector	1.52*	1.38	1.16	0.67–1.99
Medium worksite (10–49)	1.00	0.95	0.75	0.43–1.31
Large worksite (50+)	1.87*	2.05**	1.53	0.86–2.72
Unionized	1.94***	2.15***	2.05**	1.30–3.23
Light industries	0.45***	0.54*	0.44**	0.25–0.78
Heavy industries	1.05	1.31	1.51	0.75–3.04
1994	0.80	0.80	0.81	0.54–1.22
Sun protection practices				
Rural location	1.90***	1.91***	1.47	0.94–2.31
Public sector	1.98***	2.18***	1.84*	1.12–3.02
Medium worksite (10–49)	1.24	1.25	0.81	0.42–1.56
Large worksite (50+)	3.94***	4.10***	2.34*	1.05–5.22
Unionized	3.49***	3.43***	2.66***	1.69–4.17
Light industries	0.73	0.73	0.74	0.42–1.31
Heavy industries	1.15	1.16	1.34	0.77–2.33
1994	0.94	0.96	1.12	0.74–1.69
Disability access features				
Rural location	0.54***	0.51***	0.49***	0.37–0.65
Public sector	3.55***	3.19***	1.76***	1.27–2.44
Medium worksite (10–49)	1.35*	1.39*	1.09	0.80–1.49
Large worksite (50+)	2.59***	3.36***	2.96***	2.08–4.20
Unionized	2.28***	2.46***	1.47**	1.10–1.95
Light industries	0.32***	0.36***	0.45***	0.32–0.61
Heavy industries	0.20***	0.25***	0.31***	0.20–0.49
1994	1.15	1.18	1.27	0.98–1.64
Worksite health promotion program				
Rural location	0.88	0.90	0.62***	0.50–0.78
Public sector	2.58***	2.71***	2.16***	1.66–2.82
Medium worksite (10–49)	1.31*	1.31*	0.97	0.76–1.25
Large worksite (50+)	3.52***	3.43***	2.05***	1.58–2.66
Unionized	3.92***	3.95***	2.56***	2.07–3.17
Light industries	0.50***	0.49***	0.69**	0.53–0.90
Heavy industries	0.98	0.92	1.46*	1.09–1.96
1994	0.98	1.00	1.17	0.96–1.44

*0.05 > p ≥ 0.01, **0.01 > p ≥ 0.001, *** p < 0.001.

†Adjusted for sociodemographic factors: gender, age group, social disadvantage, and occupational group.

‡Adjusted for sociodemographic factors and all other industrial factors except calendar year.

gathered in four continents, suggest that the universal provision of smoke-free working conditions is far from realized, yet significant progress has been achieved since the 1980s, when workplace smoking restrictions were first introduced.[9,35] In 1985, victims of passive smoking began to receive compensation as a result of litigation.[35] By 1990, the Western Australian occupational health and safety authority adopted a policy with the ultimate goal of eliminating passive smoking in the workplace.[22]

Little is known about national and international variations in the prevalence of other healthy workplace indicators. But there are now good prospects that the situation could improve in Australia in the near future. The importance of developing and publishing national indicators of health-promoting environments in workplaces, schools, sports and arts venues, and other settings has been acknowledged in the work programs of the National Health and Medical Research Council and the Australian Institute of Health and Welfare. The National Health and Medical Research Council has instigated a series of reports defining verifiable criteria for a "health-promoting workplace," "health-promoting school," and so on, and the AIHW has reviewed options for the design of supporting systems of national surveillance. An approach based on comprehensive household survey data, rather than on separate surveys of different environmental settings, has been one of the options canvassed and is not unlike the method adopted in this research.

Role of Trade Unionism and Other Industrial Factors

Trade unionism was consistently associated with a higher level of healthy workplace attributes. With the exception of restrictive smoking policies, these associations were not explained by chance. Although the prevalence of trade unionism was higher in the public than in the private sector, at large worksites, and in service industries, adjustment for these confounders did not remove the positive effects of employment in a unionized workplace. If a causal connection exists between trade unionism and healthy workplace attributes, it could suggest that trade unions have been effective in the creation of a health-promoting workplace, and not merely the elimination of hazards arising from processes of production (i.e., a safe workplace). Alternatively, the mere presence of union activity could encourage employers to adopt healthy workplace attributes, or union activity could be no more than an indirect indicator of the overall level of social organization necessary to develop and implement healthy public policy. However, one would not expect the latter explanations to account for trade unionism having its strongest association with sun protection practices and the least effect on restrictive smoking policies.

Local knowledge is consistent with the variation in effects of trade unionism across different healthy workplace attributes. Traditionally, unions have voiced discontent at workplace health promotion activities that have blamed individual behavior or that could be used as a covert means of selecting "fit" workers.[4] Western Australian unions, and

especially those covering workers in mining and other heavy industries, have been slow to promote tobacco control policies as an occupational health and safety issue, due to the high prevalence of smoking within their constituencies and for fear of distracting attention away from potentially compensable air pollutants (dust, noxious fumes) arising from production processes. Indeed, published data in Western Australia suggest that unions still mostly address traditional work-related hazards.[36] The singular exception is that trade unions in Western Australia have been active over many years in the pursuit of work practices that limit outdoor exposure during the midday heat in summer. This history is consistent with the observations that trade unionism was least associated in this study with restrictive smoking policies and most strongly associated with sun protection practices.

The study did not measure trade unionism as a means to organize health promotion programs. Thus, the limitations of the study do not permit the conclusion that trade unions provide a means for health-promotion practitioners to achieve the creation of a health-promoting workplace. Nevertheless, it is reasonable to raise a question as to the possible greater need for health promotion practitioners to work with trade union officials, as well as employers and employees, in pursuit of environmental supports for good health. It may be relevant that the opportunity to engage the efforts of unionists is diminishing, due to the rapid decline for more than a decade in the size and influence of the trade union movement worldwide.[37]

There were effects of other industrial factors that were consistent with findings elsewhere.[38] Larger worksites are known to conduct more health promotion activities than smaller sites, probably due in part to economies of scale.[12,39,40] Data from almost 800 worksites from a multicenter community intervention trial for smoking cessation showed that manufacturing and wholesale/retail companies were less likely to offer smoking cessation activities than other type of businesses.[41] Likewise, we observed evidence of a low prevalence of healthy workplace attributes in the manufacturing, wholesale, and retail industries.

Role of Sociodemographic Factors

There were comparatively few associations found between healthy workplace attributes and sociodemographic factors after adjustment for potential confounders. High risk behaviors and other adverse health outcomes occur more often in socially disadvantaged groups.[28] Structural barriers, including lack of environmental supports for healthy behaviors, have been postulated as a causal mechanism to explain these inequalities in health. However, we found no general tendency for persons from socially disadvantaged areas to be employed in settings with a low prevalence of healthy workplace attributes. Moreover, workers from the most socially disadvantaged group had higher than average access to worksite health promotion programs and features that supported people with disabilities. Members of blue-collar occupations, however, experienced a much reduced exposure to restrictive smoking policies, a factor

that may contribute to their high prevalence of smoking and smoking-related diseases.[28]

Implications for Targeting Workplace Health Promotion Activities

Based on these results, efforts to achieve health-promoting workplaces in Western Australia should especially target small worksites in the private sector and in rural locations. These targeting parameters are the same as those applying to the need for more traditional occupational health safety measures. Small worksites are known to have higher rates of injury and ill health than larger worksites. They are considered at risk because they are disproportionately located in certain high hazard industries, employ young and inexperienced workers, and do not always offer adequate safety training and education for their employees.[40] Small worksites may also be disadvantaged by lack of infrastructure in support of some health-promoting attributes (healthy catering, fitness programs) but not others (smoking restrictions, sun protection).

There are additional reasons to suggest that the general principle of targeting workplace health promotion efforts at the small business is a good one. Among companies that provide health promotion activities, smaller companies tend to be more effective in achieving results.[38] Given that a high proportion of the workforce is employed at small worksites (38% of our respondents worked at sites with less than 10 employees and 72% reported less than 50), along with the need for a more equitable provision of healthy workplace attributes and the likely effective-

So What? Implications for Health Promotion Practitioners and Researchers

This study describes associations between several healthy workplace attributes and trade unionism, thus raising the hypothesis that the presence of a trade union could be a resource for health promotion. Depending on whether or not this hypothesis is confirmed in future research, there may be reason for health promotion practitioners, while remaining sensitive to key union concerns about the provision of safe workplaces, to seek opportunities to engage union officials in their programs. Regardless of the presence or absence of trade unions, small worksites in the private sector and in rural areas seem to be lacking in health-promoting attributes and deserve highest priority in efforts by practitioners to procure supportive workplace environments, particularly related to smoking restrictions and sun protection. Monitoring and evaluation of the achievement of the health-promoting workplace may be undertaken through the use of community surveys. These may have some advantages over the collection of data directly from worksites, because they measure practice rather than policy.[34]

ness of programs once introduced, small business represents an excellent opportunity for future health promotion activities and an important priority for further research.

References

1. Green KL. Issues of control and responsibility in workers' health. *Health Educ Q* 1988;15:473–86.
2. McLeroy KR, Bibeau D, Steckler A, et al. An ecological perspective in workers' health. *Health Educ Q* 1988;15:473–86.
3. Stokols D. Establishing and maintaining healthy environments towards a social ecology of health promotion. *Am Psychol* 1992; 47:6–22.
4. Chu C. An integrated approach to workplace health promotion. In: Chu CM, Simpson R, editors. *Ecological Public Health from Vision*

to Practice. Nathan, Queensland, Australia: Griffith University, 1994:182–94.

5. Sloan RP. Workplace health promotion: a commentary on the evolution of a paradigm. *Health Educ Q* 1987;14:181–94.

6. DeJoy DM, Southern DJ. An integrative perspective on work-site health promotion. *J Occup Med* 1993;35:1221–30.

7. Ribisi KM, Reischi TM. Measuring the climate of health at organisations. Development of the worksite health climate scales. *J Occup Med* 1993;35:812–24.

8. Muntaner C, O'Campo P.J. A critical appraisal of the demand/control model of the psychosocial work environment: epistemological social, behavioural and class considerations. *Soc Sci Med* 1993;36:1509–17.

9. Sees KL. The smoke-free workplace. *J Psychoactive Drugs* 1990;22:479–83.

10. Brigham J, Gross J, Stitzer ML, et al. Effects of a restricted work-site smoking policy on employees who smoke. *Am J Public Health* 1994;84:773–8.

11. Malmsborg T. Adapting work sites for disabled persons using advanced technology. *Int J Technol Assess Health Care* 1995;11:235–44.

12. Stokols D, Pelletier KR, Fielding JE. Integration of medical care and worksite health promotion. *JAMA* 1995;273:1136–42.

13. Pelletier KR. A review and analysis of the health and cost-effectiveness outcome studies of comprehensive health promotion and disease prevention programs. *Am J Health Promot* 1991;5:311–5.

14. Pelletier KR. A review and analysis of the health and cost-effectiveness outcome studies of comprehensive health promotion and disease prevention programs at the worksite: 1991–1993 update. *Am J Health Promot* 1993;8:350–62.

15. Veen C. Vereijken I. *Promoting Health at Work. A Review of the Effectiveness of Health Education and Health Promotion.* Utrecht: Landelijk Centrum, 1994.

16. Eggert Scott C-J, Gerberich S.G. Analysis of a smoking policy in the workplace. *Am Assoc Occup Health Nurses J* 1989;37:265–73.

17. Stillman FA, Becker DM, Swank RT, et al. Ending smoking at the John Hopkins medical institutions. *JAMA* 1990;2264:1565–9.

18. Borland R, Chapman S, Owen N, et al. Effects of work place smoking bans on cigarette consumption. *Am J Public Health* 1990;80:178–80.

19. Kinne S, Kristal AR, White E, et al. Work-site smoking policies: their population impact in Washington State. *Am J Public Health* 1993;83:1031–3.

20. Jeffrey RW, Kelder SH, Forster JL, et al. Restrictive smoking policies in the workplace: effects on smoking prevalence and cigarette consumption. *Prev Med* 1994;23:78–82.

21. Brenner H, Fleischle B. Smoking regulations at the workplace and smoking behaviour: a study from Southern Germany. *Prev Med* 1994;23:230–4.

22. Waranch HR, Wohlgemuth WK, Hantula DA, et al. The effects of a hospital smoking ban on employee smoking behaviour and participation in different types of smoking cessation programmes. *Tob Control* 1993;2:120–8.

23. Holman CDJ, Donovan RJ, Corti B. Evaluating projects funded by the Western Australian Health Promotion Foundation: a systematic approach. *Health Promot Int* 1993;8:199–208.

24. Holman CDJ, Donovan RJ, Corti B. Report of the Evaluation of the Western Australian Health Promotion Foundation. Perth: Health Promotion Development and Evaluation Program. Department of Public Health and Graduate School of Management, The University of Western Australia, 1994.

25. Corti B, Holman CDJ, Donovan RJ, et al. Using sponsorship to create healthy environments for sport, racing and arts venues in Western Australia. *Health Promot Int* 1995;10:185–97.

26. Oddy WH, Holman CDJ, Corti B, et al. Epidemiologic measures of participation in community health promotion projects. *Int J Epidemiol* 1995;24:1013–21.

27. Holman CDJ, Donovan RJ, Corti B. Evaluating projects funded by the Western Australian Health Promotion Foundation: first results. *Health Prom Int* 1996;11:75–88.

28. Hyndman JCG, Holman CDJ, Hockey RL, et al. Misclassification of social disadvantage based on geographic areas: comparison of

postcode and collector's district analyses. *Int J Epidemiol* 1995;24:165–76.

29. Rothman KJ. *Modern Epidemiology.* Boston: Little, Brown and Co., 1986.

30. Korn EL, Graubard BI. Examples of differing weighted and unweighted estimates from a sample survey. *Am Stat* 1995;49:291–5.

31. Norusis MJ. SPSS for Windows. Base System User's Guide Release 5.0. Chicago: SPSS Inc., 1992.

32. Shopland DR, Hartman AM, Repace JL, et al. Smoking behaviour, workplace policies, and public opinion regarding smoking restrictions in Maryland, *MD Med J* 1995;44:99–104.

33. Metcalf CA, Yach D. The smoking policies in the workplace in the Western Cape. S. *Afr Med J* 1992;81:23–6.

34. Koh YK, Voo YO, Tan CT. Smoking restrictions in private workplaces in Singapore. *Singapore Med J* 1994;35:245–6.

35. Holman CDJ, Corti B, Donovan RJ, et al. Tobacco control and health expectancy in Australia. *Tob Control* 1993;2:195–200.

36. Warren-Langford P, Biggins DR, Phillips M. Union participation in occupational health and safety in Western Australia. *J Ind Rel* 1993;35:585–606.

37. Kelly D. Trade unionism in 1994. *J Ind Rel* 1995;37:132–47.

38. Glasgow RE, McCaul KD, Fisher KJ. Participation in worksite health promotion: a critique of the literature and recommendations for future practice. *Health Educ Q* 1993;20:391–408.

39. Fielding JE, Piserchia PV. Frequency of worksite health promotion activities. *Am J Public Health* 1989;79:16–20.

40. Eakin JM. Weir N. Canadian approaches to the promotion of health in small workplaces. *Can J Public Health* 1995;86:109–13.

41. Glasgow RE, Sorenson G, Corbett K (for the COMMIT Research Group). Worksite smoking control activities: prevalence and related worksite characteristics from the COMMIT study, 1990. *Prev Med* 1992;21:688–700.

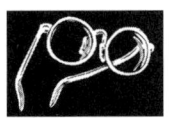 **Article Review Form at end of book.**

The results of this study indicate that, from an employee's perspective, worksite health promotion programs are _____. What are the recommendations for increasing participation in worksite health promotion programs?

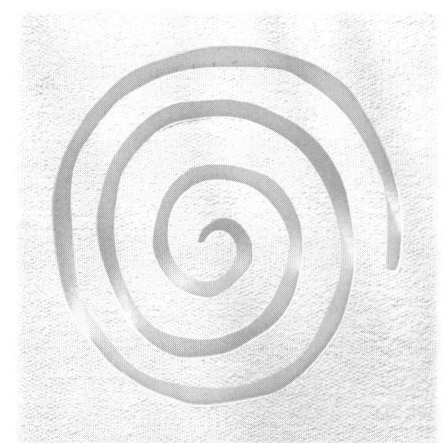

Worksite Health Promotion Programs in the U.S.: Factors Associated with Availability and Participation

James W. Grosch, Toni Alterman, Martin R. Petersen, and Lawrence R. Murphy

James W. Grosch, Toni Alterman, Martin R. Petersen, and Lawrence R. Murphy are at the National Institute for Occupational Safety and Health, Cincinnati, Ohio.

Abstract

Purpose. *To examine how the availability of and participation in worksite health promotion programs varies as a function of individual (e.g., age), organizational (e.g., occupation), and health (e.g., high blood pressure) characteristics. Availability of worksite programs was also compared to that reported in two previous national surveys of private companies.*

Introduction

During the past decade, worksite health promotion programs in the United States have grown dramatically in both number and the variety of activities that are made available to employees. It is estimated that 85% of worksites with 50 or more employees offer at least one health promotion program, which can range from nutrition education and cancer screening to aerobic classes and stress management.[1] Research on these programs has tended to focus on the experiences of a single organization or company and includes studies of cost-effectiveness,[2,3] health benefits for participants,[4,5] and impact on organizational-level variables, such as employee absenteeism, turnover, and morale.[2,4,6] Although these studies have yielded valuable insights into potential benefits and characteristics of successful health promotion programs,[7] there remains a strong need for additional data concerning the availability and use of health promotion on a national level.

In 1985 and 1992, the Office of Disease Prevention and Health Promotion of the U.S. Public Health Service conducted the National Survey of Worksite Health Promotion Activities (NSWHPA).[1,8] Both surveys involved a stratified random sample of private sector companies with 50 or more employees.[9,10] Company representatives were interviewed concerning specific health promotion activities available to employees, administrative policies used to support such activities, and perceived benefits of health promotion for employee health and well-being. The data from these two surveys provide strong evidence of the growing prevalence of health promotion programs in the U.S., and have been used as a standard to evaluate other health promotion efforts,[11,12] as well as gauge our progress toward achieving the worksite health promotion objectives outlined in Healthy People 2000.[13]

Reprinted by permission from *American Journal of Health Promotion*, September/October 1998 (Vol. 13, No. 1), pp. 36–45.

Despite the detailed information provided by the NSWHPA, a number of issues concerning health promotion on a national level remain unexplored. First, both NSWHPA surveys measured health promotion from essentially a management perspective, rather than by interviewing individual employees within a company. An important issue arises as to whether employees are aware of all the health promotion activities that are made available to them by their organization. If employees are unaware, then management needs to better communicate the availability of those activities to employees.

Second, most surveys of health promotion, including the NSWHPA, assess availability of specific programs, but not necessarily whether employees actually use them. Although participation in health promotion programs has been examined in studies involving individual companies,[14] it has not been investigated on a national level. As a result, we know little about factors that influence participation, except on a case-by-case basis.

Third, both NSWHPA surveys focused on private sector companies and, as a result, provide no information concerning worksite health promotion in the public sector. There are an estimated 3.1 million workers in the federal sector and 15.7 million in state and local government who could potentially benefit from health promotion programs.[15] Although some research has examined characteristics of programs in the public sector,[16,17] we do not know whether availability and participation in these programs is keeping up with that reported in private companies.

Finally, the design of the NSWHPA surveys did not include the collection of health-related data for individual workers who participated in health promotion activities. Information was obtained from company representatives regarding general benefits of health promotion (e.g., reduced health insurance costs), but no attempt was made to collect health data from the employees themselves. This type of information is important and would allow us to compare the health of employees participating in health promotion programs with that of employees who, despite having access to health promotion, do not participate. Previous research suggests that participants tend to be healthier and perhaps less in need of health promotion than nonparticipants,[18] although this finding is by no means universal.[19]

Given the above gaps in our understanding of worksite health promotion efforts, the present study sought to extend our knowledge by analyzing data collected as part of the 1994 National Health Interview Survey (NHIS). The NHIS is a national survey of civilian health that has been conducted continuously since 1957, and is designed to measure a broad array of respondent-assessed health variables.[20] In 1994, the NHIS asked respondents employed in worksites with at least 50 employees about several different health promotion activities, similar to those covered in the NSWHPA. Employees in both public and private organizations indicated whether these programs were made available to them at work, and whether they participated in or utilized these programs. This information provides an employee view of worksite health promotion that is

based on the employee's own experiences, rather than those of a company representative.

A major goal of the present study was to examine variables associated with the availability of, and participation in, worksite health promotion programs in the U.S. Variables examined included both individual (e.g., age, gender) and organizational (e.g., type of industry, occupation) characteristics. Since the NHIS and NSWHPA focus on a similar list of health promotion programs, but from a different perspective (i.e., employees vs. company representatives), a second goal was to compare the results of these two surveys in terms of program availability. Finally, using data from the NHIS core, the likelihood of participating in worksite health promotion programs was compared for healthy and non-healthy employees.

Methods
Design

Data for this study came from the 1994 NHIS, a national probability, household-based survey of the civilian noninstitutionalized U.S. population conducted under the supervision of the National Center for Health Statistics (note: a detailed description of the NHIS, including information concerning reliability, sampling design, and questionnaire wording, can be found in *Current Estimates from the National Health Interview Survey, 1994*[20]). The NHIS is conducted as a structured interview and provides information concerning a wide array of health-related variables, such as sociodemographic characteristics, general health, acute medical conditions, restriction of activity, and use of medical services. Based on the sampling design, data for each respondent are weighted so that unbiased estimates can be obtained for the U.S. population. The NHIS contains a core set of questions that remain fairly constant over the years. In addition, supplements are added in some years to measure health variables not covered in the core that are considered important in the public health community.

In 1994, the NHIS contained a supplement on Year 2000 Health objectives[13] that were previously established by the U.S. Department of Health and Human Services. One of the seven sections covered in the Year 2000 Supplement focused on occupational safety and health, and included questions on the availability and use of health promotion programs in companies with 50 or more employees. The Year 2000 Supplement was administered to one adult person per family in half of the households in the 1994 sample. The other half of the households was administered a supplement on acquired immunodeficiency syndrome.

Sample

National Health Interview Survey respondents were selected for this study if they had completed the safety and health section, indicated that working was their major activity, were employed during the previous 2 weeks, and worked at a location with 50 or more employees. Of the 116,179 individuals (representing 45,705 households) who were interviewed for the NHIS, 19,738 were interviewed regarding the Year 2000 Supplement. Of this number, 10,911 respondents (55%) indicated that working was their major activity and that they were

employed during the previous 2 weeks. A total of 5219 respondents (26%) met the final criterion of working at a location with at least 50 employees and formed the basis for this study. The overall household response rate for the NHIS core, excluding special sections or supplements, was 94.1%. For the Year 2000 Supplement, the response rate was 84.5%.

Based on weighted data, approximately 54% of the employees were male, with 82% classified as white, 13% black, and 5% representing other ethnic groups (Asian, Hispanic, etc.). The average age was 39.2 years and the average years of education was 13.8. Approximately 77% of respondents worked for a private company or an incorporated business, 5% for the federal government, 18% for state or local governments, and less than 1% were self-employed. Twenty-seven percent of respondents were current smokers. Although all respondents were employed in worksites with 50 or more employees, no additional information was available in the Year 2000 Supplement regarding the number of employees at the worksite.

Measures

Health Promotion Programs. The Year 2000 questions on workplace health promotion efforts focused on five areas: exercise facilities, exercise programs, health education programs, screening tests, and smoking cessation programs. For each area, employees were read a predetermined list of examples by the interviewer and were asked to indicate (1) if that particular example had been made available to them at their place of work during the past year, and (2)

whether they had participated in or used that particular example during the past year.

For instance, in the case of exercise facilities, employees were asked, "In the past year, which of these exercise facilities, if any, were made available to you by your employer?" A list, presented in Table 1, was then read, and employees responded with a simple yes or no answer. For participation, employees were asked, "In the past year, which of these facilities did you use?" Again, the list of exercise facilities was read and employees responded accordingly. Employees were asked about participation only if they indicated that a particular type of program was available.

The wording of the questions asked by the interviewer varied slightly with the area of health promotion (e.g., for exercise programs, employees were asked, "In the past year, which of these programs did you participate in?"). In all, employees responded to 33 specific examples of health promotion distributed across the five categories. A listing of the examples read by the interviewer is presented in Table 1.

Individual and Organizational Characteristics. These variables came primarily from the NHIS core questionnaire and included information concerning the employee's gender, age, ethnicity, education, occupation, industry, and type of organization. Occupation and industry were coded according to the 1990 Census codes.[21] Type of organization was coded as either private company, federal government, state or local government, or self-employed.

Health Measures. Self-reported health data for each employee were obtained from the NHIS core questionnaire and linked to data provided in the Year 2000 Supplement. The following four measures of health were selected and dichotomized into "healthy" and "nonhealthy" employee groups for logistic regression analyses: (1) General health—employees rating their overall health as good to excellent were compared to employees rating their health as fair to poor; (2) Blood pressure—employees who had not been told they had high blood pressure were compared to those who had been told; (3) Body mass index (BMI)—this measure of obesity takes into account an individual's weight and height (kilograms/meters^2).[22] Employees with a BMI less than 20% above their ideal value were compared with employees whose BMI exceeded their ideal by more than 20%; and (4) Medical conditions—this measure was based on the number of specific medical conditions an individual had experienced during the past year. Employees experiencing no medical conditions were compared to employees experiencing at least one.

Missing data in the NHIS occurred when employees were unable to answer a given question, refused to answer, or were not asked a question by the interviewer. For the individual/ organizational characteristics and health measures, missing data occurred for less than 2.5% of employees. For the health promotion program data, missing data rarely exceed 5%, with the exception of blood pressure screening (7%), cholesterol screening (8%), cancer screening (11%), and smoking cessation (19%). Most of these missing data reflect employees who did not know if a given program was available at their workplace.

Analysis

For each health promotion program, two different percentages were calculated. The availability percentage was defined as the number of employees who indicated that a specific program or facility was available at work during the past year, divided by the total number of employees who responded to that item. Employees who stated they did not know or who refused to answer were coded as missing and not used in the analysis. The participation percentage was defined as the number of employees who used a program or facility during the past year, divided by the number of employees who indicated that it was available at work. Employees who did not answer both the availability and participation questions were not included in this analysis.

Multiple logistic regression was used to compare the participation rates of healthy and nonhealthy workers. In this analysis, data for participation in a given health promotion category were used as the dependent variable, with scores on the four health measures serving as independent variables. To adjust for potential confounding variables, gender, age, ethnicity, and education of the employee were entered into the model prior to information concerning the health variable. Employees were placed in the participation group if they utilized at least one health promotion activity in a given category, whereas employees were placed in the nonparticipation group if they had access but did not participate in any type of worksite health promotion program. In addition to the five health promotion categories, a sixth was formed for participation in any of the other five. Separate analyses

were conducted for each of the four health measures and each of the six categories of health promotion programs.

All statistical analyses of NHIS data were performed with weighted values to permit extrapolation to the general U.S. population. Variance estimates, necessary for calculating standard errors and confidence intervals, were made using the with-replacement sampling method available in the SUDAAN statistical software package.[23]

Results
Availability and Participation

Overall, 82.3% of respondents indicated that at least one of the 33 health promotion programs was available at work during the past year. This percentage corresponds to an estimated 39,302,409 workers throughout the U.S. in companies with 50 or more employees who have access to some form of worksite health promotion. Of these workers, 49.6% (or 26,185,933) indicated that they had participated in or used at least one of the 33 programs. Table 1 presents the estimated availability and participation percentages for each of the 33 health promotion programs, organized by category. For each category, overall means are provided, as well as the percentage of employees who had available, and who participated in, at least one of the programs in that category. For the category of smoking cessation, this information is omitted since this category consists of only one program. Standard errors for each percentage are presented in parentheses.

As shown in Table 1, the category with the highest mean availability was smoking cessation (42.5%), followed, in order,

Table I

Estimated Availability and Participation Percentages* During the Past Year for Specific Worksite Health Promotion Programs (1994 NHIS; standard error is in parentheses)

	% Available	% Participate
Exercise facilities		
Lockers	21.3 (0.8)	42.2 (1.8)
Gym/Exercise room	19.7 (0.8)	32.4 (1.6)
Showers	19.6 (0.7)	31.0 (1.8)
Exercise equipment	17.4 (0.7)	28.3 (1.7)
Weight lifting equipment	16.6 (0.7)	27.5 (1.8)
Walking/Jogging path	14.0 (0.6)	36.1 (2.1)
Bike racks	7.4 (0.5)	9.8 (1.6)
Swimming pool	6.7 (0.5)	24.4 (2.5)
Parcourse/Fitness trails	5.2 (0.4)	12.2 (1.8)
Bike path	4.7 (0.4)	16.7 (2.6)
Mean	13.3	26.1
At least one exercise facility	34.6 (0.9)	47.5 (1.3)
Health education programs		
Job hazards/injury prevention	47.9 (1.1)	50.4 (1.4)
Stress management	40.0 (0.9)	34.7 (1.3)
Back care	38.1 (1.0)	50.2 (1.6)
Alcohol/Other drugs	33.5 (1.0)	19.4 (1.3)
Nutrition information	29.3 (0.8)	27.6 (1.4)
Weight control	28.2 (0.8)	20.5 (1.4)
Sexually transmitted diseases	25.0 (0.7)	35.8 (1.7)
Preventing off-the-job accidents	22.8 (0.7)	40.2 (1.7)
Prenatal information	14.4 (0.6)	9.5 (1.3)
Mean	31.0	32.0
At least one health education program	65.2 (1.1)	57.8 (1.2)
Exercise programs		
Aerobics class	12.2 (0.6)	14.4 (1.6)
Walking group	9.7 (0.5)	28.1 (2.5)
Partially paid membership in health club	6.5 (0.5)	18.7 (2.3)
Physical activity or exercise competition	6.3 (0.4)	26.7 (3.0)
Jogging/Running group	5.7 (0.4)	16.6 (2.5)
Weight lifting class	5.0 (0.4)	20.8 (3.3)
Nonaerobic exercise class	4.7 (0.4)	17.6 (3.3)
Biking/cycling group	3.2 (0.3)	14.6 (3.0)
Swimming class	3.2 (0.3)	10.2 (2.6)
Fully paid membership in health club	2.2 (0.2)	22.3 (3.8)
Mean	5.9	19.0
At least one exercise program	25.7 (0.8)	32.8 (1.4)
Screening tests		
Blood pressure	41.8 (0.9)	57.8 (1.3)
Cholesterol	33.9 (0.8)	50.6 (1.5)
Cancer	16.4 (0.6)	39.4 (2.1)
Mean	30.7	49.3
At least one screening test	44.3 (0.9)	58.4 (1.2)
Smoking cessation	42.5 (1.1)	4.6 (0.9)

*Availability is the percentage of all employees who have access to a health promotion program at work. Participation is the percentage of employees with access who actually use or participate in a health promotion program. Percentages are based on the responses of 5219 NHIS respondents, who represent an estimated population of 52,776,573 employees.

Table 2

Estimated Availability and Participation Percentages[†] During the Past Year for Five Different Categories of Health Promotion, According to Gender, Age, Ethnicity, and Education (1994 NHIS)

	Exercise Facilities		Exercise Programs		Health Education Programs		Screening Tests		Smoking Cessation		Overall Mean[‡]	
	% Available	% Participate	% Available	% Participate	% Available	% Participate	% Available	% Participate	% Available	% Participate	% Available	% Participate
Gender												
Male	36.1*	50.3*	25.0	30.9	64.6	56.5	44.4	61.4*	43.9	3.9	39.9	40.6
Female	32.9	43.8	26.5	34.8	65.9	59.3	44.2	55.0	40.9	5.6	39.4	39.7
Age												
18–24	22.7**	51.9*	19.8*	33.1	50.5**	48.2**	27.2**	42.4**	22.1**	2.1*	26.4	35.5
25–39	35.7	50.6	25.7	33.3	66.1	57.8	43.5	58.4	41.4	7.7	39.7	41.6
40–54	36.7	45.3	28.0	34.2	68.8	60.6	49.1	60.7	47.7	2.8	43.7	40.7
55+	33.2	38.3	22.8	23.9	61.2	53.9	45.5	57.6	45.5	2.2	38.6	35.2
Ethnicity												
Black	29.8	44.4	21.4	42.0	61.0	62.5*	46.4	64.4	40.9	10.2	39.9	44.7
White	35.5	48.0	26.3	31.6	65.9	57.7	44.1	57.3	42.7	3.8	42.9	39.7
Other	32.6	44.9	27.1	32.7	65.5	47.1	41.6	61.3	43.8	5.3	42.1	38.3
Education												
0–11 years	20.0**	51.5	12.0**	34.0	46.9**	59.7**	30.9**	52.4	24.1**	1.4	24.6	39.8
H.S. degree	28.7	49.2	20.3	29.4	60.2	61.6	39.2	62.3	36.9	6.1	34.5	41.9
Some college	36.7	50.8	27.9	33.7	68.3	63.3	44.9	59.2	46.2	3.9	41.9	42.2
College or more	43.9	43.4	33.9	34.3	73.6	49.7	53.4	55.5	51.0	4.0	48.8	37.4

[†]Availability is the percentage of all employees who have access to a health promotion program at work. Participation is the percentage of employees with access who actually use or participate in a health promotion program.

[‡]Overall mean is the average for the five categories of health promotion programs.

*$p \leq 0.05$ for at least one difference in a set of comparisons, **$p \leq 0.01$ for at least one difference in a set of comparisons.

by health education programs, screening tests, exercise facilities and exercise programs. In terms of having access to at least one program in a category, employees rated health education programs highest (65.2%), with screening tests second. For participation, screening tests had the highest mean percentage (49.3%), followed by health education programs, exercise facilities, exercise programs, and smoking cessation programs.

Role of Individual Characteristics

Table 2 presents availability and participation percentages according to the gender, age, ethnicity, and education of the respondents. All percentages were cal-culated in terms of whether at least one program was available or used for each of the five categories of health promotion covered in the NHIS. The final two columns of the table provide means for availability and participation across the five categories. For presentation purposes, standard errors are not provided in the table, but are available upon request from the authors.

Gender. Overall mean availability and participation for men and women (see final two columns of Table 2) were very similar, differing by .5% and .9%, respectively. However, participation by gender varied slightly with the category of health promotion, with men significantly more likely to use exercise facilities and screening tests. Availability for men and women was almost identical for the five categories, with the exception of exercise facilities, where men reported a higher percentage.

Age. Availability and participation generally followed a curvilinear pattern, with the 18 to 24 age group usually having the lowest values. Specifically, availability and participation increased for the 25 to 39 and 40 to 54 age groups, and then decreased slightly for workers 55 and over. Differences among age categories were usually larger for availability than for participation.

Ethnicity. Blacks reported the lowest level of availability for four of the five categories of worksite health promotion.

Table 3

Estimated Availability and Participation Percentages† During the Past Year for Five Categories of Health Promotion, According to Type of Organization, Occupational Group, and Industrial Group (1994 NHIS)

	Exercise Facilities		Exercise Programs		Health Education Programs		Screening Tests		Smoking Cessation		Overall Mean‡	
	% Avail- able	% Partic- ipate	% Avail- able	% Partic- ipate	% Avail- able	% Partic- ipate	% Avail- able	% Partic- ipate	% Avail- able	% Partic- ipate	% Avail- able	% Partic- ipate
Type of organization												
Private company	31.7**	46.5	24.7**	31.3	63.1**	58.5	43.6**	59.7*	42.2**	5.1	40.5	40.2
Federal government	45.7	49.0	39.0	42.5	80.9	53.0	60.0	63.0	63.6	3.1	56.4	42.1
State and local government	44.6	49.2	26.6	34.7	70.0	56.2	43.7	51.1	37.4	2.8	44.1	38.8
Occupational group												
Professional/Managerial/ Technical	44.3**	42.1**	35.5**	32.6*	75.0**	54.8**	55.0**	57.4	51.7**	4.4	49.8	38.3
Sales/Clerical	27.7	43.3	22.1	36.9	60.3	52.3	36.5	54.6	39.3	3.9	34.5	38.2
Service	37.3	62.3	18.8	40.5	60.9	66.9	38.1	58.1	27.7	15.7	34.5	48.7
Operatives/Laborers/ Craftsmen	25.4	55.1	17.1	23.3	57.1	65.4	38.2	64.4	37.8	3.1	32.3	42.3
Industry group												
Manufacturing	33.9**	46.8	25.3**	30.1	64.7**	60.7*	47.3**	62.8	47.5**	5.0	43.7	41.1
Utilities/Transportation/ Communications	31.5	48.6	22.7	28.6	65.8	59.2	42.5	61.1	52.2	2.2	42.9	39.9
Wholesale/Retail	17.2	55.9	11.4	34.5	49.2	56.1	19.3	54.4	21.4	9.1	23.7	42.0
Financial/Real Estate/ Insurance	29.3	34.7	31.9	41.8	64.0	44.9	47.7	56.7	50.4	5.1	44.7	36.6
Service	43.4	47.7	31.9	33.8	72.0	57.3	50.9	54.9	44.2	3.5	48.5	39.4
Agriculture/Mining/ Construction	27.8	49.7	12.8	24.4	64.1	67.0	41.6	70.6	32.3	8.5	35.7	44.0

†Availability is the percentage of all employees who have access to a health promotion program at work. Participation is the percentage of employees with access who actually use or participate in a health promotion program.

‡ Overall mean is the average for the five categories of health promotion programs.

*$p \leq 0.05$ for at least one difference in a set of comparisons, **$p \leq 0.01$ for at least one difference in a set of comparisons.

Although none of these differences attained statistical significance, this pattern suggests an overall lower rate of availability for blacks. In terms of participation, blacks had the highest percentages for four of five categories, with participation in screening programs attaining significance. The overall mean for participation confirms this pattern, with blacks having the highest percentage.

Education. Availability increased with each level of education for all five categories of health pro-

motion. In each category, employees with a college degree or more reported about twice as much availability as employees having less than a high school degree. Participation, however, differed very little across education levels, with the overall mean percentage lowest for employees having at least a college degree.

Role of Organizational Characteristics

Table 3 presents availability and participation data according to organizational characteristics for

each of the five categories of health promotion.

Type of Organization. Employees in the federal government had the highest availability for all categories of health promotion. With the exception of smoking cessation, employees in private companies reported the lowest availability, with state and local government employees falling in the middle. Participation differed only slightly with organizational type, with no group having consistently higher percentages than the other two.

Occupational Group. Workers in professional/managerial/technical occupations had the highest availability, while operatives/laborers/craftsmen usually had the lowest. Again, participation differed very little across groups, with service workers generally having the highest participation, followed by operatives/laborers/craftsmen.

Industry Group. With the exception of smoking cessation, service sector workers reported the highest level of availability for all categories. Workers in wholesale/retail and agriculture/mining/construction consistently had the lowest availability. Participation was fairly similar over these groups, with no consistent pattern emerging across the five categories.

Comparing the NSWHPA (1985, 1992) and NHIS (1994)

A comparison of data from the NSWHPA and NHIS is presented in Table 4. The Year 2000 objective, if available, is also displayed for each health promotion activity. Only availability data are presented since participation was not measured in the NSWHPA. For this comparison, analysis of the NHIS data was limited to employees working in private companies, since this was the focus of the two previous NSWHPA surveys.

Table 4 shows that availability in private companies has continued to increase across the three national surveys for several health promotion activities, including back care, smoking policies, screening tests, and weight control. Availability of other activities, such as stress management, smoking cessation, and nutrition education, has remained

| Table 4 | Percentage of the Private Sector Workforce with Access to Selected Health Promotion Activities According to Three National Surveys and Year 2000 Objectives |

Health Promotion Activity	NSWHPA* (1985)	NSWHPA* (1992)	NHIS† (1994)	Year 2000 Objective
Back care	29	32	40	50
Smoking policy	27	86	92	75
Stress management	27	37	37	40
Nutrition education	17	31	29	50
Weight control	15	24	28	50
Blood pressure screening	17	32	41	NA‡
Cholesterol screening	9	20	34	NA
Cancer screening	6	12	17	NA
Job hazards/Injury prevention	NA	64	48	NA
Smoking cessation	NA	40	42	NA
Alcohol/Other drugs	NA	36	32	NA
At least one health promotion activity§	66	81	78	85
At least one exercise/ fitness program‖	22	42	40	NA

*NSWHPA is the National Survey of Worksite Health Promotion Activities (1985, n = 1360 companies; 1992, n = 1507 companies).

†NHIS is the National Health Interview Survey (1994, n = 5219 employees).

‡NA, not available.

§Health promotion activity is based on the definition used in the 1985 NSWHPA and includes: weight control, stress management, screening tests, off-the-job accident prevention, back care, nutrition education, and exercise/fitness programs.

‖Exercise/fitness program includes both exercise programs and exercise facilities. The list of programs respondents were asked about varied slightly across the three national surveys.

similar to that reported in the 1992 NSWHPA. The most noticeable declines since 1992 occurred for job hazards/injury prevention (16%) and alcohol/drug programs (4%). Of the programs for which Year 2000 goals were set, only the goal for smoking policy has been met.

Participation Differences between Healthy and Nonhealthy Employees

The adjusted odds ratios (ORs) from multiple logistic regression comparing participation in health promotion programs for healthy and nonhealthy employees are presented in Table 5. The ORs are calculated so that a value above 1.0 indicates that healthier employees were more likely to participate in worksite health promotion whereas a value below 1.0 indicates that healthier employees were less likely to participate. The upper and lower ORs for the 95% confidence interval are presented in parentheses.

Only two of the 24 ORs presented in Table 5 were statistically significant at the $p \leq .05$ level, after adjusting for gender, race, age, and education. Unfortunately, the two significant ORs are contradictory with regard to whether healthier employees are

Table 5 Adjusted Odds Ratios[†] for Participation in Worksite Health Promotion Programs According to Four NHIS Measures of Health

NHIS Health Measure	At Least One Exercise Facility	At Least One Exercise Program	At Least One Health Education Program	At Least One Screening Test	Smoking Cessation	At Least One Program/ Facility of Any Kind
General health	0.60	0.66	1.15	1.07	1.01	1.11
	(0.26–1.39)	(0.21–2.02)	(0.73–1.80)	(0.53–2.17)	(0.19–5.33)	(0.73–1.68)
Blood pressure	1.43**	1.55*	0.97	0.94	2.99	1.02
	(1.01–2.03)	(0.96–2.49)	(0.77–1.23)	(0.65–1.37)	(0.73–12.27)	(0.83–1.25)
Body mass index (BMI)	1.29	1.46*	0.81*	0.86	1.55	0.83**
	(0.92–1.79)	(0.98–2.19)	(0.65–1.01)	(0.64–1.16)	(0.59–4.06)	(0.69–1.00)
Medical conditions	0.78*	1.13	0.95	1.23	1.14	0.97
	(0.60–1.01)	(0.79–1.61)	(0.80–1.14)	(0.94–1.61)	(0.53–2.45)	(0.84–1.12)

[†]Odds ratios were calculated by using each of the four dichotomized NHIS health measures to predict participation in separate logistic regressions. All odds ratios have been adjusted for gender, age, ethnicity, and education. Odds ratios above 1.0 indicate that healthy workers have greater participation than non-healthy workers. Odds ratios below 1.0 indicate that healthy workers have lower participation than nonhealthy workers.

*$p \leq 0.10$, **$p \leq 0.05$.

more likely to participate in worksite health promotion. Workers not reporting high blood pressure were more likely to use exercise facilities than workers with high blood pressure. By contrast, workers with a BMI less than 20% above their ideal were less likely to participate in at least one health promotion program or facility of any kind than workers whose BMI exceeded 20%. Table 5 also indicates that four additional ORs were marginally significant at $p \leq$ .10. However, these ORs do not follow a consistent pattern, in that two are above 1.0 and two are below 1.0. The remaining nonsignificant ORs also show little consistency, with almost an even split between values above and below 1.0.

Discussion

The results of this study indicate that, from an employee's perspective, worksite health promotion programs are widespread within both public and private sector organizations. The most widely available programs are those in

the areas of health education, screening tests, and smoking cessation. Exercise programs and facilities, which usually require the greatest investment of resources, are also the least common. In terms of availability, the 1994 NHIS data reveal a picture of health promotion fairly similar to that in the 1992 NSWHPA, with some programs showing modest increases (e.g., screening tests, back care) and others showing declines (e.g., injury prevention, alcohol/drug programs). Interpreting these changes, however, must be done cautiously in light of the differences in measures and samples existing between the three surveys. In the case of declining availability, one contributing factor may be that employees are simply unaware of the health promotion activities that management is making available to them. In other words, the availability of certain programs, like those focusing on injury prevention and alcohol/drugs, may need to be better communicated and advertised to workers. It may also be that recent pressures

on organizations to downsize and increase efficiency have resulted in some health promotion programs being discontinued or deemphasized by management. Clearly, additional research is needed to more carefully identify the different factors responsible for any recent changes in the availability of worksite health promotion programs.

The importance of individual and organizational characteristics appears greater in predicting availability of health promotion programs than in predicting participation (see Tables 2 and 3). For example, availability of worksite health promotion is higher for employees who are well-educated, white, between the ages of 25 and 54, and who work as professionals or managers in a public sector organization. Unfortunately, availability is lowest for blacks and the less educated, two groups that may have the most to gain from access. Participation follows a much more complex pattern, and differences between groups are typically smaller for participation than for availability. These findings suggest that participation is less dependent on individual or organizational variables, and determined more by other factors in the workplace, such as organizational culture, management commitment, incentives for participation, or qualities of the actual health promotion activities. This conclusion is consistent with previous studies indicating that environmental or contextual factors in the workplace (e.g., organizational culture, marketing of program) are important determinants of participation.[17,24–26] Future research needs to more systematically examine these contextual factors and discover how they may be linked to participation in health promotion activities.

To the degree that individual and organizational characteristics are important, the results of the present study should add to and help clarify findings from previous research that has tended to focus on health promotion practices within a single organization. For example, although evidence exists that women are more likely than men to participate in most health promotion activities,[27] not all studies report such a difference.[18,28] The present study found that, although overall gender differences were small, women were less likely to use exercise facilities and screening tests than men. For education and age, which previous research suggests are not consistently related to participation,[14,18] the present study found a curvilinear relationship. Employees in the middle age and education groups tended to have the highest participation. For ethnicity, the finding that blacks displayed a pattern of slightly higher participation contradicts a previous report indicating that blacks have lower participation.[19] Although there may be conditions

in a given organization that lead to greater participation by whites, this doesn't appear to be the case on a general basis. In terms of organizational variables, the finding regarding the high level of access to health promotion for public sector employees is particularly noteworthy, since this group has not been studied before on a national level.

This study failed to find consistent support for the position that only healthier workers are likely to participate in health promotion activities. There were few, if any, systematic differences in participation for workers with healthy attributes (e.g., good to excellent general health) compared to workers with nonhealthy attributes (e.g., fair to poor general health). This finding suggests that participation is a complex process involving factors that overshadow a simple consideration of a worker's health. Such a conclusion, however, needs to be verified by prospective research, since differences between participants and nonparticipants may be confounded with any benefit that occurs from actually participating in a health promotion activity.[29]

It is important to note that participation in a health promotion program should be kept separate from the issue of its effectiveness. Low participation in a program, such as in the case of smoking cessation, which is utilized by fewer than 5% of employees, tells us little about the cost-effectiveness or health impact for participating employees. Participation in a program may be low for a number of reasons, including the fact that some programs focus on health risks experienced by a minority of workers (e.g., smoking, alcohol abuse). The amount of participa-

tion may provide some insight into which programs are most popular with employees, but the issue of effectiveness is one that cannot be adequately addressed by the cross-sectional data available in the NHIS.

Other limitations of the present study include the lack of detail in the NHIS concerning health promotion activities made available to workers. Some activities may have involved workshops or classes over several weeks, while others may have been limited to brief presentations or, in the case of health education programs, distribution of relevant brochures and handouts. Participants may have varied with regard to their level of participation, and some may have used health promotion programs outside of work. For example, one possible explanation for the comparatively low level of participation among professional and managerial workers (see Table 3) is that these employees, having higher disposable incomes, were more likely to belong to health clubs or utilize health-related activities not sponsored by their organizations.

All three national surveys relied on self-reports that may be subject to recall biases. The precise wording of questions varied across the three surveys, as did the range of information collected from the respondents. Although the NHIS collected extensive health-related data from employees, no information concerning organizational size was collected in the Year 2000 Supplement, beyond the minimum requirement of 50 or more employees. As a result, this study's findings apply only to organizations with at least 50 employees. Organizational size has been found to be positively associated with availability,[1] and

So What? Implications for Health Promotion Practitioners and Researchers

This study indicates that worksite health promotion programs are available for approximately 82% of workers in U.S. companies with 50 or more employees. Participation in these programs appears to vary widely and is only minimally related to factors such as an employee's age, gender, ethnicity, occupation, and health. If these findings hold true, attempts to increase participation should include consideration of contextual factors in the workplace, such as management commitment and incentives for participation, that can be used to make worksite health promotion programs a more attractive option for workers.

additional data on size might help explain differences in availability reported in Table 3 for type of organization (i.e., public vs. private) and industry group.

Despite these limitations, this study provides the first systematic analysis of availability and participation from an employee's perspective. The data presented indicate that worksite health promotion programs are not equally available to all groups (e.g., nonprofessionals, less educated, blacks) and that participation varies widely across programs, with organizational and individual variables playing, at best, a small role. These findings highlight the need to provide better access to health promotion programs and to more completely understand the circumstances within organizations that encourage participation, so that health promotion can become a more attractive opportunity for workers.

References

1. McGinnis J. 1992 national survey of worksite health promotion activities: summary. *Am J Health Promot* 1993;7:452–64.

2. Golaszewski T, Snow D, Lynch W, et al. A benefit-to-cost analysis of a work-site health promotion program. *J Occup Med* 1992;34:1164–72.

3. Pelletier KR. A review and analysis of the health and cost-effective outcome studies of comprehensive health promotion and disease prevention programs at the worksite: 1993–1995 update. *Am J Health Promot* 1996;10:380–8.

4. Spilman MA, Goetz A, Schultz J, et al. Effects of a corporate health promotion program. *J Occup Med* 1986;28:285–9.

5. Holt MC, McCauley M, Paul D. Health impacts of AT&T's total life concept (TLC) program after five years. *Am J Health Promot* 1995;9:421–5.

6. Lechner L, de Vries H, Adriaansen S, et al. Effects of an employee fitness program on reduced absenteeism. *J Occup Environ Med* 1997;39:827–31.

7. Heaney CA, Goetzel RZ. A review of health-related outcomes of multi-component worksite health promotion programs. *Am J Health Promot* 1997;11:290–308.

8. Fielding J, Piserchia P. Frequency of worksite health promotion activities. *Am J Public Health* 1989;79:16–20.

9. Office of Disease Prevention and Health Promotion, US Department of Health and Human Services, 1985 National Survey of Worksite Health Promotion Activities: Executive Summary, Washington DC: Public Health Service, 1987.

10. Office of Disease Prevention and Health Promotion, US Department of Health and Human Service, 1992 National Survey of Worksite Health Promotion Activities: Executive Summary, Washington DC. Public Health Service, 1992.

11. Eickhoff-Shemek JM, Ryan KF. A comparison of Omaha worksite health promotion activities to the 1992 national survey with a special perspective on program intervention. *Am J Health Promot* 1995;10:132–9.

12. Centers for Disease Control and Prevention. Worksite health promotion—N.H. *MMWR* 1993;42:28–37.

13. US Department of Health and Human Services. Healthy People 2000: National Health Promotion and Disease Prevention Objectives. Washington, DC: Public Health Service, 1991.

14. Glasgow RE, McCaul KD, Fisher KJ. Participation in worksite health promotion: a critique of the literature and recommendations for future practice. *Health Educ Q* 1993;20:391–408.

15. *The American Almanac: Statistical Abstract of the United States.* Washington, DC: The Reference Press Inc., 1995.

16. Carter WB, Omenn GS, Martin M. et al. Characteristics of health promotion programs in federal worksites: Findings from the federal employee worksite project. *Am J Health Promot* 1995;10:140–7.

17. Crump CE, Earp JAL, Mozma CM, et al. Effect of organizational-level variables on differential employee participation in 10 federal worksite health promotion programs. *Health Educ Q* 1996;23:204–23.

18. Conrad P. Who comes to work-site wellness programs? A preliminary review. *J Occup Med* 1987;29:317–9.

19. Strange KC, Strogatz D, Schoenbach VJ, et al. Demographic and health characteristics of participants and nonparticipants in a work site health-promotion program. *J Occup Med* 1991;33:474–8.

20. Adams PF, Marano MA. Current estimates from the National Health Interview Survey, 1994. National Center for Health Statistics. *Vital Health Stat* 1995;10:193.

21. US Bureau of the Census. 1990 Census of the Population. Alphabetical Index of Industries and Occupations. Washington, DC: US Bureau of the Census, 1992.

22. National Institutes of Health Consensus Development Panel on the Health Implications of Obesity. Health implications of obesity. *Ann Intern Med* 1985;103:1073–7.

23. Shah BV. Software for Survey Data Analysis (SUDAAN) Version 7.10. Research Triangle Park, North Carolina: Research Triangle Institute, 1996.

24. Strange KC, Streaker VJ, Schoenbach VJ, et al. Psychosocial predictors of participation in a work site health-promotion program. *J Occup Med* 1991;33:479–85.

25. Lechner L, De Vries H. Participation in an employee fitness program: determinants of high adherence, low adherence, and dropout. *J Occup Environ Med* 1995;37:429–36.

26. Allen RF, Allen J. A sense of community, a shared vision and a positive culture: core enabling factors in successful culture based health promotion. *Am J Health Promot* 1987;1:40–7.

27. Spilman MA. Gender differences in worksite health promotion activities. *Soc Sci Med* 1988;26:525–35.

28. Lynch WD, Golaszewski TJ, Clearie A, et al. Characteristics of self-selected responders to a health risk appraisal: generalizability of corporate health assessments. *Am J Public Health* 1989;79:887–8.

29. Heaney CA, Inglish P. Are employees who are at risk for cardiovascular disease joining worksite fitness centers? *J Occup Environ Med* 1995;37:718–24.

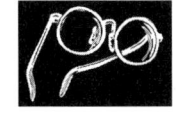 **Article Review Form at end of book.**

Is the renewed interest in health promotion and disease prevention really buoyed up by better health and cost outcomes data and research? How has managed care impacted worksite health promotion?

A Review and Analysis of the Health and Cost-Effective Outcome Studies of Comprehensive Health Promotion and Disease Prevention Programs at the Worksite:

1993–1995 Update

Kenneth R. Pelletier

Kenneth R. Pelletier, PhD, MD (hc), Stanford University School of Medicine, Stanford, California.

Mark Twain once quipped that he "discovered he had been speaking 'prose' for his entire life." Today, health promotion and disease prevention programs are also being "discovered" because they play a vital role in managed care by providing quality services that may decrease inappropriate or excessive use of medical care. Managed care organizations appear in myriad forms, but when such an organization is financially at risk regarding use, health promotion and disease prevention are discovered. Increasingly, it is evident that the self-insured, self-administered health and medical plans of large corporations, with their emphasis on health promotion and disease prevention, were and are prototypes of managed health care.[1,2]

During the recent national debate, the term "managed care" emerged as though it was a radical and untested approach lacking in precedent and evaluation.[3] Rather than viewing managed care as either a threat or a panacea, it is important to recognize that the 51 studies cited in the two earlier articles[4] in this series; the 26 studies cited in this article, an ongoing annotation compiled by Larry S. Chapman of Corporate Health Designs,[5] and a vast number of

Reprinted by permission from *American Journal of Health Promotion,* May/June 1996 (Vol. 10, No. 5), pp. 380–388 and from Dr. Kenneth R. Pelletier, Clinical Associate Professor of Medicine, Director—Stanford Corporate Health Programs, Stanford University School of Medicine.

rigorous, randomized clinical trials conducted outside the worksite focus on this article,[6,7] clearly demonstrate a substantial and growing body of research demonstrating that health promotion and disease prevention within managed health care are both health- and cost-effective.[8] For this article and grid, the focus is limited to those articles that contain both health and cost outcomes of worksite-based comprehensive health promotion and disease prevention. Briefly, three important definitions are used throughout this review. "Cost-effectiveness" refers to the unit cost of providing a service or for achieving a specific health outcome. In discussing a possible reduction in actual medical care costs, the term "cost savings" is appropriate. "Cost benefit analysis" compares the savings from a program compared with the cost of providing that program. All three types of outcomes are evidenced in the studies cited here and the specific type of cost outcome is specified in the table or grid where each individual study is cited. In some instances a study in which cost-effectiveness is not part of the formal outcomes analysis but is strongly inferred is included in this review. All cited research has been published in peer-reviewed, professional journals.

Surely many other worksite programs, such as the ongoing "Working Well" project of the National Cancer Institute, focused on worksite nutrition programs to reduce cancer incidence in 114 worksites involving more than 25,000 employees;[9,10] a study of highly effective childhood immunizations is a large corporation;[11] and an overview of 44 exercise interventions indicating an annual savings of $61 to $450 per employee per year plus coronary heart disease risk reduction benefits ranging from $75 to $300 per employee annually[12] that are not included in this review because analyses of cost-effectiveness or strongly inferred cost-effectiveness have not formally been conducted in their published research. Overall, most research involving health promotion and disease prevention in the worksite and other clinical sites indicates that such interventions are both health- and cost-effective. From a purely medical perspective, a recent study from Duke University, "Five-Hundred Life-Saving Interventions and Their Cost-effectiveness," concluded overall that primary prevention is actually more cost-effective than secondary or tertiary prevention. Primary prevention was found to be cost-effective at an approximate average of $5000 per life per year saved.[13] It is increasingly evident that the issues of the cost-effectiveness of health promotion and disease prevention depend on the specificity of the intervention, the characteristics of the patients, and the appropriate level of intervention for a specific condition.[14]

Is the renewed interest in health promotion and disease prevention really buoyed up by better health and cost outcomes data and research? In a word, no! During this decade of fiscal frugality, the driving question is simply whether prevention is cost-effective. Even within a traditional fee-for-service model, health promotion and disease prevention are both health- and cost-effective as exemplified by the fact that an immunization program for measles, mumps, and rubella can save approximately $14 for every dollar spent.[15,16] A program to increase the use of bicycle safety helmets can yield an estimated net savings of more than $200 million each year.[17] Screening mammograms for women 50 to 70 years old every 2 years is highly cost-effective at $4050 per year of life saved.[17] Programs that target smoking during pregnancy can save more than $6 for every dollar spent.[18] A survey of both employers and health care providers by the U.S. Department of Health and Human Services indicated that the "work setting represents the single most important channel to systematically reach the adult population through health information and health promotion programs."[19] Among the reasons for the increasing frequency of such programs are that they are popular with employees, supply management with positive yet low-cost benefits for employees, improve both health and productivity in the short term, and reduce medical expenditures in the long term. However, the essence of the reinvigorated interest in prevention is driven by the accelerating movement toward "capitated managed care" and away from fee-for-service models.

Within fee-for-service systems, to be simplistic, the more services that are performed, the more the provider is paid. This same provider also determines both the demand and supply of those services while a remote "third party payor" pays for the self-perpetuating and self-serving transaction. Beyond the economic consequences of such an approach is the abundant documentation of excessive and/or inappropriate services, including unnecessary inpatient days of hospitalization ranging from a low of 43% unnecessary days in Seattle to a high of 69% in New York with an approximate nationwide average of 59% in such cities as Cleveland, Denver, Los

Angeles, Oklahoma City, San Francisco, and Tampa;[20] inappropriate prescription of medication to approximately 40% of the elderly residents in 12 nursing homes in Los Angeles,[21] unnecessary transfusions ranging from 18% to 25%; extensive documentation in numerous studies of excessive use of diagnostic imaging technologies;[22] the common and long-standing documentation of unnecessary cesarean sections and hysterectomies;[23] increasing acceptance that an "estimated 50% of coronary angiography currently undertaken in the United States is unnecessary;"[24] and on and on. These are literally only a few of the most recent studies to document excessive and inappropriate use under a fee-for-service structure. This is not to castigate fee-for-service care per se[3] but simply to underscore that the hue and cry that managed care will lead to denial of appropriate care, rationing, and suboptimal clinical services is virtually lacking in documentation, whereas evidence of excessive care is overwhelmingly evident.[25] What is a legitimate issue is appropriate levels of care that ensure neither overutilization nor underutilization.

Managed care, with its renewed attention to health promotion and disease prevention, is not a panacea. It does, however, militate against the perverse incentive of excessive or inappropriate services to generate revenues or, in some instances, to pay for the investment in a new technology or the politics of empire building by having a hospital or other provider dependent on the revenues derived from a particular medical service or individual practitioner. Within managed care, "capitation" dominates because a provider system and the practitioners within that system receive a fixed amount of money per person per year (i.e., "capitated"). This gives them the incentive to manage the care for that group within the global annual budget. Among the best and most comprehensive analysis of the promise and pitfalls of managed care is a report written for Volpe, Welty & Company by Dr. Jason M. Rosenbluth, called "Integrated Delivery Systems: The Battle Among Payers, Hospitals, and Physicians"[1] and is essential reading for the coming decade. One of the earliest and still best documented studies of such an approach characterized by a Preferred Provider Organization (PPO) with a Point of Service (POS) option was conducted in conjunction with Southwestern Bell Corporation[26] and Metropolitan Insurance Company.

Managed care is in the process of evolving, and it is certain that its ultimate forms, because many variants do exist, will "resemble neither the model espoused by proponents of managed competition nor the models advocated by proponents of more government controls."[27] Writing in *Health Affairs*, Dr. Jonathan E. Fielding and Dr. Thomas Rice of the UCLA School of Public Health have clearly considered both the applications and limitations of managed care to resolve the national medical care and expenditure crisis. With all due acknowledgement to these well-articulated caveats, the variants of managed care most evident to date in large corporations, health maintenance organizations (HMOs) and their variants, as well as newly emerging models of preferred provider organizations (PPOs) and similar systems, do represent a potent solution for a significant portion of both the clinical care and fiscal crisis so clearly evident at the national, state, community, and individual level.

Within the new systems of managed care and their capitated budget, a renewed emphasis is on health promotion and disease prevention. Presumably, both primary and secondary prevention will have the effect of reducing the necessity of later and more costly interventions for diseases and disorders that have progressed in severity. In addition, a growing power of consumer or patient demand and satisfaction have emerged because individuals have the option to re-enroll in competing plans on an annual basis.[28] If patients perceive or are denied access to appropriate care, they are likely to change plans, and such a turnover is undesirable to a capitated plan. Given the strong and growing interest of the general public in health promotion and disease prevention, one way to steer between the "Scylla and Charybdis" of demand versus denial is to manage the patient's demands by providing health promotion programs that appear to satisfy the individual's need for services at a more appropriate, earlier, and less costly stage of demand so that access to such services does not have to be denied.[29] This innovation has been termed "demand management" and is exemplified by the earliest and still the most well-documented research conducted by Dr. James F. Fries of the Stanford University School of Medicine under the "Healthtrac" Company and Foundation.[30–32] This and other research appears to demonstrate that responsible "demand management" is both health- and cost-effective while satisfying the individual need for earlier preventive care without imposing denial to appropriate access or rationing of care. Although this is not proven now, it does provide a note of optimism amid the dire pronouncements of impending doom. Most important, it is a model that is amenable to sophisticated, longitudinal, randomized clinical trails that will enable us to empirically determine whether such an approach is health- and cost-effective while maintaining, or perhaps even enhancing, the subjective satisfaction and quality of life of the individual patient.

Because managed care/demand management is such a powerful model, why is it not more evident? That literally depends to a large degree on where you live. An insightful analysis from the University Hospital Consortium has separated the current health care market into five stages while citing specific cities characterizing each stage.[33] At stage 1, which is "unstructured" little or no managed care exists in cities such as Shreveport. At the other extreme of stage 5 or "endgame" is a theoretical market of "true partnerships and networks" nationwide. Between these ends of the continuum are varying degrees of managed care penetration such as stage 2 or "loose framework" in Miami, Atlanta, Cleveland, St. Louis, Dallas/Fort Worth, and Philadelphia. Stage 3 or "consolidation" is the first stage in which managed care actually becomes the dominant model in cities exemplified by Portland, San Francisco, Oakland, Denver, Boston, Salt Lake City, Seattle, Houston, Chicago, and Washington, D.C. At stage 4 or "managed competition" more than 50% HMO penetration and other forms of managed care are as well developed as they can be at present characterized by "em-

ployer coalitions," "little fee-for-service," "a few large dominant providers," "providers and insurers strongly align," "doctors not in groups pushed out," "eliminate hospital beds," "shift in physician supply," "use of specialists and their fees driven down dramatically," "network develop full continuum of care," and "providers and insurers organize to serve covered (i.e., capitated) lives." Cities characterizing stage 4 are San Diego, Minneapolis, Los Angeles, and Worcester. This mature, stage 4 market clearly represents a graphic prototype of the future look of managed care with both the pluses and minuses in play. Whether we like or agree with this model, it is increasingly dominant and its national persuasiveness is inexorable. It is simply a function of time and geographic location and, indeed, the mountain will come to you.

Focusing specifically on the issue of cost-effectiveness, two remaining issues need to be addressed. One is a methodological one weighing in to support health promotion and disease prevention interventions. The other is an obvious point that not all such programs are cost-effective. With regard to methodology, Dr. Paul M. Kingery and his colleagues addressed the issue of "high-cost analysis" methodology in the *Journal of Occupational Medicine.* Their observation is that medical claims data are highly skewed and violate the statistical assumption of normality. Because a small percentage of employees incur the largest percentage of medical costs, the standard deviation is large and skews the claims data to the right of the normal curve. As a result, the mean is generally much higher than the median. This "inappropriate use of means in cross-sectional studies under-

estimates sample bias, overestimates the descriptive difference in cost for high-risk and low-risk employees, and underestimates the statistical significance of large differences observed between the means for the two groups."[34] These worksite studies engender the problems mentioned above and two additional ones. Using statistical measures of arithmetic means assumes that an intervention that appears to lower costs for participants achieved a small effect among all high-risk participants. It may in fact have substantially reduced the costs for a small number of participants at high risk and had little effect on costs for the other. Practically speaking, this potential of the most cost savings concentrated in a small number of high-risk employees, the failure to target high-risk employees dilutes the cost-effectiveness of the intervention. Although "comprehensive" programs will and should continue, it is increasingly clear that programs of secondary prevention focused on high-risk individuals, such as the Stanford Coronary Risk Intervention Program, will be increasingly important in managed care.

Not all health promotion and disease prevention programs in the worksite are health- and/or cost-effective.[35] Negative results and methodologic limitations of studies were included and extensively discussed in both earlier reviews and in this one as well.[4] Advocacy for health promotion and disease prevention programs is neither naive nor uncritical. Two recent studies, both focused on heart disease, did not demonstrate positive health impacts. In 1994, the "Staff Healthy Heart Project" was established at the Royal Prince Alfred Hospital and five nearby hospitals in Sydney,

Cost-Effectiveness Grid

Study	Purpose of Evaluation	Sample Size	Types of Workers	Comparison Group	Evaluation Period
Textile plants (1992)[46]	Examine relationship between workplace health promotion and medical claims	38 textile plants	All	No	1 yr
Traveler's insurance (1992)[47]	Analyze the benefit/cost ratio of a comprehensive HP/DP program for 1986–1990 with projections to the year 2000	Total of 36,000 employees and retirees nationwide	All	No	4 yr and projected over 15 yr
Bank of America (1993)[48]	Determine both health- and cost-effectiveness of a health promotion program for retirees of Bank of America	4712 retirees	All	Yes	2 yr (followed for 3 yr from April 1987–March, 1990)
Thirty–two (32) worksites (1993)[49]	Effect of worksite smoking cessation and weight control on absenteeism in 32 Minneapolis-St. Paul companies	32 sites of 200 employees each = 6400	All	Yes	2 yr
Utility company (1993)[50]	Effect of worksite health promotion on sick days and medical care use	Nine (9) divisions of the company	All (mostly men between 30 and 49 yr old)	No	1 yr
California county (1993)[51]	Health- and cost-effectiveness of a back injury prevention program	205 (six divisions)	Blue collar	No	1 yr
Montreal, Quebec (1993)[52]	Evaluate a worksite alcohol awareness program	322	Blue collar	Yes (within one site of 813 workers with 199 participants)	3 yr
General Motors (1993)[53]	Health- and cost-effectiveness of worksite health promotion in reducing CVD	1880	Auto workers	Yes by worksite	3 yr
DuPoint (1993)[54]	Assess impact of worksite health promotion program on 7 behavioral risks and self-reported sick days	7178 and time lagged comparison group of 7101	All	Yes (time lagged, nonequivalent comparison group)	2 yr

Intervention and Outcome Measures	Evaluation Design	Subject Self-Selection	Findings
Number of medical claims per worker	Cross-sectional analysis with a linear regression	Yes	Claims per worker varied threefold. In a linear regression, age: sex, race, plant product, and medical access explained 23% of variance in medical claims. Health promotion (in interaction with plant product) explained 54% of claims (controlling for race, sex, and access variables).
"Taking Care" program of lifestyle management, health risk appraisal, medical self-care book, newsletter, and videotapes. Total program costs from 1986–1990 projected at 5% inflation/year to year 2000. Determine impact on pension liability by use of proxy measures.	Program costs tracked and benefits calculated to reflect decreases in medical costs, absenteeism, life insurance claims, and increases in productivity. Different econometric modeling used for costs in each of these areas and then totaled.	Yes	Study indicated a positive return of $1:$3.4 for 1986–2000. Program reached a positive benefit/cost in the first year with a positive balance of $330,000. A net cumulative benefit of more than $146 million (for a $60 million investment) projected to accrue over the 15-yr period.
Health risk appraisal scores (Healthtrac) and medical care costs. Participation rates of 57% at 1 yr and 47% at 2 yr.	Randomized with 3 groups: (1) with individual HRAs, recommendation and materials; (2) HRA but no recommendation until year 2; and, (3) control	No	HRA improves 11.7% in group 1 vs 1% in group 2 for year 1 and 2; HRA improved 23% in group 1 and 19% in group 2. First year medical costs reduced by 20% in group 1 or $164 average decrease vs combined increase of $15 in groups 2 and 3. Full program cost (group 1) was $30/person/yr.
Absenteeism (reported sick days). Intervention was a series of behavior change classes repeated 4 times over 2 yr.	Randomly assigned 32 worksites. Both cohort and cross-sectional analysis.	No	Absenteeism decreased 4.5% in the intervention by cohort and 3.5% by cross-sectional analysis. Smoking was associated with sick days but weight loss program was not. Authors conclude that savings are accrued due to reduced absenteeism
Doctor visits, hospitalization, and reported injuries. A "low" intensity program of access to health resource center and self-care booklet; "medium" with classes and team for group support; and "high" with all of the above plus environmental improvements and targeted high risk participants.	Longitudinal pre-post design	Yes	Only the "high-intensity" group showed declines in doctor visits, hospitalizations, and injuries. Both high- and medium-intensity groups showed declines in sick days. Cost-effectiveness is inferred but not analyzed.
Overall, 77% or 205 of the targeted employees participated for 1 yr. Classes consisted of an HRA, education classes, training, physical fitness and ergonomics improvement.	Six divisions randomized into 4 interventions and 2 controls. Pre-post analysis on HRA and back disability claims.	No	Modest reduction in intervention sites in back pain, significant increase in employee satisfaction and reduction in risky behavior. Net benefit of $161,108 and ROI of 179%.
Two worksite sessions on "responsible drinking" given to small groups of workers in 5 organizations in both private and public sectors	Pre-post based on cycles of written reports/memos with surveys	Yes	Alcohol health promotion in the worksite is complex but feasible. Cost-effectiveness considered but not analyzed.
CHD risks and per employee program costs in 4 interventions: (1) A: control; (2) B: staffed fitness facility; (3) C: outreach and individual counseling; and, (4) D: counseling outreach, plus organized activity at work	Pre- and postlongitudinal design	No	Sites A and C increased exercise; site B decreased; more employees with CVD exercised 3 or more times/week in C and D than other sites. Site B gained an average of 2.5 lb and hypertensive patients under control decreased. Sites C and D had most impact. Per employee costs in B, C, and D were $39.28, $30.96, and $33.57. Least expensive programs (C and D) were most effective.
Worksite program of: (1) HRAs; (2) coordinators; (3) on-site classes; (4) environmental changes such as smoking policy and cafeteria; and (5) recognition. Effects on 7 behavioral risks and self-reported illness days.	Pre- and postintervention group with 2-yr follow-up and a time lagged, nonequivalent comparison group	No	Number and level of behavioral risk factors improved over 2 yr in the intervention. Employees with 3 or more risk factors decreased by 14% and self-reported illness decreased by 12%. Risk levels most improved (4.5% to 79%) for 6 or 7 factors among high-risk individuals. Reduction in illness days may imply cost-effectiveness but not analyzed.

Cost-Effectiveness Grid (continued)

Study	Purpose of Evaluation	Sample Size	Types of Workers	Comparison Group	Evaluation Period
Utility company (1993)[55]	Determine health and cost outcomes of a worksite health promotion program on medical costs	1188	All	Yes	1 yr
BlueCross/Blue Shield of Indiana (1993)[56]	Determine whether employee participation in a comprehensive worksite health promotion program was associated with reduced employee medical care costs	743 men and women	All	No	7 yr
City of Mesa, Arizona (1994)[57]	Assess the impact of a mobile, comprehensive worksite health promotion program on medical costs	1325	All	Yes (340 age and and sex matched)	2 yr
Johnson & Johnson (1994)[58]	Analyze the incremental effectiveness of a blood pressure control program entitled "IMPACT"	80 (in 5 sites in California, Florida, Georgia, and Texas)	All	Yes (79 controls)	1 yr
Chicago Companies (1994)[59]	Examine data collected 2 yr after the onset of a medical worksite smoking intervention program in 38 Chicago companies	38 companies	All	Yes	2 yr
Cal PERS (1994)[60]	Cost reduction of a mail-delivered intervention (Healthtrac) delivered to California retirees	54,902	All	Yes	1 yr
First Chicago Bank (1994)[61]	Analyze the medical and disability costs of depressive disorders within a comprehensive, worksite HP/DP program	Varying number of claims per year	All	No	4 yr
Duke University (1994)[62]	Effects of the "Live for Life" program offered to Duke University employees	15,500 (30% participation rate)	All	No	3 yr
Metropolitan Toronto (1994)[63]	Improve detection of hypertension in blue-collar workers	7856 (545 with blood pressure >90–114) mg Hg	Blue collar	No	At 40 days and at 1 yr
Johnson & Johnson (1995)[64]	Evaluate effectiveness of a deliberately designed low-cost, worksite cholesterol reduction program (IMPACT)	4 worksites	All	Yes	1 yr
Small worksites (42) in Colorado, Minnesota, Missouri, and Washington (1995)[65]	Study conducted by the Centers for Disease Control and Prevention (CDC) to determine health and cost outcomes of a worksite nutritional program after cholesterol screening	42 worksites	All	Yes	6 and 12 mo

Intervention and Outcome Measures	Evaluation Design	Subject Self-Selection	Findings
4 different health promotion programs of different levels of intensity; focus on behavior change workshops of risk factors	Pre- and post intervention	No	Strong association between intervention and reduction in medical costs, hospital days, based on cost estimates. With increasing intensity there was increased benefit from $145/person in group 1 to $421/person in group 4. Cost/benefit analysis indicated that "medium" intensity of group 3 had greatest level of cost reduction per dollar expended.
4 independent study groups (2 intervention, 2 controls) engaged the BC/BS program with 2 yr of preprogram medical cost data and 5 yr of postprogram data	Pre- and post longitudinal design with 2 interventions and 2 controls. Pre- and post employee medical care costs.	No	Program participation was not associated with reduced medical costs.
Participant vs control group medical costs based on data from their carrier, CIGNA Healthplan	Participant and medical costs 2 yr before and 2 yr after the program	Yes	Medical costs decreased in both groups, with 16% for the intervention and 7% for controls. Specific reduction in general sickness, outpatient and inpatient claims, and total claims. No change in psychologic, substance abuse, or emergency care. Benefit/cost ratio of $1:$3.6.
Pre- and post blood pressures adjusted for age, sex, and baseline blood pressures. Low-intensity and low-cost intervention of monthly, 10-minute counseling sessions at work, monthly mailings, and incentives.	Pre- and post	No	Intervention designed to be low impact and low cost and to determine health efficacy before proceeding to cost analysis. Data consistent with cost-effectiveness but not analyzed in this study.
Workers randomized to 2 groups with both receiving self-help manuals and a 20-day TV series over 3 wk. In addition, 1 group received 6 classes and social support over 12 mo.	Pre- and post	No	24 mo after pretest, 30% of the participants in the full program had quit vs 19.5%. A program that demonstrates significant differences at 2 yr after the initial intervention, appears to be cost-effective.
A randomized control trial with periodic risk assessments, doctor visits, hospital days, sick days, and claims data from Blue Shield of California. Participants were Cal PERS (21,170), non-Medicare eligible (8316), and Medical Supplement (25,416).	Pre- and post randomized, quasi-experimental design	No	Reduced HRA scores, reduced self-report of medical use, and decrease in claims relative to controls. Annual claim costs were in the range of $3.2 to $8 million less than expected.
Introduction of EAP in 1985 and tracked annually up to 1989 for changes in number of depressive diagnoses and number of days per event	Quasi-experimental, longitudinal	Yes	Depressive disorders accounted for the largest medical plan costs of all behavioral diagnoses with greatest length of disability and relapse. Higher prevalence in women. Significant reductions in depressive events and costs after introduction of the EAP.
Voluntary, free program with HRA, smoking, weight, stress, nutrition, fitness, and blood pressure components	Longitudinal with absenteeism as the primary outcome	Yes	Absenteeism increased for participants and nonparticipants from 9.4 hr to 13.5 hr over 3 yr. Participants less than nonparticipants with an average of 4.6 fewer absentee hours. Cost-effectiveness inferred but not analyzed.
After screening, employees randomized to a physician for usual care (1 stage) or scheduled for another screening in 2 wk (2 stage)	Randomized trial to determine cost-effectiveness of one-stage vs. two-stage blood pressure screening at the worksite.	Yes	Blood pressure declined in both groups by 8.5 mg/Hg after 1 yr. Cost-effectiveness of the two groups did not differ significantly. One-stage screening is preferred and appears more cost-effective.
After screening, 127 randomized into IMPACT (information and counseling) and 125 to regular screening and referral	Randomized, control trials. At 1 yr, 118 in IMPACT and 116 controls for follow-up evaluation.	No	IMPACT had 16.6 mg/dl decline vs 10 mg/dl in controls. Difference not significant at the .05 level because of small group size. Cost-effectiveness of this low-cost intervention inferred but not analyzed.
After cholesterol screening, 42 worksites randomized into "usual" intervention of 5 min of counseling vs "special" of a 2-hr behavior change class in nutrition	Randomized, control trial. Cholesterol and medical cost at 6 and 12 mo.	No	Total cost was $50/person/yr. Cholesterol unchanged at 6 mo. At 12 mo, "special" intervention had 6.5% drop vs 3.0% in "usual" group. Concluded that "low-cost" nutrition program is effective in reducing cholesterol. Cost-effectiveness discussed but not analyzed.

Australia. It was a worksite cholesterol reduction intervention based on dietary interventions in a randomized, controlled trial. Cholesterol reduction was not achieved, and this failure was attributed to poor ongoing participation rates by the hospital's employees.[37] A second study reported in 1995 entitled "Take Heart" evaluated the short-term effects of a low-intensity worksite heart disease risk reduction program using a matched pair design with the worksite as the unit of analysis. Twenty-six heterogeneous worksites of between 125 and 750 employees per site were randomized into early or delayed interventions. After 18 months, no improvements in risk beyond the secular trends were observed in the control sites.[37] Because neither study demonstrated health outcomes, the issue of cost-effectiveness is moot. Although many possible reasons why these two interventions did not demonstrate effects exist, it is evident in reading the description of the actual interventions that they were quite limited in their intervention sophistication given the effectiveness of similar interventions. They failed to address issues of motivation and compliance, and with an intervention of such minimal intensity these were predictable failures.

The usual litany of why such studies fail and/or do not demonstrate cost-effectiveness has been studied.[37] Not only have these previous reviews[4] fully acknowledged such limitations, but these methodologic limitations are applicable to most, if not all, areas of research whether conducted in the worksite or not. Many studies do suffer from methodologic and practical limitations. In reporting the results of the "Take Heart" in-

tervention, the researchers observed that many interventions have been tested by evaluating only employees who self-select to participate in programs, and participation rates are often low. Only rarely is the effect of the intervention assessed in terms of change among all employees. Another problem is that studies comparing treatment and control worksites often include only two or, at most, a few sites. Even when sites are randomly assigned to condition, evaluation designs typically do not permit use of the worksite, as opposed to employees, as the unit of analysis. Another supposed limitation of many worksite studies is the reliance on intensive, highly structured, and expensive interventions delivered by highly trained research staff, a set of conditions that may be difficult to replicate. Another cited limitation is the difficulty in differentiating intervention effects from other variables, such as secular trends, other contextual factors including state or local health policy changes such as indoor air acts, and medical insurance. Finally, many worksite interventions are relatively short and do not address the challenge of how to support long-term maintenance of employee behavior change. To some degree this frequently recanted, rote litany is applicable to all research and surely applies to worksite evaluations of other programs. Although the previous reviews of this literature have fully acknowledged these limitations and more, they have been misinterpreted as an uncritical advocacy of worksite health promotion and disease prevention programs.[38] For the record, that is not the case. It remains accurate, however, that despite the limitations most of the research to date

does (1) indicate favorable health and cost outcomes; (2) more recent and more rigorously designed research tends to support rather than refute earlier and less rigorously designed studies;[39–41] and (3) rather than interpreting the methodologic flaws and diversity as presumptively negative, it is equally indicative of a robust phenomena evident in many types of worksites, with diverse employees, different interventions, and varying degrees of methodologic sophistication.[42–44] In any case, even the most rigorous methodology cannot compensate for predictably, unsophisticated interventions that do not take into account more than 15 years of increasingly multifactorial, effective interventions.

Given "business as usual" in the U. S. Congress, which translates into a virtual paralysis except in matters of re-election, raising their own salaries, and dismantling the policies of the previous administration, it is important to note that these national trends are due predominantly to private initiatives by major insurers, large corporations, coalitions of insurers and corporations, a few hints of state government innovation, and literally nothing out of Washington, D.C. No one is waiting breathlessly for Congress to act. It is precisely because national and state health care reform is being determined by the private sector that the particular studies cited in this article and the previous two in this series are so important. Their outcomes represent documented, viable, ongoing, replicable, and demonstrably effective managed care programs delivered to hundreds of thousands, and collectively to millions, of active employees, dependents, and retirees. Collectively, these projects represent positive models of the future of managed care and responsible demand management. Surely, many unanswered questions and issues remain, particularly regarding the persistent plight of the disadvantaged, racial and ethnic minorities, disabled, and the growing elderly population where prevention strategies are even less well developed or tested. Most important, as Dr. Steven A. Schroeder, president of the Robert Wood Johnson Foundation, has pointed out, "The shift from fee-for-service practice to the many variants of managed care will undoubtedly increase the prevalence of implicit rationing by queue and other administrative means. In addition, the continuing pressure to reduce Medicare expenditures may erode the current high level of medical care received by the elderly in the United States. For now, we must recognize that rationing already occurs in the United States, although less systematically than in other countries, and certainly much less frequently among the elderly."[45] Through the prudent and effective use of demand management, a major objective is to reduce the excessive demands and expenditures inherent in late-stage disease interventions through early detection and free up crisis intervention for all who truly need such measures.

References

1. Rosenbluth JM. *Integrated delivery systems: the battle among prayers, hospitals, and physicians.* San Francisco: Volpe, Welty & Company, March 3, 1995.
2. Stokols D, Pelletier KR, Fieldings JE. Integration of medical care and worksite health promotion. *JAMA* 1995;273:1136–42.
3. Miller RH, Luft HS. Managed care plan performanced since 1980: a literature analysis. *JAMA* 1994;271:1512–9.
4. Pelletier KR. A review and analysis of the health and cost-effective outcome studies of comprehensive health promotion and disease prevention programs at the worksite: 1991–1993 update. *Am J Health Promot* 1993;8:50–62.
5. Chapman LS. *Proof positive: an analysis of the cost-effectiveness of wellness.* 2nd ed. Seattle: Corporate Health Designs, 1995.
6. Kahn KL, Keeler EB, Sherwood MJ, et al. Comparing outcomes of care before and after implementation of the DRG-based prospective payment systems. *JAMA* 1990;264:1984–8.
7. Terborg JR, Glasgow RE. Worksite interventions: a brief review of health promotion programs at work. In: Baum A, McManus C, Newman S, Weinman J, West R, eds. *Cambridge handbook of psychology, health and medicine.* London, England:1992.
8. Naditch MP, Matarazzo JD, Weiss SM, Herd JA, Miller NE, eds. *Behavioral health: a handbook of health promotion and disease prevention.* New York, Plenum, 1984.
9. Abrams DB. Cancer control at the workplace: the working well trail. *Prev Med* 1994;23:15–27.
10. Hunt MK, Hebert JR, Sorensen G, et al. Impact of a worksite cancer prevention program on eating patterns of workers. *Ann Behav Med* 1993;25:236–44.
11. Fielding JE, Cumberland WG, Pettitt L. Immunization status of children of employees in a large corporation. *JAMA* 1994;271:525–9
12. Shephard RJ. Exercise and reduced health-care costs: a substantial dividend of primary preventive programs? *J Cardiopulmonary Rehabil* 1994;14:161–5.
13. Tengs TO, Adams ME, Pliskin JS, Safran DG, Siegel JE, Weinstein MC, et al. *Five hundred life saving interventions and their cost effectiveness.* Duke University (Preprint), July 25, 1994.
14. Woo B, Cook EF, Weisberg M, Goldman L. Screening procedures in the asymptomatic adult: comparison of physicians' recommendations, patients' desires, published guidelines and actual practice. *JAMA* 1985;254:1480–4.
15. US Preventive Services Task Force. *Guide to clinical preventive services: an assessment of 169 interventions: report of the US preventive services task force.* Baltimore: Williams & Wilkins, 1989.
16. Effectiveness in disease and injury prevention: comprehensive delivery of adult vaccination: Minnesota. 1986–1992. *MMWR Morbid Mortal Wkly Rep* 1993;42:768–9.
17. Newhouse JP. *Free for all: lessons from the Rand Health Insurance Experiment.* Cambridge Mass: Harvard University Press, 1993:45–7.
18. McKinlay JB, McKinlay SM. The questionable contribution of medical measures to the decline of mortality in the United States in the twentieth century. In: William SJ, ed. *Issues in health services.* New York: John Wiley & Sons, 1980:3–16.
19. Lewis CE. Disease prevention and health promotion practices of primary care physicians in the United States. *Am J Prev Med* 1988;4(suppl):9–16.
20. Axene DV, Doyle RL, Milliman & Robertson Inc. Analysis of medically unnecessary inpatient services. July 1994.
21. Gurwitz JH. Suboptimal medication use in the elderly: the tip of the iceberg. *JAMA* 1994;272:316–7.
22. Black WC, Welch GH. Advances in diagnostic imaging and overestimations of disease prevalence and the benefits of therapy. *N Engl J Med* 1993;328:1237–43.
23. Berstein SJ, Bernstein SJ, McGlynn EA, Siv AL, Roth CP, Sherwood MJ, Keesey JW, et al. The appropriateness of hysterectomy: a comparison of care in seven health plans. *JAMA* 1993;269:2398–402.
24. Graboys TB, Biegelsen B, Lampert S, et al. Half of all angiographies are unnecessary. *JAMA* 1992;268:2537–40.
25. Rubenstein LV, Kahn KL, Reinisch E, et al. Changes in quality of care for five diseases measured by implicit review, 1981 to 1986. *JAMA* 1990;264:1974–9.
26. Goetzel R, Thorpe K, Fielding J, Pelletier K. Behind the scenes of a POS program. *J Health Care Benefits* 1992;March/April:33–7.
27. Fielding JE, Rice T. Can managed competition solve the problems of market failure? *Health Affairs* 1993;(suppl):216–28.
28. Navarro F. Accounting for physician labor hours: the role of patient health care attitudes and behaviors in shaping demand. *Managed Care Issues/Trends* 1995;March:1–4.
29. Navarro F. Managing capitated populations: the role of health care attitudes and behaviors in predicting and managing risk. *Managed Care Issues/Trends* 1995;April:1–4.
30. Fries J, Harrington H, Edwards R, Richardson N. Randomized controlled trial of cost reductions from a health education program: the California Public Employees' Retirement System (PERS) study. *Am J Health Promot* 1994;8:216–23.
31. Fries J, Bloch D, Harrington H, Richardson N, Beck R. Two-year results of a randomized controlled trial of a health promotion program in a retiree population. *Am J Med* 1993;94:455–62.
32. Lorig K, Mazonson P, Holman H. Evidence suggesting that health education for self-management in patients with chronic arthritis has sustained health benefits while reducing health care costs. *Arthritis Rheum* 1993;36:439–46.
33. How markets evolve. *Hospitals Health Networks,* 1995;April 15:10.
34. Kingery PM, Ellsworth CG, Corbett BS, Bowden RG, Brizzolara JA. High-cost analysis: a closer look at the case for worksite-site health promotion. *J Occup Med* 1994;36:1341–7.

35. Lovato CY, Green LW, Stainbrook GL. *Benefits anticipated by industry in supporting health promotion programs in the worksite.* Champaign, Illinois: Human Kinetics Publishers, 1994, 3–31.

36. Barratt A, Reznick R, Irwig L, Cuff A, Simpson JM, Oldenburg B, et al. Worksite cholesterol screening and dietary intervention: the staff healthy heart project. *Am J Public Health* 1994;84:779–81.

37. Glasgow RE, Tefborg JR, Hollis JF, Severson HH, Boler SM. Take heart: results from the initial phase of a work-site wellness program. *Am J Health Promot* 1995;8:209–16.

38. Glasgow RE, McCaul KD, Fisher, KJ. Participation in worksite health promotion: a critique of the literature and recommendations for future practice. *Health Educ Q* 1991;20:391–408.

39. Erfurt JC, Foote A, Heirich MA. Worksite wellness programs: incremental comparison of screening and referral along, health education, follow-up counseling, and plant organization. *Am J Health Promot* 1991;5:438–48.

40. Henritze J, Brammell H, Phase II cardiac wellness at the Adolph Coors Company. *Am J Health Promot* 1989;4:25–31.

41. Jeffery RW, Forster JL, French SA, et al. The healthy worker project: a worksite intervention for weight control and smoking cessation. *Am J Health Promot* 1993;8:395–401.

42. Harvey MR, Whitmen RW, Hilyer JC, Brown KC. The impact of a comprehensive medical benefits cost management program for the city of Birmingham: results at five years. *Am J Health Promot* 1993;7:296–303.

43. Emont SL, Choi WS, Novotny TE, Giovino GA. Clean indoor air legislation, taxation, and smoking behavior in the United States: an ecological analysis. *Tobacco Control* 1991;2:13–7

44. Biglan A, Glasgow RE. The social unit: an important facet in the design of cancer control research. *Prev Med* 1991;20:292–305.

45. Schroeder SA. Rationing medical care: a comparative perspective. *N Engl J Med* 1994;331:1089–91.

46. Wheat JR, Graney MJ, Schachtman RH, Ginn GL, Patrick DL, Hulka BS. Does workplace health promotion decrease medical claims? *Am J Prev Med* 1982;8:110–4.

47. Golaszewski T, Snow D, Lynch W, Yen L, Solomita D, Fries JF, et al. A benefit-to-cost analysis of a worksite health promotion program. *J Occup Med* 1992;34:1164–72.

48. Fries JF, Bloch DA, Harnington H, Richardson N, Beck R. Two-year results of a randomized controlled trial of a health promotion program in a retiree population: the Bank of America study. *Am J Med* 1993;94:455–62.

49. Jeffery RW, Forster JL, Dunn BV, French SA, McGovern PG, Lando HA. Effects of worksite health promotion on illness related absenteeism. *J Occup Med* 1993;35:1142–6.

50. Shi L. Worksite health promotion and changes in medical care use and sick days. *J Health Behav Educ Promot* 1993;17:9–17.

51. Shi L. A cost-benefit analysis of a California county's back injury prevention program. *Public Health Rep* 1993;108:204.

52. Towers AM, Kishchuk N, Sylvestre M, Peters C, Bourgault C. A qualitative investigation of organizational issues in an alcohol awareness program for blue-collar workers. *Am J Health Promot* 1994;9:56–64.

53. Heirich MA, Foote A, Erfurt JC, Konopka B. Worksite physical fitness programs: comparing the impact of different program designs on cardiovascular risks. *J Occup Med* 1993;35:510–7.

54. Bertera RL. Behavioral risk factor and illness day changes with workplace health promotion: two-year results. *Am J Health Promot* 1993;7:365–72.

55. Shi L. Health promotion, medical care use, and costs in a sample of worksite employees. *Eval Rev* 1993;12:475–87.

56. Sciacca J, Seehafer R, Reed R, Mulvaney D. The impact of participation in health promotion on medical costs: a reconsideration of the Blue Cross and Blue Shield of Indiana Study. *Am J Health Promot* 1993;7:374–84

57. Aldana SG, Jacobson BH, Harris CJ, Kelley PL, Stone WJ. Influence of a mobile worksite health promotion program on health care costs. *Am J Prev Med* 1994;9:378–82.

58. Fielding JE, Knight K, Mason T, Klesges RC, Pelletier KR. Evaluation of the IMPACT Blood Pressure Program. *J Occup Med* 1994;36:743–6.

59. Salina D, Jason LA, Heckker D, Kaufman J, Lesondak L, McMahon SD, et al. A follow-up of a media-based, worksite smoking cessation program. *Am J Commun Psychol* 1994;22:257–61.

60. Fries JF, Harrington H, Edwards R, Kent LA, Richardson N. Randomized controlled trial of cost reductions from a health education program: the California Public Employees' Retirement System (PERS) study. *Am J Health Promot* 1994;8:xxx–x.

61. Conti DJ, Burton WN. The economic impact of depression in a workplace. *J Occup Med* 1994;36:981–3.

62. Knight KK, Goetzel RZ, Fielding JE. An evaluation of Duke University's Live for Life health promotion program on changes in worker absenteeism. *J Occup Med* 1994;36:533–6.

63. Edward E, Koblin W, Irvine JM, Legare J, Logan AG. Small, blue collar work site hypertension screening: a cost effectiveness study. *J Occup Med* 1994;36:346–55.

64. Fielding JE, Mason T, Knight K, Klesges R, Pelletier KR. A randomized trial of the IMPACT Worksite Cholesterol Reduction Program. *Am J Prev Med* 1995;11:120–3.

65. Byers T, Mullis R, Anderson J, Dusenbury L, Gorsky R, Kimber C, et al. The cost and effects of a nutritional education program following work-site cholesterol screening. *Am J Public Health* 1995;85:650–5.

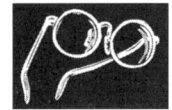 **Article Review Form at end of book.**

What are the two primary types of employee assistance programs (EAPs)? What are the benefits of each type of EAP?

Costs of Employee Assistance Programs:

Findings from a National Survey

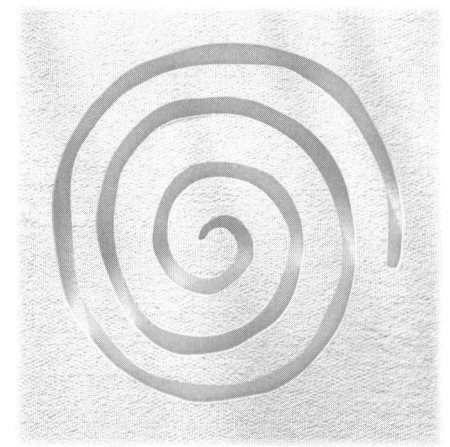

**Michael T. French,
Gary A. Zarkin, Jeremy W. Bray,
and Tyler D. Hartwell**

Michael T. French, PhD, University of Miami. Gary A. Zarkin, PhD, Jeremy W. Bray, MA, Tyler D. Hartwell, PhD, Research Triangle Institute, Research Triangle Park, North Carolina.

Purpose

Partly in reaction to heavy alcohol use and illicit drug use by some workers,[1,2] many employers have created employee assistance programs (EAPs) to address the variety of problems posed by substance use. Although the initial impetus for establishing EAPs often comes from the need to deal with substance-abuse problems, the mission of EAPs has grown much larger and now encompasses a much broader range of employee problems.[3]

Numerous studies[3,4] have examined the EAP process in terms of service delivery and core technologies. This literature provides a rich understanding of the types of workers who obtain help from EAPs and the range of problems addressed.[5,6] However, few studies[3,7–10] have evaluated the costs and effectiveness of EAPs. In particular, no study has estimated the per-employee annual cost of operating an EAP across a large number of worksites drawn from a national probability sample. Using data from a nationally representative survey of EAPs, this article presents findings on the annual cost per eligible employee for EAP services by type of EAP, worksite characteristics, and other factors.

Methods

Design

The National Survey of Worksites and Employee Assistance Programs (NSWEAP) was conducted by the Research Triangle Institute between October 1992 and March 1993.[11] A stratified random sample was used, and data were collected through a computer-assisted telephone interview protocol. To ensure that the findings would be comparable to earlier worksite surveys,[12,13] the study was designed with a similar target population and sample stratification.

Sample

The target population consisted of all private non-agricultural worksites in the United States with 50 or more full-time employees. The sampling frame was constructed by using the Dun's Market Identifiers database from Dun's Marketing Services. A worksite is defined as any business location with a unique, separate, and distinct operation, including headquarters units within an enterprise. The sampling frame included approximately 421,000 worksites and the final stratified sample contained 6488 worksites, of which 3204 were eligible responding worksites. Sampling weights were computed on the basis of the selection probability of the worksite within the sampling stratum and adjusted to

Reprinted by permission from *American Journal of Health Promotion*, January/February 1997 (Vol. 11, No. 3), pp. 219–222.

compensate for nonresponse. Detailed information on the sampling frame, the stratification scheme, and the development of the sampling weights can be found in the study by Boyle et al.[14]

Measurement

The introductory section of the survey instrument confirmed that the correct worksite was contacted and the worksite was eligible to participate in the survey. The typical respondent at each worksite was the director of human resources and/or the EAP director for internal EAPs. If the worksite had an active EAP, then 130 questions were administered on worksite demographics, EAP characteristics, EAP services provided, EAP costs, and employee benefits. For worksites without an EAP, only information on worksite demographics and employee benefits was collected.

Analysis

Two primary types of AP settings or models exist: internal and external. Internal EAPs are typically staffed by company employees and located at the worksite or a short distance away. External EAPs provide services to worksite employees on a contract basis, and their offices are typically located away from company property. Given these operational differences between internal and external EAPs, the two models were distinguished throughout the descriptive analysis.

Because worksite size varies widely in the United States, the annual cost *per eligible employee* was analyzed.[1] This variable was calculated from data on the total annual cost of the EAP and the number of eligible employees. Eligible employees were defined as all employees eligible for EAP services at all worksites served by the EAP. Relative to total cost estimates, analyzing the cost per eligible employee is a better way to compare EAPs of varying sizes.

The relationships between per-employee EAP cost and worksite characteristics such as firm size, geographic region, and industry were examined. All statistics are weighted population estimates, which account for complex sampling designs when variance estimates are computed.[15]

Results

The survey interviewers contacted 3204 eligible responding worksites and obtained an overall response rate of 90%. Financial data were collected from 878 responding worksites.

EAP Prevalence and Service Provision

It is estimated that 53,500 worksites nationwide with 50 or more full-time employees (i.e., 33%) have an EAP. Of the worksites with an EAP, 16.7% have an internal EAP, 81.1% have an external EAP, and 2.6% have both an internal and an external EAP.[2] Because the NSWEAP instrument lists only one cost figure per worksite, it was impossible to determine if the cost reported for worksites with multiple EAPs applied to their internal or their external EAP. For this reason, worksites with both an internal and an external EAP were excluded from the cost analysis.

EAP costs are presumably related to program services. Table 1 presents a summary of the services that are usually provided by internal and external EAPs. For every service listed except short-term counseling, internal EAPs were more likely to offer the service than external EAPs. The last row of Table 1 reports the average number of services provided by each type of EAP. It is clear that internal EAPs offer significantly more services than external EAPs, on average.

EAP Cost

The survey data showed that a few worksites reported a per-employee annual cost of $0 for either an internal or external EAP, and some worksites reported a per employee annual EAP cost that was implausibly high (e.g., $200 per employee) on the basis of case studies of existing programs and expert opinion.[8] These outliers are probably coding mistakes or gross miscalculations by respondents. Rather than performing a rigorous outlier analysis on the full data set, we defined an outlier criterion and observations that failed this test were deleted. Specifically, any observation that reported per-employee costs below $1 or above $150 per year was deleted from the cost analysis file. A total of 31 observations from the original sample failed this outlier test and were removed from the cost analyses.

Table 2 shows that the mean EAP cost per eligible employee was $26.59 for internal EAPs and $21.47 for external EAPs. The median values were about 18% lower, $21.84 for internal EAPs and $18.09 for external programs.[3] While these data indicate that internal EAPs are generally more costly than external EAPs, part of the differential is probably caused by differences in service provision. Indeed, as shown in Table 1, internal EAPs in the sample offer 1.5 more services than external EAPs, on average.

The results in Table 2 show that median internal EAP cost displays a U-shaped relationship with the size of the worksite: the median EAP cost initially decreases as firm size increases, but eventually increases slightly for larger firms. With regard to differences across EAP types, the median cost is similar for internal and external EAPs in all size categories except those firms with more than 1000 employees.

The range across industries in median internal EAP cost is considerable, with a low of $11.72 for manufacturing and a high of $37.20 for mining and construction. With the exception of wholesale and retail trade, external EAPs display a much smaller range in EAP cost across industries.

For internal EAPs, the regional differences in median cost range from a low of $15.74 in the West to a high of $28.44 in the Northeast. For external EAPs, regional differences in median cost are small.

The last part of Table 2 reports the mean and median cost per eligible employee for EAPs that offer a particular service compared to EAPs that do not offer that service. No significant differences were found between EAPs that offer a specific service and those that do not. Furthermore, no consistent pattern is evident in the differences in the median cost estimates. For example, external EAPs that provide consultation with supervisors have a higher median cost than those that do not provide this service, but the opposite is true for internal EAPs. Both internal and external EAPs that provide short-term counseling have higher costs than those that do not. Also, both internal and external EAPs that provide assessment and referral have lower costs than those that do not. While the service-related findings are informative, it is important to remember that these

Table I	National Estimates of EAP Service Provision by Type of EAP		
Services Usually Provided by the EAP		**Internal**	**External**
Consultation with supervisors*		87.84% (2.93)	58.19% (2.74)
Participation in constructive confrontations with employees*		62.50 (5.03)	29.58 (2.78)
Short-term counseling*		75.61 (4.52)	90.77 (1.73)
Assessment and referral		92.06 (2.83)	90.35 (1.82)
Contact providers to determine progress of EAP clients in treatment		77.19 (4.78)	74.57 (2.86)
Contact supervisors to determine success of clients after treatment*		64.69 (4.90)	39.80 (3.15)
Involvement in health promotion activities*		67.77 (4.94)	36.09 (2.77)
Average number of services provided†		5.22 (0.12)	3.74 (0.09)

Note: Data are weighted to reflect population statistics. Standard errors are shown in parentheses.

*Significant differences between internal and external EAP distributions at the 0.01 level based on a x^2 test.

†Significant differences between internal and external EAPs at the 0.01 level based on a t-test.

bivariate descriptive cross tabulations do not control for the potentially confounding effects of providing multiple services.

Discussion
Summary and Interpretation of Results

This study represents the first attempt to generate national estimates of EAP costs. On the basis of data from a 1992–1993 national survey of worksites, the estimated mean cost per eligible employee for internal EAPs was $26.59; the median was $21.84. Within internal EAPs the cost estimates were U-shaped in moving from smaller to larger worksites, and variation was moderate to high on the basis of industry and region. The estimated mean cost per employee for external EAPs was $21.47, with the median $18.09. Within external EAPs the cost estimates were fairly stable

across most factors with the exception of primary industry. In a comparison of EAP types, the median costs of internal and external EAPs were significantly different across a wide range of worksite characteristics: internal EAPs were generally more expensive. As noted earlier, most of the cost differentials can probably be attributed to greater service provision by internal EAPs.

Significance

The findings have at least two important uses. First, EAP coverage among worksites is growing rapidly, but many firms have yet to implement such programs. In recent analyses, Hartwell et al.[11] found that 9% of those worksites without an EAP were seriously considering starting a program in the next year. The cost estimates presented in this article can serve as guidelines for the range of costs that firms can anticipate as

Table 2
Annual EAP Cost Per Eligible Employee by Worksite Characteristics, EAP Services, and Type of EAP

	Internal EAPs		External EAPs		Unweighted
	Mean	Median	Mean	Median	N
All Worksites[†]	$26.59 (2.22)	$21.84	$21.47 (1.31)	$18.09	878
Worksite Characteristics					
Number of Employees					
50–99	$28.01 (7.38)	$21.30	$24.32 (4.33)	$18.16	116
100–249	$22.78 (3.80)	$19.94	$19.21 (1.24)	$18.01	236
250–999	$25.63 (3.65)	$19.98	$22.52 (1.70)	$17.99	308
> 1000[‡]	$32.04 (3.48)	$29.37	$20.56 (1.79)	$16.95	218
Industry					
Manufacturing	$22.01 (5.22)	$11.72	$21.24 (1.53)	$17.23	184
Wholesale/Retail Trade	$21.36 (5.77)	$25.77	$15.69 (1.95)	$7.95	121
Communications/Utilities/Transportation	$28.77 (5.10)	$21.91	$26.51 (2.63)	$21.28	176
Financial/Real Estate/					
Insurance	$19.40 (2.26)	$16.70	$19.22 (1.35)	$17.28	163
Mining/Construction[‡]	$49.64 (10.47)	$37.20	$26.53 (3.21)	$20.90	77
Services	$31.38 (3.72)	$24.50	$26.71 (5.54)	$20.30	157
Region					
Northeast[†]	$31.84 (3.67)	$28.44	$21.02 (1.99)	$19.33	185
Midwest	$26.28 (5.04)	$21.75	$20.42 (1.55)	$17.75	218
South[†]	$24.51 (3.05)	$19.98	$18.36 (1.33)	$15.73	308
West	$25.10 (6.11)	$15.74	$28.15 (4.72)	$21.17	167
Services Usually Provided by the EAP					
Consultation with supervisors					
Yes	$26.54 (2.49)	$21.75	$22.16 (1.23)	$19.97	509
No	$27.03 (3.03)	$24.97	$22.45 (2.81)	$17.43	331
Participation in constructive confrontations with employees					
Yes	$28.43 (3.43)	$21.74	$22.48 (1.59)	$19.58	331
No	$23.47 (1.94)	$21.32	$22.78 (1.87)	$19.00	495
Short-term counseling					
Yes	$28.11 (2.79)	$22.12	$22.22 (1.43)	$18.74	745
No	$21.97 (2.90)	$19.96	$20.15 (2.83)	$17.30	108
Assessment and referral					
Yes*	$26.30 (2.28)	$21.87	$21.26 (1.44)	$18.09	774
No	$30.50 (8.50)	$23.18	$23.65 (2.53)	$19.42	82
Contact providers to determine progress of EAP clients in treatment					
Yes[†]	$28.45 (2.46)	$23.55	$22.17 (1.25)	$18.91	546
No	$20.06 (4.65)	$11.73	$25.95 (5.67)	$20.12	154
Contact supervisors to determine success of clients after treatment					
Yes	$25.87 (2.84)	$20.85	$22.47 (1.55)	$19.36	354
No	$27.95 (3.65)	$24.85	$22.02 (2.03)	$18.61	455
Involvement in health promotion activities					
Yes*	$27.51 (2.60)	$23.57	$21.32 (1.40)	$18.23	397
No	$24.81 (4.27)	$19.78	$21.97 (2.01)	$18.74	453

Note: Data are weighted to reflect population statistics. Standard deviations are shown in parentheses.

[†]Significant differences between medians for internal and external EAPs at the 0.10 level based on a test by Williams and Perritt[18]

[‡]Significant differences between medians for internal and external EAPs at the 0.05 level based on a test by Williams and Perritt[18]

*Significant differences between medians for internal and external EAPs at the 0.01 level based on a test by Williams and Perritt[18]

they begin to explore EAP options. Second, considerable attention is currently focused on state and federal health care reform and especially on the role of employers. An understanding of the costs associated with EAPs will help policy makers in their efforts to estimate the resources necessary for employment-based health promotion programs.

Limitations

Several limitations of this research should be acknowledged. First, the cost estimates are differentiated by type of EAP, but they are not service specific. Because internal EAPs generally offer a greater number of service components compared to external programs,[16] it is predictable that internal EAPs were somewhat more costly than external EAPs. Second, the self-reported data were collected through a computer-assisted telephone interview. The 90% response rate is certainly commendable, but self-reported data raise questions about content validity. In addition, the telephone survey approach limited the types of questions that could be asked and the depth of the information. Third, a worksite representative (e.g., human resources director) is not always the best person to provide information regarding their external EAP. And last, changes may have occurred in the prevalence and cost of EAPs since these data were collected in 1992 and 1993, which would limit the generalizability to contemporary worksites.

Notes

1. While almost all EAPs provide services for dependents as well as employees, the telephone interviewers were unable to obtain reliable data on the number of dependents covered to estimate the cost *per eligible person.*

2. For a detailed presentation of EAP prevalence findings and other results from the national survey, see references 11, 16, and 17.
3. As suggested by an anonymous reviewer, EAP costs were also estimated with an outlier criterion of less than $10 and greater than $60 per eligible employee. Under this criterion, internal EAPs had a mean (median) cost per eligible employee of $27.57 ($24.93) and external EAPs had a mean (median) cost of $23.92 ($21.23). These results are very similar to those based on the original outlier criterion.

References

1. Kopstein A, Gfroerer J. Drug use patterns and demographics of employed drug users: data from the 1988 household survey. In: Gust SW, Walsh JM, Thomas LB, Crouch DJ, editors. *Drugs in the workplace: research and evaluation data,* Rockville, Maryland: National Institute on Drug Abuse 1990. NIDA Research Monograph 100, vol 2:25–44.
2. Substance Abuse and Mental Health Services Administration (SAMHSA). National household survey on drug abuse: main findings 1991. Rockville, Maryland: Substance Abuse and Mental Health Services Administration, 1993.
3. Normand J, Lempert RO, O'Brien CP, editors. *Under the influence? Drugs and the American work force National Research Council/Institute of Medicine (NCR/IOM).* Washington, DC: National Academy Press, 1994.
4. Roman PM, Blum TC. Drugs, the workplace, and employee-oriented programming. In: Gerstein DR, Harwood HJ, editors. *Treating drug problems,* Institute of Medicine. Washington, DC: National Academy Press. 1992, vol. 2, Committee for the Substance Abuse Coverage Study. pp. 197–244.
5. Blum TC, Martin JK, Roman PM. A research note on EAP prevalence, components and utilization. *Journal of Employee Assistance Research* 1992;1:209–29.
6. Blum TC, Roman PM. A description of clients using employee assistance programs. *Alcohol Health and Research World.* 1992;16:120–8.
7. French MT, Zarkin GA, Bray JW. A methodology for evaluating the costs and benefits of employee

assistance programs. *Journal of Drug Issues* 1995;25:451–70.
8. Bray JW, French MT, Bowland BJ, Dunlap LJ. The cost of employee assistance programs (EAPs): findings from seven case studies. *Employee Assistance Quarterly.* 1996:11.
9. Walsh DC. Employee assistance programs. *Health and Society* 1982;60:492–517.
10. Decker JT, Starrett R, Redhorse J. Evaluating the cost-effectiveness of employee assistance programs. *Social Work* 1986;31:391–3.
11. Hartwell TD, Steele P, French M, Potter FJ, Zarkin GA, Rodman NF. Prevalence, cost, and characteristics of employee assistance programs (EAPs) in the US. *Am J Public Health.* [In press].
12. Bureau of Labor Statistics. Survey of employer anti-drug programs. Report 760, US Government Printing Office, January, 1989.
13. Hayghe H. Anti-drug programs in the workplace: Are they here to stay? *Monthly Labor Review* 1991:(April):26–8.
14. Boyle KE, Potter FJ, Rush M, Snodgrass J. Sample selection and survey methodology for the 1992/1993 national survey of worksites and employee assistance programs. Unpublished manuscript. Research Triangle Park, North Carolina. Research Triangle Institute, 1994.
15. Shah BV, Barnwell BG, Hunt PN, LaVauge LM. SUDAAN user's manual, Release 5.50. Research Triangle Park, North Carolina: Research Triangle Institute. 1991.
16. Potter FJ, Boyle KE, Steele PD, Rush M. Characteristics of employee assistance programs (EAPs) in the US during 1993. Unpublished manuscript. Research Triangle Park, North Carolina. Research Triangle Institute, 1995.
17. Hartwell TD, Steele PD, Rodman NA, French MT. Prevalence and characteristics of alcohol and other drug testing programs in the US *Monthly Labor Review.* [In press].
18. Williams RL, Perritt RL. The weighted median test for finite population samples. Presented at 1986 American Statistical Association Joint Statistical Meetings.

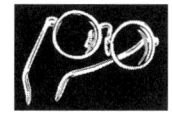

Article Review Form at end of book.

Studies have found links between unemployment and such behaviors as _____. Describe underemployment.

Health and Unemployment

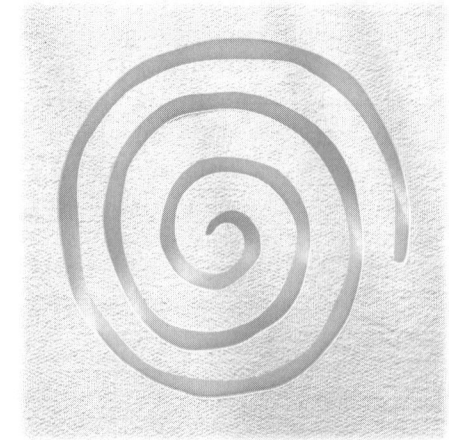

David Dooley[1], Jonathan Fielding[2], and Lennart Levi[3]

[1]School of Social Ecology, University of California, Irvine,
[2]Schools of Public Health and Medicine, University of California, Los Angeles,
[3]Karolinska Institutet, Solna, Sweden

Abstract

This paper reviews the relationship between health and inadequate employment, especially unemployment. Poor physical or mental health can lead, via poor work performance, to job loss; however, studies that control for such selection effects are still scarce except for a few health outcomes. For example, aggregate-level studies typically find a positive association between unemployment and suicide rates over time. At the individual level of analysis, panel surveys of laid-off workers tend to find increased psychiatric problems such as depression and substance abuse. Few studies have evaluated interventions to prevent or reduce the adverse health effects of job loss. There have been even fewer studies of the health effects of other types of inadequate employment such as the increasingly prevalent forms of underemployment.

Introduction

This paper is intended to review the relationship of health and unemployment, and possible initiatives to promote the health of workers who have lost jobs or who experience various kinds of underemployment.

The present restructuring of the world economy has given many American employees reason to fear the loss of their jobs in the next few years. The health consequences of unemployment and resulting special health needs have received little attention.

According to recent OECD analyses, over 33 million people were unemployed in the developed countries in 1993, with an increase to 35 million in 1994 (84, 101). As of August 1995, in the United States, there were 7,457,000 unemployed people (5.6% unemployment rate), down somewhat from a year earlier (104). Unemployment falls unevenly on different population subgroups. Typically, young people and ethnic minorities face the highest rates, with those of black youth being chronically extremely high (103). Data on underemployment are less widely available, in part because of the lack of standardization of the term. One of several categories of underemployment is that of involuntary part-time employment. In June 1994, there were 8.6 million Americans who regarded themselves as full-time workers but who were working less than 35 hours per week for economic or noneconomic reasons (103).

Key Terms
Unemployment

Unemployment may refer either to a community's aggregate unemployment rate or an individual's personal unemployment experience. According to the official measure used in the United States, the unemployment rate is the number of people who have recently been seeking work divided by the number of people who are in the labor force, i.e. either employed or seeking work. Some analysts consider this definition flawed because individuals who want work but who have given up seeking work, the so-called discouraged workers, are not counted as officially unemployed. Sometimes called the "subunemployed," they are grouped in official labor statistics with others such as fulltime students and certain groups of retirees as out of the labor force (OLF). Paradoxically, the official unemployment rate could decrease even in bad times if many job seekers became discouraged. Another unemployment measure, the number of people receiving unemployment compensation, is an even poorer indicator. It underestimates the number of people who are unemployed since not every worker has unemployment insurance and because unemployment insurance runs out after a period of time whether new employment is found or not. Neither of these measures reliably discriminates the unemployed who cannot find work at their preferred wage level (called the reservation wage) from those who can find no work at any wage.

Individual-level personal unemployment may result from losing a job or from entering the workforce but failing to find a job. Job loss usually includes a sequence of stressful events from anticipation of job loss (e.g. after the announcement of plant closure), through the layoff itself, to job search and training and finally, to reemployment. The link between aggregate and personal unemployment is seldom studied but appears to be complex and warrants further research (13). Moreover, the new job found after job loss may well be one of the increasingly common variety termed underemployment.

Health

Just as the presumed stressor of employment status is complex, so the presumed outcome of health has been categorized in a variety of ways: physical health, mental health, and well-being or role functioning. Suspected physical

health responses to unemployment have ranged from self-reported physical illness (61) to mortality, especially suicide (9). Suspected mental health effects of unemployment have included admissions to mental hospitals (7) and incidence of surveyed clinical mental disorders (32).

The category of well-being and role functioning is an umbrella term for other psychosocial outcomes. Well-being includes measures of psychological and psychophysiological or somatic symptoms (e.g. the General Health Questionnaire, or GHQ) (107) that reflect distress short of psychiatric diagnosis. The distinction between a symptom score reflecting subclinical demoralization and a score that meets the criterion for a clinical case (e.g. anxiety disorder) may be only one symptom above an arbitrary cutpoint. However, ordinary symptom counts and the risk of having clinically high symptom levels appear to move together in response to unemployment (33, 62). The other element of this third type of outcome measure, role functioning, includes behaviors that are considered disruptive or antisocial behaviors such as child abuse.

Such different kinds of health outcomes probably involve varying etiologic and pathogenic processes, and some may be strongly influenced by sociocultural factors. Unemployment may also affect some illness processes indirectly by causing loss of health insurance, but this mechanism goes beyond the scope of the present analysis.

Mechanisms

There exist a number of pathways by which a downturn in the economy might produce this variety of potential outcomes (30). One mechanism is a direct effect of ag-

gregate unemployment on people regardless of employment status (13, 81). A downturn in the economy may lead to restructured job routines that bring increased stress (41). Decreased job opportunities may force people to stay in or move to unsatisfying and insecure jobs, at too few hours, at too low wages, or with a too heavy work load ("lean production," or more overtime work).

Most of the unemployment research, at the individual level, has focused on the indirect effect of aggregate unemployment via personal unemployment on the health of the job loser. Personal unemployment is usually viewed as a stressor that involves loss of financial resources and possibly of psychosocial assets such as goal and meaning in life, time structure, status, and social support (57). Whether adverse psychosocial outcomes of unemployment can only be remedied by reemployment is of practical significance because it could guide interventions other than the obvious, i.e. finding and/or creating new jobs—either income maintenance alone or additional assistance targeted at replacing the psychosocial functions of employment. The answer to this question probably varies across social contexts and different types of people. For example, controlling for financial loss, unemployment is more difficult for people with high employment commitment than those with low psychological orientation to work (107). On the other hand, providing a social safety net of unemployment benefits has been credited with reducing the adverse effects of job loss (94).

Although most studies of personal unemployment have limited their assessment of health consequences to the job loser, several studies report social contagion from the job loser to dependents, particularly the spouse (75, 91). Less is known about the social contagion effects on the children of job losers, and virtually nothing is known about the social contagion from underemployment, but the total impact of unemployment surely goes beyond directly affected workers. Finally, a host of variables may moderate the effect of personal unemployment, including both personal characteristics such as coping repertoire, hardiness, social support, education, or ethnicity, and social environmental factors such as the prevailing economic climate in which the unemployed live.

Inferential Problems and Research Design

The varying strength of association in research studies on the health effects of unemployment may be due in part to the instability of the unemployment/health relationship across eras, locales, and types of people. Studies may show no adverse outcomes from unemployment because of a generous social safety net. Some studies actually show improvement following job loss for especially proactive people (45). Different findings may also reflect the variable nature of occupations and work environments. Employment imposes health risks in its own right, including job stress (63, 71, 72), worksite pollution, and occupational accidents (82). Leaving an especially stressful job may bring relief (110). Interventions to return the unemployed to the workplace must balance the potential gains and health risks from reemployment, especially of the underemployment type.

Aggregate-Level Methods

The aggregate method studies the effect of community level unemployment on community level pathology over time, e.g. correlating annual psychiatric admissions with manufacturing employment (7). Such methods risk the ecological fallacy of drawing incorrect individual-level interpretations from aggregate-level data (90). They have also provoked a statistical debate about the proper way to model time series (15, 26, 47).

Individual-Level Methods

Relying on the cross-sectional, individual approach risks the danger of reverse causation (43). In contrast, the various longitudinal, individual or panel approaches avoid such reverse causation by controlling for the health status of people before they experience joblessness. The closing-factory method follows workers beginning when they learn that their plant will close, continuing through their actual layoff and beyond (3, 25, 73, 74). Another panel method surveys a general population over time and thus requires a large initial sample in order to yield enough unemployed people (76). A related method begins with high school students and follows them into the workforce to determine the effects of finding or not finding employment (49, 111). Each of these approaches has found adverse effects of unemployment, but most of these individual-only studies omit the effect of community economic conditions.

Cross-Level Methods

Cross-level studies combine measures of the economic climate with personal economic stressors and health outcomes and thus can explore the direct and moderating effects of the aggregate economy simultaneously with the indirect effect of the economy via the personal unemployment of individuals. There are some indications of both direct effects (33) and interaction effects (27) of the aggregate economy, but other studies have not replicated these effects (32).

Findings on Unemployment and Health

Reviews of the unemployment and health literature are numerous. These include the school-leaver unemployment literature (40, 87, 111) and reviews of unemployment among adults (3, 16, 35, 42, 46, 50, 51, 53, 57, 58, 60, 88, 96, 108). One of the key features of the unemployment literature is the association of research design type with the outcome studied (31). Such low-incidence phenomena as suicide and mental hospitalization have been studied mainly through archival records giving aggregate rates, but these time-series analyses risk the ecological fallacy and controversy about statistical procedure. On the other hand, self-reported symptoms of physical illness or psychological wellbeing are usually studied at the individual level using sample survey questionnaires. The resulting literature has produced only a few areas with numerous replications using similar designs and measures. Because of the risks of type I error and nonpublication of valid nonsignificant results (92), small numbers of studies reporting an adverse effect of unemployment on a health outcome may be considered insufficient evidence on which to base policy decisions. The present paper tries to characterize those subareas of the literature with a substantial body of work rather than noting every health outcome appearing in an unemployment study. However, the relationship between health and unemployment occurs in both directions. That people in mental or physical ill health are at more risk for selection into the ranks of the unemployed has been well documented (43). As just one example, among people who were employed at the first interview of one large-scale epidemiological survey, those who had ever been diagnosed with alcohol disorder were over twice as likely as those not so diagnosed to become unemployed a year later (32). As a result, the best-designed studies of the social costs of unemployment adjust for the confounding effects of preexisting health status.

Physical Health

Most evidence supports the generally assumed negative effects of unemployment on physical and mental health and well-being. In one of the best studies of effects of job loss on biochemical factors, a longitudinal Swedish plant closure study reported evidence for consistent significant increases in cortisol, prolactin, growth hormone, cholesterol, and HDL-cholesterol, and decreased immune reactions (3, 4, 10, 74). However, there have been few efforts to replicate these and other biochemical outcomes. Most individual-level studies rely on self-reported symptoms or events linked to stress associated with job loss or chronic unemployment. One cross-level study found that self-reported incidence of illness or accident was related

indirectly to the aggregate economy via the incidence of personal job and financial life events (19). There have been relatively few studies of specific medical diagnoses or other objective health outcomes, e.g. dyspepsia and joint swelling (59) and corticoid production (99).

Unemployment has been shown to lead to an increase in unhealthy behaviors such as alcohol (32, 48) and tobacco consumption (68), diet, exercise, and other health-related behaviors, which, in turn, might lead to subsequently increased risk for disease or mortality. Unfortunately, there have been rather few replications to establish with confidence the net impact of unemployment on such risk factors, and the effect is likely to be highly moderated. For example, naturally active persons might take advantage of their unemployment to increase their exercise, while their more sedentary counterparts might well decrease their exercise. The literature does offer some aggregate studies correlating unemployment rates with overall (56) and cardiovascular-renal disease mortality (9), infant mortality (8, 22, 112), low birthweight (23), highway fatalities (69), and ischemic heart disease mortality (6, 12). Aside from the small number of their replications, these mortality studies share the problems common to all aggregate-only analyses. Even the interpretation that recession—unless it is extreme, as in the former USSR (93, 100)—causes added mortality is debatable, albeit likely.

Of all of the physical health outcomes, suicide has produced the largest literature, consisting mainly of aggregate time-series studies [see Platt (88) for the most detailed review including parasui-

cide or nonfatal suicide attempts]. By 1986, at least 20 such studies (31) had appeared, most of which came to the conclusion that unemployment and suicide were positively correlated over time. One exception was Pierce's (86) finding that economic change per se (i.e. either up or down, following Durkheim) (39) led to increases in suicide, but that conclusion was challenged on reanalysis (80). Another exception occurred in the United Kingdom where the suicide rate fell while unemployment was rising between 1962 and 1971, but this pattern was attributed to the coincident detoxification of domestic gas during that time period (65). These and other negative findings (34) point up the importance of making interpretations only on the basis of well-designed and replicated studies.

Mental Health and Behavior

As a "life change" event, job loss might be expected to provoke both other kinds of life change events and certain kinds of mental health disorders such as adjustment disorder. Some early research measured the association between recently experienced unemployment and other types of life events of the kind included on such scales as the social readjustment rating scale of Holmes & Rahe (52). In one such study, elevated unemployment rates in the community were associated with elevated risk of undesirable job or financial life events in middle socioeconomic status respondents more than for either high or low status respondents. Those respondents who experienced such undesirable job or financial events were in turn more likely to report recent illness or injury health events (19). Such job and nonjob stressful life events are in turn associated with elevated psychological symptoms such as demoralization (37). The magnitude of the effect of unemployment on mental health measures varies from report to report, depending on the population under study and the disorder being measured. For example, in analyses based on the NIMH Epidemiologic Catchment Area project, becoming unemployed was associated with a doubling of the risk of increased symptoms of depression (36), but with no increased risk of symptoms of anxiety disorder. In contrast, in the same data set, unemployment was associated with a ninefold increase in the risk of having clinical alcohol disorder (32). Individual- and cross-level studies have seldom been able to survey enough respondents to study low-incidence psychiatric admissions regardless of diagnosis. However, a study of 677 bricklayer union members found that the risk of admission to a psychiatric facility was significantly higher for those unemployed more than half the time in the past year (67). One problem with admissions studies is that it is possible that community-level economic stress leads to increased use of mental health services by uncovering or revealing existing cases of disorder rather than by provoking or triggering new cases (17). An alternative is to study self-reported help-seeking with controls for actual symptoms, and one such cross-level survey found multiple pathways between the aggregate economy and help-seeking (20).

The largest part of the unemployment-mental health literature consists of time-series studies of aggregate economic change and mental hospitalization rates (at least 15 such reports by 1986) (31). One potential prob-

lem with such aggregate admissions studies is that community economic change can lead to changes in the supply of public psychiatric services that, in turn, might moderate the covariation between unemployment and admission rates (95). Although many of these studies report the expected positive correlation of unemployment and admissions, there are numerous exceptions. In one of the earliest studies of this type, Brenner (7) reported both positive coefficients for some subgroups and negative coefficients for others. While he found, in general, that inpatient admissions increased with worsening economic times, others found just the opposite (28) or a mixture of a few significant associations among numerous nonsignificant ones (5). Efforts to replicate Brenner's work have succeeded sometimes (79) but failed other times (20, 38, 78). The net effect in these aggregate studies of psychiatric admissions is one of great complexity, with patterns that seem highly time- and place-specific rather than robustly stable.

A few studies have also found links between unemployment and such behaviors as increased drinking (32), aggression (21), divorce (97), and child abuse (98). Other studies have dealt with behaviors that have an indirect bearing on health such as criminal deviance (9), and at least one such study has linked community underemployment to high arrest rates for young adults (1).

Well-Being and Behavior

Most of the individual- and cross-level unemployment literature and virtually all of the minuscule underemployment literature fo-

cuses on self-reported subclinical symptoms such as depression, anxiety, self-esteem, and demoralization. Among adults, factory-closing studies have reported the lowest level of well-being in the anticipation phase before the job loss itself (3, 4, 25, 74), suggesting a multistage model in which symptoms rise and fall at different times in the unemployment process. Panel surveys of adults tend to find that becoming unemployed is associated with a worsening in psychological symptoms such as depression, somatization, and anxiety (76). In contrast, school-leaver studies tend to find that young people who fail to find satisfactory jobs (111) do not experience decreases in self-esteem but rather fail to gain as much as their more happily employed counterparts [however, see (49)]. Seven relatively recent studies from the Nordic countries (2, 49, 54, 55, 58, 66, 109) all find evidence of adverse effects on well-being.

In sum, most individual-level studies have detected a statistically significant adverse effect of unemployment on psychological symptoms, but the magnitude of this effect has tended to be relatively modest, consistent with an adjustment of many job losers to their unemployment.

Directions for Research to Guide Interventions
Stress Buffering Mechanisms

Research could usefully identify those types of persons who are most and least vulnerable to economic stress, as well as causal processes that transmit or moderate their stress reactions. While there are hints as to the kinds of people who are more vulnerable (e.g. those with a psychological commitment to work) (107), the literature has not established a well-replicated set of such risk factors.

Social Contagion

A few studies have documented the adverse effects of the wage earner's unemployment on the spouse or children within a family system (29), but very little work has followed up the research hints that unemployment may play a role in child abuse (98) or infant mortality (22,23). Findings from such research could target unemployment interventions, not just at the job loser but also at other family members.

Underemployment and Reemployment

The majority of job leavers do so to move to a better job or to relocate geographically. Involuntary joblessness can, as indicated above, have adverse health effects. Although some studies report that finding a new job is an antidote to the toxic experience of this type of unemployment (62), for some proportion of the employed the new job that follows unemployment (particularly involuntary unemployment) may be hazardous, unsatisfactory, insecure, low-paid, or stressful (83). Interventions predicated on reemployment may need to be reconsidered in light of the new research on underemployment and its potentially adverse effects. What facets of a job are restorative to the newly reemployed—the salary, the security, the psychological satisfaction of the work itself—and how shall we assure that new jobs include these characteristics (84, 85)?

School-Leavers

If one were to target unemployment interventions based on un-employment rates, the most vulnerable age segment would certainly be recent school-leavers, especially drop-outs from school and minority youth. Interventions in this area will need to deal with such complexities as the interface of secondary education and the job market as well as the culture of poverty, but there may be useful guidance in European approaches to the school-to-work transition.

Immigrant Unemployment

Often drawn by or pushed to low-pay, low-benefit jobs, undocumented workers may have the least employment security and the least-developed social safety net in case of job loss. Research on the occupational risks of employed immigrants is scarce (105), and research on the health impact of their unemployment or underemployment is virtually nonexistent.

Interventions to Reduce Adverse Effects of Unemployment

An appropriate extension of interest in the health effects of unemployment is what interventions can reduce adverse consequences for the small but important job terminations that are involuntary. The unemployment intervention literature has been summarized mainly in program descriptions (89) or bibliographies (RH Price & L Bronfman, unpublished paper), and it has not received a comprehensive review in recent years [the closest approximation being Koziowski et al (64)]. Interventions are usually expensive and lengthy, infrequently funded, and when they do take place, often described in unpublished technical reports. Unemployment programs may be categorized along various dimensions including the time of intervention (before or after job loss) and the level of intervention (macro versus individual) (18). However, there is no consensus among economists on the advisability of public policy interventions to prevent unwanted job loss or the effectiveness of localized efforts to stimulate employment, including many targeted to the newly unemployed. More constructive approaches may include attempts by the social parties on the labor market to enhance lifelong employability by promoting lifelong learning at the workplace or outside it.

Rising unemployment rates usually entail massive economic costs in the form of lost income taxes and depleted unemployment insurance accounts and social welfare funds. On the other hand, unemployment increases are sometimes regarded as a means of preventing inflation, which explains why the stock and bond markets sometimes react bullishly to rising joblessness. Proposals to lower unemployment by raising government spending are typically challenged as aggravating the federal deficit and imposing an unfair debt on future generations. The economics of unemployment are complex; age and social class groups of the population are affected differently by the same employment policies.

Health and social researchers have usually contributed indirectly to the unemployment policy debate through basic epidemiologic research documenting the health effects of economic stress (14). This strategy was attempted in the 1970s in the United States when scholarly support for federally guaranteed full-employment legislation was mustered by research (commissioned by the Joint Economic Committee of Congress) showing the social costs of unemployment (9). Although endorsing full employment in principle, Congress never provided the budgetary support to implement the policy. Perhaps the basic research on the adverse effects of unemployment has not been convincing. Or perhaps some of the actors on the labor market were unwilling to listen, in spite of strong evidence.

Helping Workers Cope

Most developed countries have some form of safety net of public assistance such as unemployment insurance and access to health care. These programs vary in their coverage of the population and the duration and type of assistance provided. Many western European countries provide a more comprehensive safety net than does the United States. Some studies that have found no association between unemployment and well-being have attributed this result to the effectiveness of such national programs [e.g. for Dutch school-leavers, see (94)].

Some unemployed workers manage to cope effectively on their own or with the help of friends and family. This may explain, in part, the low utilization rates reported by many unemployment counseling programs, and the natural coping processes of the most resilient workers could give clues to improving more formal, participative, interventions (44). The less resilient unemployed can seek professional services at any time, including those of clergy, marriage counselors, psychiatrists, psychologists, general practice medical doctors, or others. One recent study capitalized on the closing

of a number of General Motors plants to survey a panel of 1597 workers (11). Controlling for prior use of mental health service, unemployment status did not predict increased usage of specialty mental health services, although depression and nonfinancial stressful events did. Surprisingly, the use of mental health services was associated with a decrease in mental well-being. This perplexing finding warrants further research, but it does not necessarily address the effectiveness of mental health interventions custom-tailored to the needs of dislocated workers. In Norway, attempts have been made to encourage primary health workers to help unemployed people both to regain health and reenter the labor market (24).

One such program was offered to the workers at the closing General Motors plant in Southgate, California (77). The dislocated workers who voluntarily participated reported elevated levels of distress. Those in retraining felt higher levels of worry (39 vs 2%), depression (27 vs 15%), and anger (20 vs 7%) than those not in training (i.e. seeking only job placement), suggesting that stress may come with training. However, common to most such programs, emotional support was offered without complementary tangible support or empowerment. This may explain why so relatively few of those offered psychosocial assistance accepted such help. Just 112 individual and family therapy clients received treatment on an ongoing basis out of 2000 workers over a one-year period, and the outcome of this treatment was not evaluated. More workers accepted other kinds of assistance such as screening for hypertension [407], job search workshops

that included health promotion techniques [302], and support groups dealing with the stress of relocation [126]. These utilization findings highlight the resistance of blue-collar workers to potentially stigmatizing purely mental health-oriented interventions.

Another type of intervention was offered to a group of women workers as part of a Swedish plant closing study (10, 74). The aim of this program was to stimulate structured daily activities such as various courses, and coffee meetings to serve as substitutes for the latent functions lost through unemployment such as time structure and social engagement. Unfortunately, there were no statistically significant benefits of this program on mental or physical well-being, possibly because unemployment is best dealt with by creating or finding a new and satisfactory job.

The best-designed American unemployment intervention in recent years was conducted by the Michigan Prevention Research Center (106). Unemployed workers were recruited while waiting in line at state employment offices, and those interested in receiving an intervention were randomly assigned to a two-week, eight-session experimental program or a self-guided booklet control condition. Of the 752 persons assigned to the experimental condition, 440 (59%) never came. Participants were those who attended at least one session (mean sessions attended = 6.2). The experimental program covered such topics as preparing resumes, using social networks to find jobs, learning problem-solving processes, and accepting social support. The outcomes included benefits both in becoming reemployed and on mental health variables such as anxiety and depression. When the participants' outcomes were compared with those estimated for the controls who would have participated, the results showed significant benefits for the participants in reemployment and mental health, and follow-up analyses suggested that the persons who most needed the program self-selected themselves into it (106).

Conclusion

Workers can experience the economy in a variety of employment roles ranging on a continuum from unemployment through underemployment to adequate or even overemployment. This paper summarized the adverse health effects of the various less-than-adequate employment conditions and the kinds of health promotion interventions that might be initiated in response to these conditions.

Although its serious economic and social consequences are known, unemployment's health effects are not yet fully understood despite over a century of research. Aggregate-level studies have typically found significant positive associations over time between unemployment and suicide, the most frequently studied physical health outcome. Aggregate-level studies of mental health have produced mixed findings for the most commonly studied outcome of psychiatric treatment rates. But such aggregate-level studies cannot be interpreted at the individual level as evidence that personal unemployment raises the risk of suicide or mental disorder, and some of these time-series analyses have used controversial statistical methods. Most individual- and cross-level studies have focused

on measures of well-being such as symptoms of physical and/or mental distress or dysfunctional behaviors, and typically find adverse effects of personal unemployment on the job loser. However, many questions remain unanswered about the mechanisms of the unemployment-health relationship, the restorative effects of reemployment in the restructured workforce with its rising underemployment, and the impact of unemployment on special groups such as school-leavers, dependents of job losers, and immigrants.

Most studies on the relation between unemployment status and health have contrasted just two conditions—employment vs unemployment. But in recent years, increasing numbers of American workers have found themselves in various types of underemployment, including involuntary part-time employment, poverty-wage employment, and insecure employment (i.e. intermittent unemployment). For example, the rate of involuntary part-time employment increased from 2.8% in 1967 to 4.8% in 1985 (70), and the share of full-time workers making poverty wages increased from 12% in 1979 to 18% in 1992 (102). Because these underemployment statuses share some of the more stressful features of unemployment (e.g. decreased income, status, or time structure), it seems plausible that they could produce adverse effects on health similar to those reported above for unemployment. It follows that future research in this area might usefully explore the health correlates of these increasingly common statuses that fall between adequate employment and unemployment on the employment continuum.

Literature Cited

1. Allan EA, Steffensmeier DJ. 1989. Youth, underemployment, and property crime: differential effects of job availability and job quality on juvenile and young adult arrest rates. *Am. Sociol. Rev.* 54:107–23
2. Angelöw B. 1988. *Att Berövas Sitt Arbete (To Be Deprived of One's Job)* Räviunda/Stockholm: Fri Press/Symp.
3. Arnetz B, Brenner S, Hjelm H, Levi L, Petterson, et al. 1988. *Stress reactions in relation to threat of job loss and actual unemployment: physiological, psychological, and economic effects of job loss and unemployment.* Stress Res. Rep. No. 206. Stockhom: Karolinska Inst.
4. Arnetz B, Brenner S-O, Levi L, Hjelm R, Petterson I-L, et al. 1991. Neuroendocrine and immunologic effects of unemployment and job insecurity. *Psychother Psychosom.* 55:76–80
5. Barling P, Handal P. 1980. Incidence of utilization of public mental health facilities as a function of short term economic decline. *Am. J. Community Psychol.* 8:31–39
6. Brenner MH. 1971. Economic changes and heart disease mortality. *Am. J. Public Health* 59:1154–68
7. Brenner MH. 1973. *Mental Illness and the Economy.* Cambridge. MA: Harvard Univ. Press
8. Brenner MH. 1973. Fetal, infant, and maternity mortality during periods of economic stress. *Int. J. Health Serv.* 3:145–59
9. Brenner MH. 1976. *Estimating the social costs of economic policy: implications for mental and physical health and criminal aggression.* Pap. No. 5, Rep. Congr. Res. Serv. Libr. Congr. Joint Econ. Comm. Congr. Washington, DC: US GPO
10. Brenner S-O. Starrin B. 1988. Unemployment and health in Sweden: public issues and private troubles. *J. Soc. Issues* 4:125–44
11. Broman CL, Hoffman WS, Hamilton VL. 1994. Impact of mental health services on subsequent mental health of autoworkers. *J. Health Soc. Behav.* 35:80–94
12. Bunn AR. 1979. Ischaemic heart disease mortality and the business cycle in Australia. *Am. J. Public Health* 69:772–81
13. Burchell B. 1992. Towards a social psychology of the labour market: Or why we need to understand the

labour market before we can understand unemployment. *J. Occup. Organ. Psychol.* 65:345–54

14. Cahill J. 1983. Structural characteristics of the macroeconomy and mental health: implications for primary prevention research. *Am. J. Community Psychol.* 11:553–71

15. Catalano R. 1981. Contending with rival hypotheses in correlation of aggregate time-series (CATS): an overview for community psychologists. *Am. J. Community Psychol.* 9:67–79

16. Catalano R. 1991. The health effects of economic security. *Am. J. Public Health* 81:1148–52

17. Catalano R, Dooley D. 1979. Does economic change provoke or uncover behavioral disorder? A preliminary test. In *Mental Health and the Economy*, ed. L Ferman, J Gordus, pp. 321–41. Kalamazoo, MI: Upjohn Inst.

18. Catalano R, Dooley D. 1980. Economic change in primary prevention. In *Prevention in Mental Health: Research, Policy, and Practice*, ed. RH Price, RF Ketterer, BC Bader, J Monohan, pp. 21–40. Beverly Hills, CA: Sage

19. Catalano R, Dooley D. 1983. Health effects of economic instability: a test of economic stress hypothesis. *J. Health Soc. Behav.* 24:46–60

20. Catalano R, Dooley D, Jackson R. 1985. Economic antecedents of help seeking: reformulation of time-series tests. *J. Health Soc. Behav.* 26:141–52

21. Catalano R, Dooley D, Novaco R, Wilson G. Hough R. 1993. Using ECA survey data to examine the effect of job layoffs on violent behavior. *Hosp. Community Psychiatr.* 44:874–79

22. Catalano R, Serxner S. 1992. Neonatal mortality and the economy revisited. *Int. J. Health Serv.* 22:275–86

23. Catalano R, Serxner S. 1992. The effect of ambient threats to employment on low birthweight. *J. Health Soc. Behav.* 33:363–77

24. Claussen B. 1992. *Arbeidsledighet og Helse. (Unemployment and Health).* Oslo: Helsedirektoratet

25. Cobb S, Kasi SV. 1977. *Termination: the consequences of job loss.* Rep. No. 76–1261. Cincinnati, OH: DHEW (NIOSH)

26. Cohen LE, Felson M. 1979. On estimating the social costs of national economic policy: a critical examination of the Brenner study. *Soc. Indicators Res.* 6:251–59

27. Cohn RM. 1978. The effect of employment status change on self-attitudes. *Soc. Psychol.* 41:81–93

28. Dear M, Clark G, Clark S. 1979. Economic cycles and mental health care policy: an examination of the macro-context for social service planning. *Soc. Sci. Med.* 13:43–53

29. Dew MA, Penkower L, Bromet EJ. 1991. Effects of unemployment on mental health in the contemporary family. *Behav. Modif* 15:501–42

30. Dooley D, Catalano R. 1980. Economic change as a cause of behavioral disorder. *Psychol. Bull.* 87:450–68

31. Dooley D, Catalano R. 1986. Do economic variables generate psychological problems? Different methods, different answers. In *Economic Psychology: Intersection in Theory and Application*, ed. AJ MacFadyen, HW MacFadyen, pp. 503–46. Amsterdam: Elsevier

32. Dooley D, Catalano R, Hough R. 1992. Unemployment and alcohol disorder in 1910 and 1990: drift versus social causation. *J. Occup. Organ. Psychol.* 65:277–90

33. Dooley D, Catalano R, Rook KS. 1988. Personal and aggregate unemployment and psychological symptoms. *J. Soc. Issues* 11:107–23

34. Dooley D, Catalano R, Rook KS, Serxner S. 1989. Economic stress and suicide: multilevel analyses. Part 1: Aggregate time-series analyses of economic stress and suicide. *Suicide Life Threat. Behav.* 19:321–36

35. Dooley D, Catalano R, Serxner S. 1988. The economy as stressor. In *Location and Stigma: Contemporary Perspectives on Mental Health and Mental Health Care*, ed. CJ Smith, JHA Giggs, pp. 134–51. Boston: Unwin Hyman

36. Dooley D, Catalano R, Wilson G. 1994. Depression and unemployment: panel findings from the Epidemiologic Catchment Area Study. *Am J. Community Psychol.* 22:745–65

37. Dooley D, Rook K, Catalano R. 1987. Job and non-job stressors and their moderators. *J. Occup. Psychol.* 60:115–32

38. Dowdall GW, Marshall JR, Morra WA. 1990. Economic antecedents of mental hospitalization: a nineteenth-century time-series test. *J. Health Soc. Behav.* 31:141–47

39. Durkheim E. 1897. *Suicide: A Study in Sociology.* Transl. J Spaulding, G Simpson. 1966. New York: Free Press

40. Feather NT. 1990. *The Psychological Impact of Unemployment.* New York: Springer-Verlag

41. Fenwick R, Tausig M. 1994. The macro-economic context of job stress. *J. Health Soc. Behav.* 35:266–82

42. Fineman S. 1983. *White Collar Unemployment: Impact and Stress.* New York: Wiley

43. Fruensgaard K, Benjaminsen S, Joensen S, Heistrup K. 1983. Psychosocial characteristics of a group of unemployed patients consecutively admitted to a psychiatric emergency department. *Soc. Psychiatr.* 18:137–44

44. Fryer D, Fagan R. 1993. Coping with unemployment. *Int. J. Polit. Econ.* 23:95–120

45. Fryer D, Payne R. 1984. Proactive behaviour in unemployment: findings and implications. *Leis. Stud.* 3:273–95

46. Gordus JP, McAlinden SP. 1984. *Economic change, physical illness, mental illness, and social deviance.* A study for the Subcomm. Econ. Goals Intergov. Policy Joint Econ. Comm. Congr. Washington, DC: US GPO

47. Gravelle HS E., Hutchinson G, Stern J. 1981. Mortality and unemployment. A critique of Brenner's time-series analyses. *Lancet* ii:675–79

48. Halford WK, Learner E. 1984. Correlates of coping with unemployment in young Australians. *Aust. Psychol.* 19:333–44

49. Hammarström A. 1986. *Youth unemployment and ill health. Results from a two-year follow-up study.* Doctoral diss. Stockholm: Karolinska Inst.

50. Hartley J, Fryer D. 1984. The psychology of unemployment: a critical appraisal. *Prog. Appl. Soc. Psychol.* 2:3–30

51. Hayes J, Nutman P. 1981. *Understanding the Unemployed: The Psychological Effects of Unemployment.* New York: Tavistock

52. Holmes TH, Rahe RH. 1967. The social readjustment rating scale. *J. Psychosom. Res.* 11:213–18

53. Horwitz AV. 1984. The economy and social pathology. *Annu. Rev. Social.* 10:95–119

54. Isaksson K. 1990. *Arbetslöshetoch Mental Hälsa Bland Unga Manliga Socialtjänstklienter. (Life Without Work. Unemployment and Mental Health in Young Male Clients of Social*

Welfare). Stockholm: Univ. Stockholm

55. Iversen L. 1990. *Virksomhedslukninger, Arbeodslöshed og helbred. (Closures of Enterprises, Unemployment and Health.* Copenhagen: FADL's Forlag

56. Iversen L, Andersen O, Andersen PK, Christoffersen K, Keiding N. 1987. Unemployment and mortality in Denmark 1970–80. *Br. Med. J.* 295:879–84

57. Jahoda M. 1982. *Employment and Unemployment: A Social Psychological Analysis.* New York: Cambridge Univ. Press

58. Janlert U. 1991. *Work deprivation and health: consequences of job loss and unemployment.* Doctoral diss. Luleä/Sundbyberg: Karolinska Inst.

59. Kasl SV, Gore S, Cobb S. 1975. The experience of losing a job: repeated changes in health, symptoms, and illness behavior. *Psychosom. Med.* 37:106–22

60. Kaufman HG. 1982. *Professionals in Search of Work. Coping with the Stress of Job Loss and Underemployment.* New York: Wiley

61. Kessler RC, House JS, Turner JB. 1987. Unemployment and health in a community sample. *J. Health Soc. Behav.* 28:51–59

62. Kessler RC, Turner JB, House JS. 1988. Effects of unemployment on health in a community survey: main, modifying, and mediating effects. *J. Soc. Issues* 44:69–85

63. Kompier M, Levi L. 1994. *Stress at Work: Causes, Effects, and Prevention.* Dublin: Eur. Found.

64. Kozlowski SWJ, Chao GT, Smith EM, Hedlund J. 1993. Organizational downsizing: strategies, interventions, and research implications. *International Review of Industrial and Organizational Psychology*: 1993. New York: Wiley

65. Kreitman N, Platt S. 1984. Suicide, unemployment and domestic gas detoxification in Britain. *J. Epidemiol. Community Health* 38:1–6

66. Laheima E. 1989. Unemployment, reemployment and mental well-being. A panel survey of industrial jobseekers in Finland. *Scand. J. Soc. Med.* 43 (suppl.)

67. Lajer M. 1982. Unemployment and hospitalization among bricklayers. *Scand. J. Soc. Med.* 10:3–10

68. Lee AJ, Crombie IK, Smith WCS, Tunstall-Pedoe HD. 1991. Cigarette smoking and employment status. *Soc. Sci. Med.* 33:1309–12

69. Leigh JP, Waldon HM. 1991. Unemployment and highway fatalities. *J. Health Policy* 16:135–56

70. Leppel K, Cain SH. 1988. The growth in involuntary part-time employment of men and women. *Appl. Econ.* 20:1155–66

71. Levi L, ed. 1981. *Society, Stress and Disease: Working Life.* Oxford/New York/Toronto: Oxford Univ. Press

72. Levi L. 1984. *Stress in Industry: Causes, Effects and Prevention.* Geneva: ILO

73. Levi L. 1992. Intervening in social systems to promote health. In *Aging, Health, and Behavior*, ed. MG Ory, RP Abeles, PD Lipman, pp. 276–95. Newbury Park, CA: Sage

74. Levi L, Brenner S-O, Hall EM, Hjelm R, Salovaara H, et al. 1984. The psychological, social, and biochemical impacts of unemployment in Sweden. *Int. J. Ment. Health.* 13:18–34

75. Liem R, Liem JH. 1988. Psychological effects of unemployment on workers and their families. *J. Soc. Issues* 44:87–105

76. Linn MW, Sandifer R, Stein S. 1985. Effects of unemployment on mental and physical health. *Am. J. Public Health* 75:502–06

77. Maida CA, Gordon NS, Farberow NL. 1989. *The Crisis of Competence: Transitional Stress and the Displaced Worker.* New York: Brunner/Mazel

78. Marshall JR, Dowdall GW. 1982. Employment and mental hospitalization: the case of Buffalo, New York, 1914–1955. *Soc. Forces* 60:843–53

79. Marshall JR, Funch DP. 1979. Mental illness and the economy: a critique and partial replication. *J. Health Soc. Behav.* 20:282–89

80. Marshall JR, Hodge RW. 1981. Durkheim and Pierce on suicide and economic change. *Soc. Sci. Res.* 10:101–14

81. Martin R. 1987. The effect of unemployment upon the employed: a new realism in industrial relations. In *Unemployment: Personal and Social Consequences*, ed. S. Fineman, pp. 219–34. London: Tavistock

82. McKenna SP, McEwen J. 1987. Employment and health. In *Unemployed People: Social and Psychological Perspectives*, ed. D Fryer, P Ullah, pp. 174–93. Philadelphia: Open Univ. Press

83. OECD. 1993. *OECD Employment Outlook.* Paris: OECD

84. OECD. 1994. The OECD Jobs Study. OECD *Econ. Outl.* 55:1–4

85. OECD. 1994. The OECD *Jobs Study. Facts, Analysis, Strategies.* Paris: OECD

86. Pierce A. 1967. The economic cycle and the social suicide rate. *Am. Sociol. Rev.* 32:457–62

87. Petersen AC, Mortimer JT, eds. 1994. *Youth Unemployment and Society.* New York: Cambridge Univ. Press

88. Platt S. 1984. Unemployment and suicidal behavior: a review of the literature. *Soc. Sci. Med.* 19:93–115

89. Popay J. 1985. Responding to unemployment at a local level. In *Health Policy Implications of Unemployment*, ed. G. Westcott, PG Svensson HFK Zollner, pp. 383–99. Copenhagen: WHO, Reg. Off. Eur.

90. Robinson WS. 1950. Ecological correlations and the behavior of individuals. *Am. Soc. Rev.* 15:352–57

91. Rook K, Dooley D, Catalano R. 1991. Stress transmission: the effects of husbands' job stressors on the emotional health of their wives. *J. Marriage Fam.* 53:165–77

92. Rosenthal R. 1979. The "file drawer problem" and tolerance for null results. *Psychol. Bull.* 86:638–41

93. Russian Ministry of Health. 1994. *Towards a Healthy Russia. Policy for Health Promotion and Disease Prevention: Focus on Major Noncommunicable Diseases.* State Res. Cent. Prevent. Med., Moscow (From Russian)

94. Schaufeli WB, Van Yperen NW. 1992. Unemployment and psychological distress among graduates: a longitudinal study. *J. Occup. Organ. Psychol.* 65:291–305

95. Searight HR, Handal PJ, McCauliffe TM. 1989. The relationship between public mental health admission rates, institutional constraints, and unemployment. *Admin. Policy Ment. Health* 17:33–42

96. Seidman E, Rapkin B. 1983. Economics and psychological dysfunction: toward a conceptual framework and prevention strategies. In *Preventive Psychology: Theory, Research and Practice*, ed. RD Felner, LA Jason, JN Moritsugu, SS Faber. New York: Pergamon

97. Stack S. 1981. Divorce and suicide: a time series analysis. 1933–1970. *J Fam. Issues* 2:77–90

98. Steinberg L, Catalano R, Dooley D. 1981. Economic antecedents of child abuse and neglect. *Child Dev.* 52:260–67

99. Theorell T. 1974. Life events before and after the onset of premature myocardial infarction. In *Stressful Life Events: Their Nature and Effect*, ed. BS Dohrenwend, BP Dohrenwend, pp. 101–17. New York: Wiley

100. UNICEF. 1994. *Crisis in Mortality, Health and Nutrition*. Florence: UNICEF Int. Child Dev. Cent.

101. United Nations. 1995. *Draft Declaration of Heads of States and Governments, World Summit for Social Development (revised Oct. 26, 1994)*. Copenhagen: UN Inf. Cent. Nord. Ctries.

102. US Bur. Census. 1994. The earnings ladder: Who's at the bottom: Who's at the top? *Stat. Brief*, SB/94–3. Washington, DC: US GPO

103. US Dep. Labor 1994. *Employment and Earnings* 41:7

104. US Dep. Labor 1995. *Employment and Earnings* 42:9

105. Vaughan E. 1993. Chronic exposure to an environmental hazard: risk perceptions and self-protective behavior. *Health Psychol.* 12:74–85.

106. Vinokur AD, Price RH, Caplan RD. 1991. From field experiments to program implementation: assessing the potential outcomes of an experimental intervention program for unemployed persons. *Am J. Community Psychol.* 19:543–62.

107. Warr P, Jackson P, Banks M. 1988. Unemployment and mental health: some British studies. *J. Soc. Issues* 44:47–68

108. Warr P, Parry G. 1982. Paid employment and women's psychological wellbeing. *Psychol. Bull.* 19:498–516

109. Westin S. 1990. *Unemployment and Health: Medical and Social Consequences of a Factory Closure in a Ten-Year Controlled Follow-Up Study:*
A Study from General Practice. Trondheim: Tapir

110. Wheaton B. 1990. Life transitions, role histories, and mental health. *Am. Sociol. Rev.* 55:209–23

111. Winefield AH, Tiggemann M, Winefield HR, Goldney RD. 1993. *Growing Up with Unemployment: A Longitudinal Study of Its Psychological Impact*. London: Routledge

112. Winter JM. 1983. Unemployment, nutrition and infant mortality in Britain: 1920–1950. In *Influence of Economic Instability on Health*, ed. J John, D Schwefel, H Zollner, pp. 169–99. Berlin: Springer-Verlag

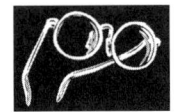 **Article Review Form at end of book.**

WiseGuide Wrap-Up

- Small worksites in the private sector and in rural areas seem to be lacking in health-promoting attributes and deserve highest priority in efforts by practitioners to procure supportive workplace environments.

- Although the availability of worksite health-promotion programs remains high, participation by employees in specific types of programs can vary widely. Attempts to increase participation should look beyond individual health and organizational variables to specific features of the work environment that encourage involvement in health-promotion activities.

- Most research involving health promotion and disease prevention at the worksite and other clinical sites indicates that such interventions are both health- and cost-effective.

- Employee assistance programs were created to provide a safe environment for employees to seek help with emotional, behavioral, and social problems. EAPs can function as either internal or external programs. Internal programs are staffed by company employees and located at the worksite. External programs provide services to worksite employees on a contractual basis, and their offices are typically located away from the company.

- Workers can experience the economy in a variety of employment roles ranging on a continuum from unemployment through underemployment to adequate or even overemployment. There are many adverse health effects associated with the various less-than-adequate employment conditions. There are numerous health-promotion interventions that could be initiated in response to these conditions.

R.E.A.L. Sites

This list provides a print preview of typical **Coursewise** R.E.A.L. sites. (There are over 100 such sites at the **Courselinks**™ site.) The danger in printing URLs is that web sites can change overnight. As we went to press, these sites were functional using the URLs provided. If you come across one that isn't, please let us know via email to: webmaster@coursewise.com. Use your Passport to access the most current list of R.E.A.L. sites at the **Courselinks** site.

Site name: Federal Interagency Committee on Worksite Health Promotion and Disease Prevention

URL: http://nhic-nt.health.org/wsintage.htm

Why is it R.E.A.L.? The Federal Interagency Committee on Worksite Health Promotion and Disease Prevention provides a forum for federal agencies to exchange information and ideas about worksite health-promotion issues, including research, policy development, programs, and projects.

Key topic: worksite health promotion

Try this: Review the list of participating agency members to see the scope of worksite health promotion.

Site name: Year 2000 Worksite Health Promotion and Disease Prevention Objectives

URL: http://nhic-nt.health.org/wsobject.htm

Why is it R.E.A.L.? This site provides the Year 2000 Worksite Health Promotion and Disease Prevention Objectives.

Key topics: worksite health promotion, disease prevention

Try this: Review the objectives. Note the recommendations for specific target populations.

section

4

Learning Objectives

- To examine the current system of public health and to consider improvements for the year 2000

- To assess the impact of Medicaid on managed care

- To explore the impact of Medicaid on public health responsibilities

- To examine the community-based approaches for the prevention of ATOD problems

- To review the use of prevalence data to unite the community in prevention programs

- To explore a commentary addressing whether community or commodity is the focus of public health

- To examine the appropriate "how-to" in order to conduct community needs assessment

Community Health Promotion

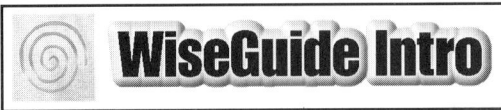 **WiseGuide Intro**

Traditional community health brings to mind images of public health departments. Those local health departments were charged with maintaining infection control records, providing immunizations, and offering some environmental controls. Today, community health has expanded to include not only local health departments but also numerous social service agencies, not-for-profit agencies directed at specific health concerns, parish nursing programs, grassroots coalitions, and sophisticated collaborations.

In this section, we will examine several community health programs. Suggestions for improving public health, the impact of Medicaid managed care on local health departments, community approaches to ATOD (alcohol, tobacco, and other drugs) prevention, the use of prevalence data in prevention programming, and community needs assessments will be examined.

Bernard J. Turnock and Arden S. Handler (both at the University of Illinois at Chicago) present "From Measuring to Improving Public Health Practice." Recent assessments suggest that the system of public health practice must be improved to achieve the targets of effectiveness established for the year 2000.

Liza Corso, Grace Gorenflo, and Carol Brown (all of the National Association of County and City Health Officials), Thomas Richards and Zachary Taylor (both at the Centers for Disease Control), and Patricia Gadow (Madison Department of Public Health) collaborate on "Assessing the Impact of Medicaid Managed Care on TB Activities in Local Health Departments." Three in-depth case studies were conducted to explore the impact of Medicaid managed care on local health department prevention activities. Tuberculosis was selected as the sentinel issue. Many suggestions for areas to monitor, possible collaborative opportunities, and mechanisms to assure continued TB prevention and control are discussed.

John Lumpkin, Laura Landrum, Angela Oldfield, Patti Kimmel, Michael Jones, and Conny Mueller Moody (all at the Illinois Department of Public Health) and Bernard J. Turnock (University of Illinois at Chicago) present "Impact of Medicaid Resources on Core Public Health Responsibilities of Local Health Departments in Illinois." This study highlights how critical it is for the entire public health community to become involved in the policy-making process to ensure the integration of public health approaches with those of managed care.

Marilyn Aguirre-Molina (Robert Wood Johnson Foundation) and D.M. Gorman (Rutgers) present "Community-Based Approaches for the Prevention of Alcohol, Tobacco, and Other Drug Use." This paper summarizes what is known about community-based approaches for the prevention of ATOD problems and how the current practices in the field reflect these approaches.

Bernard Healey (Kings College) presents "The Use of Prevalence Data to Unite the Community in Prevention Programs." This study examined the prevalence of cigarette smoking in a three-county area of northeastern Pennsylvania. The results of the study were used to unite the health community in a number of prevention initiatives.

Toby Citrin (University of Michigan) presents "Topics for Our Times: Public Health—Community or Commodity? Reflections on *Healthy Communities*." In response to the Institute of Medicine report *Healthy Communities*, a discussion of community versus commodity of public health is presented. The impact of managed care is also examined.

Virginia Pearson (Baton Rouge Health Forum) presents "Community Assessment: A Model 'How-To' Based on Two Communities' Experience." If done correctly, a community health needs assessment is a systematic method for identifying the unmet human needs of particular populations at risk within a defined community or geographic area. This article examines a model based on the experiences of two communities.

? Questions ?

Reading 18. Services that would result from each local health department carrying out its functions include three categories; list them. Why should the "functions" of public health change whenever the system responds to changing conditions with a new set of services?

Reading 19. List the five issue areas that are "important" to local health departments (LHDs). Discuss the difficulties the LHDs faced in obtaining reimbursements from managed care organizations.

Reading 20. An estimated _____ would be needed to offset core public health productivity reductions associated with each 1 million in Medicaid funding losses. Discuss one of the three key steps for assessing the impact of Medicaid managed care on core public health responsibilities of Illinois local health departments.

Reading 21. What is "community empowerment"? Compare the role mass media outlets play in community-based intervention programs with the role of community organizations.

Reading 22. About half of all smokers die in middle age, resulting in a loss of _____ of potential life. What does the study show regarding gender and smoking?

Reading 23. How does Citrin define *community*? Citrin states that, by following this path, public health will become the next significant societal enterprise to be converted into a commodity. Describe the "path."

Reading 24. If done correctly, a community health needs assessment will identify _____. Differentiate between the coalition-building process and the collaboration-building process.

Services that would result from each local health department carrying out its functions include three categories; list them. Why should the "functions" of public health change whenever the system responds to changing conditions with a new set of services?

From Measuring to Improving Public Health Practice

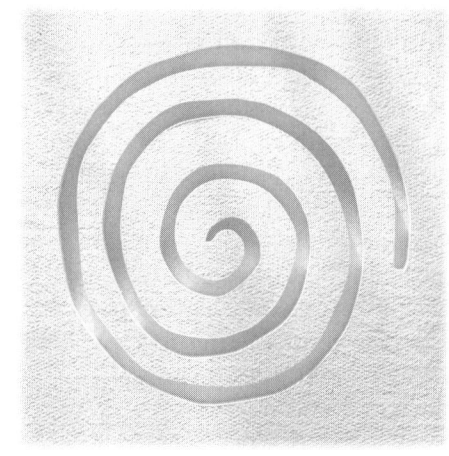

Bernard J. Turnock
and Arden S. Handler

Division of Community Health Sciences, School of Public Health, University of Illinois at Chicago.

Abstract

Efforts to measure public health practice have taken on various forms and focused on different aspects of the system of public health practice over the past century. Before 1990, measurement was primarily based on a series of self-assessment instruments initiated under the auspices of the Committee on Administrative Practice of the American Public Health Association. These instruments emphasized measurement of immediate results of local public health services although they also provided information on local resources and capacity to perform. Following the Institute of Medicine's report in 1988, efforts began to focus on performance related to public health's core functions. These more recent assessments suggest that the system of public health practice must be improved to achieve the targets of effectiveness established for the year 2000. Ultimately, a comprehensive national surveillance system for public health practice will need to both measure and examine the relationships among inputs (resources, capacity, etc), core function-related processes, outputs (services) as well as outcomes.

Introduction

In the nearly ten years since the Institute of Medicine (IOM) reported on the state of public health in the United States, the mission, substance, and core functions of public health have been re-articulated (19); important and achievable national health objectives have been established for the year 2000 (39, 58); exciting opportunities afforded by better integration of our public health and medical care activities have emerged (8); and new approaches for improving results throughout the public health system have gained momentum (9, 21, 22). Although the sad state of affairs decried in the IOM report has undergone considerable change over the past ten years, it is much less clear whether these changes have led to improvements in public health practice or, more importantly, in the results of public health practice—health outcomes. This chapter describes efforts to measure the extent and effectiveness of public health practice in the United States since 1900, and examines the approaches, findings, and implications of these activities for future efforts toward improving health outcomes through the public health system.

A basic tenet of improving systems is that results reflect the systems that produce them. As is often stated, "Every system is perfectly designed to achieve exactly the results it gets" (9). This simple aphorism unmasks the major challenge confronting efforts to improve the results of public health practice: improving health outcomes calls for improving the system of public health practice itself. But, as some additional improvement wisdom warns, to improve something we must be able to control it; to control it we must be able to understand it; and to understand it we must be able to measure it (18). Public health professionals would be quick to add an even more basic need: Before we measure something, we must be able to define it operationally. Defining, measuring, understanding, and controlling are the essential elements of the improvement agenda for the public health system.

There is ample evidence that the public health community has been wrestling with this agenda for the greater part of this century. Unfortunately, past efforts to measure public health practice lacked an adequate conceptual framework for defining the public health system. As a result, these efforts focused on measuring aspects of the public health system that only indirectly or partially characterized the functions embodied in public health practice. Consequently, opportunities for understanding, controlling, and improving public health practice and health outcomes were limited. Still, these efforts set the stage for developments since the 1988 IOM report and the even greater opportunities that lie ahead.

Eras of public health practice performance measurement can be conveniently separated by the IOM report's appearance in 1988. Importantly, an examination of measurement issues is part and parcel of an examination of what public health practice is, what it does, and how it does what it does. Over much of this century, the purpose and functions of public health (what it is and what it

does) were confused with how it carries out its purpose and functions through the delivery of specific community services. As a result, public health, like many other enterprises, has become known more by its deeds than by whether it is achieving its intent. Likewise, efforts to measure public health practice have been in accord with the prevailing perceptions as to what constituted public health practice at different points in time. In light of these considerations, what follows examines both the measurement of local public health practice as well as its conceptualization.

Efforts to Describe What Local Public Health Practice Does
Measurement of Local Public Health Services: 1915–1987

Efforts to characterize and measure public health practice in the United States date back more than 80 years. It is tempting to speculate that early efforts were designed primarily to describe and count resources and services rather than to measure performance relative to established standards. This interpretation, however, is not completely accurate.

Much of the early activity focused on local public health practice, although the earliest attempt in 1914 targeted state health departments. At that time Chapin completed a survey of state health agencies for the American Medical Association to describe the services of those agencies and their role in fostering the development of local health departments. Chapin concluded that state public health agencies were "mostly ill-balanced. Much of what is done counts little for health and

much is left undone which would save many lives" (57). In response, he formulated relative values for various preventive services and scored the state agencies on each service and in the aggregate. This quantitative approach was later incorporated into local public health practice appraisal initiatives orchestrated by the American Public Health Association (APHA).

In 1921, the First Report of APHA's Committee on Municipal Health Department Practice (1, 2) called for the collection of information on local public health practice to provide the basis for the development of standards of organization and achievement for local health departments (LHDs) serving the nation's largest municipalities. The Committee concluded that "few standards are available to the health officers who would pattern their departments after those which predominate in American practice or achieve most satisfactory results" (2). A survey instrument was developed and applied to 83 cities through site visits involving various committee members, including public health giants Winslow (committee chairman), Chapin, and Frost (2).

The Committee soon saw the need to examine local public health practice more broadly and in 1925 was reconstituted as APHA's Committee on Administrative Practice. The new Committee developed the first version of an Appraisal Form (3, 4), which was designed to provide "a reasonably accurate picture of the health services performed in a city" (4) and to focus

. . . not on money expended or personnel employed, which indicate resources rather than performance. Nor was it to be based on mortality rates, which are affected by so many racial and industrial factors as to make comparisons between various cities misleading. The idea was rather to measure the immediate results attained—such as statistics properly obtained and analyzed, vaccinations performed, infants in attendance at instructive clinics, physical defects of school children discovered and corrected, tuberculosis cases hospitalized, laboratory tests performed—with the confidence that such immediate results would inevitably lead on to the ultimate end of all public health work, the conservation of human life and efficiency (4).

The Appraisal Form was to be used as a self-appraisal tool by local health officers with a focus on all public health work—"that performed by official agencies . . . and that performed by unofficial agencies as well" (4). Successive iterations appeared throughout the 1920s and 1930s, and were generally well received by LHDs, although there were occasional concerns that quantity was being emphasized over quality (59). Local health officers were able to compare their ratings with other agencies and submit their assessment to the Health Conservation Contest and its successor, the National Honor Roll. The basis for comparison was a numerical rating score based on aggregated points awarded across key administrative and service areas. Comparative ratings were to be used to improve health programs, advocate for resources, summarize health agency activities in annual reports, and engage other health interests in the community (4). Agency ratings often attracted considerable media interest, resulting in both good and bad publicity for local agencies as "newspapers devoured the results. National magazines interested in the public health field

commented extensively on it. More important still, the cities concerned took steps to make the improvements needed" (43). Despite the initial intent to emphasize "immediate results," the major focus of the ratings remained on measuring some of the more concrete aspects of public health practice such as staff, financial resources, and clinic sites (6, 15).

In 1943, the Appraisal Form was replaced by a new, and still vital instrument, the Evaluation Schedule, which was scored centrally by the APHA Committee on Administrative Practice. The Evaluation Schedule attempted to measure "first, problems or needs; second, available resources; and third, as objectively as possible, the degree of success in applying appropriate resources to those various needs" (6). The National Honor Roll was discontinued in 1943 and succeeded by the National Reporting Area for Health Practices and "Health Practice Indices" (6, 14). No longer was the focus on good or bad scores; the indices presented scores for health agencies of varying size and type so that individual LHDs could directly compare their performance in meeting community needs with that of their peers (5). These new initiatives placed even greater emphasis on measuring results rather than resources and activities while broadening the unit of analysis from the health department to the community as a whole (15).

In order to develop a blueprint for a national network of local public health departments that would provide every American with coverage by a local health department, the Committee on Administrative Practice established a Subcommittee on Local

Health Units chaired by Emerson. The Emerson Report (14) of 1945 served as a landmark for recommendations regarding local public health practice and virtually became the post war plan for public health in the United States. The report gave increased prominence to six basic services believed to represent local government's public health responsibilities to its citizens. These "basic six" services were: vital statistics, communicable disease control, environmental sanitation, public health laboratory services, maternal and child health services, and public health education (14). This was essentially the same package of services that had been considered the standard of practice among LHDs for several decades and which had been assessed since the early years of the Appraisal Form. Over time, these services have been widely known as the basic six "functions" of LHDs. Because of the Emerson Report, however, they became the cornerstone for restructuring local public health agencies. Although the report's extensive recommendations never became national public policy, they stimulated change in many states (48).

During the height of its efforts the APHA Committee on Administrative Practice stimulated considerable interest in local public health practice; this interest persisted until several years after the Committee's demise in 1956, when its functions were split among several association committees. A series of APHA policy statements from 1950–1970 illuminate "the search for mission redefinition" (48) for local public health practice. In a 1950 APHA statement on local health department services and responsibilities, the basic six were presented as desirable minimal services while a new list of "optimal" responsibilities was unveiled: recording and analysis of health data, health education and information, supervision and regulation, provision of direct environmental health facilities and area-wide planning and coordination (48). A 1970 APHA policy expanded these concepts to call for increased involvement of state and local health departments in coordinating, monitoring, and assessing the adequacy of health services in their jurisdictions. Nonetheless, beginning in the 1950s, APHA's intensive interest in local public health practice and its measurement diminished as the association took on national health policy concerns, especially gaps in the medical care system.

The changing expectations for local public health practice after World War II emerged as a major issue for LHDs (32). Lack of medical care was identified as an significant impediment to promoting and improving community health, and LHDs became increasingly called upon to fill a safety net function. A 1947 study by Terris & Kramer (51) concluded that health departments had advanced beyond the traditional basic six model and were increasingly involved in administering general medical services. Myers and colleagues, in concert with PHS and the Association of State and Territorial Health Officials (ASTHO), completed a similar examination in 1966; however, they concluded that LHDs were not emerging as leaders within their communities in integrating medical and community health services (34). The movement into medical care appears to have been controversial from its inception.

Hanlon in examining the future of LHDs in 1973 called for official public health agencies to withdraw from the business of providing personal health services (whether preventive or therapeutic) and instead "concentrate upon its important and unique potential as community health conscience and leader" in promoting the establishment of sound social policy (17). A series of studies by Miller and colleagues during the 1970s and 1980s (10, 13, 24–26) provided new insights into the public health infrastructure and the effect of various forces on LHDs. Despite Hanlon's call, these studies largely supported the need for LHDs to provide personal health care services within their communities.

Measurement of Core Public Health Functions: 1988–2000

The picture of the state of the public health system painted in the IOM report was more dismal than many had expected. After all, the infrastructure of the national public health system had grown substantially throughout the century, especially in terms of LHD coverage of the population. There was widespread acceptance of an expanded package of community services that added chronic, disease prevention and medical care to the "basic six." And, more importantly, health status had never been better. Yet, the tragic face of the AIDS epidemic had appeared, and there was no shortage of intractable health and social issues now being placed on the public health agenda. Resources to meet these challenges were greatly limited due in part to the insatiable appetite of the medical care delivery system for every available health dollar. Somehow these forces had acted together to dissipate public appreciation and support for public health, and the IOM feared that public health would not be able to meet these challenges without a new vision that would engender the support of the public, policy makers, the media, the medical establishment, and other key stakeholders.

The vision articulated in the IOM report was founded in a broader view of public health functions than had existed in the past. In part, the IOM built upon the concept of a governmental presence at the local level that emerged in the planning of the initial model standards process (40). Throughout earlier decades, the services provided by public health agencies had come to be viewed as public health's "functions." In characterizing three core functions (assessment, policy development, and assurance), the IOM report suggested that the function "to serve"— whether termed services, assurance, or something else—is an inadequate characterization of the unique role of public health in our society. Why should the "functions" of public health change whenever the system responds to changing conditions with a new set of services? Services should be viewed as the output of carrying out public health's core functions rather than as the "functions" themselves. When the focus shifts from services to functions, greater attention can be directed to the operational aspects of those in ways that allow for their performance to be improved. As a result, it becomes possible to measure inputs (e.g. budgets, staff), operational aspects of the core functions themselves (practices or processes), and to relate these to the outputs (e.g. services) provided, and ultimately to health status in the community.

The IOM report was soon followed by a series of initiatives to facilitate operationalization by LHDs of the core function framework, especially its assessment and policy development components. New national health objectives were established for the year 2000 based on a decade's experience with the year 1990 national health objectives (58). Broader participation in their design and better tools for their implementation in community settings distinguished the year 2000 objectives from the earlier effort. An updated version of the Model Standards document was created with the specific aim of linking it with the year 2000 health objectives (39). Several community needs assessment instruments—all using the same basic steps and fostering community participation—were promoted by various health organizations. The national public health organization developed understandable guidance to facilitate the use of these tools as a means of operationalizing public health's core functions within the community (39).

In addition, for the first time ever, a national health objective for coverage of the population by an effective local public health presence was developed. By the year 2000, Objective 8.14 called for 90% of the population to be served by a LHD that was effectively carrying out public health's core functions in that community (58). Despite little consensus as to what was meant by "effectively" addressing the core functions of public health, the implication was clear that counting the number of LHDs or even "immediate" results would no longer be sufficient.

One of the most important of these new initiatives was the de-

velopment of the Assessment Protocol for Excellence in Public Health (APEXPH) by the National Association of County and City Health Officials (NACCHO) in collaboration with other national public health organizations (38). APEXPH provided a tool for organizational self-assessment and improvement for LHDs as well as a simple and effective community needs assessment process. Since its appearance in 1990, APEXPH has been well accepted among LHDs; nearly one half of all LHDs had utilized it as of mid-1996. Use of the APEXPH framework has been credited with significant change in LHD practice patterns in Illinois, Washington State, and elsewhere (41, 55).

The Center for Disease Control (CDC)'s Public Health Practice Program Office stimulated several research activities related to the new Objective 8.14. These projects sought to design and test public health practice measures related to the core functions of public health both for the purpose of measuring progress toward Objective 8.14 and for assessing the operational aspects of the core functions (practices). A framework using ten organizational practices as operational definitions for the three core functions was used to evaluate local public health performance (16, 27–31, 55, 56); this was initially used to assess LHD practice performance patterns in six states (12, 44, 45) as well as in a national sample of LHDs in an effort to benchmark progress toward Objective 8.14 (56), and to relate LHD personnel expenditures to core functions (49).

The findings from these various studies provided little comfort to the public health community as to the adequacy of the public health system in address-

ing its core functions. One recent study (49) found that 89% of the manpower hours of one large LHD were expended in carrying out practices related to the assurance function. Nine percent of the total manpower hours were devoted to the assessment function while only two percent were devoted to policy development. When the various practices and functions were related to specific programs and services, primary care and communicable disease programs consumed three fourths of the LHD's resources (49).

Several studies used similar measures of core function-related practice performance to examine mean LHD performance scores (the percent of practice performance measures fulfilled). In one study of a national sample of 208 LHDs in 1993, the mean performance score on a panel of ten measures was 50% (56). In another 1993 study of 370 LHDs in six states, the mean performance score was 56% based on a panel of 26 items (44). The use of this same 26-item panel with a group of 14 LHDs that have been longitudinally followed since the 1970s produced similar performance patterns (30). These findings are consistent with results from NACCHO's 1992/93 profile of LHDs(37), which found similar levels of performance using questions that were comparable to many of those used in these various studies.

During the formulation of the Clinton Health Security Act proposal in 1994, federal officials sought to integrate public health practice into the health reform proposal. A set of core public health functions was identified and received widespread attention despite creating some confusion with the IOM report core functions. PHS established a national working group to develop a single characterization of public health practice in view of confusion surrounding the IOM core functions, health reform's core functions, CDC's ten public health practices, and NACCHO's blueprint for healthy communities (36). The result was a single statement that characterized what public health does for external constituencies and how it does those things for more internal constituencies. The list of ten has become known as the ten essential services of public health (8), although it is comprised of inputs, processes, and outputs (services) (52).

Efforts to Measure Public Health Structure

Both before and after the IOM report, efforts were made to assess the overall national public health system. These efforts have focused primarily on structural aspects of the system (such as the presence or absence of a LHD in a jurisdiction and the full or part-time availability of health officers), but have not necessarily related these inputs to public health's functions. During the period 1914–1988, several examinations described below tracked increases in the number of LHDs, the number of full-time LHDs, and the population served by those categories of LHDs.

After 1915, the growth in the number of LHDs occurred primarily among county-based agencies. The number of counties with full-time public health services increased from 14 in 1915 to 762 in 1935 to 2088 in 1950 (23, 46). Since some of these agencies served more than one county, and because some were organized at the municipal, district, or other level, the number of LHD units actually

grew from 886 in 1935 to 1348 in 1950 (46). The proportion of the population served by full-time LHDs increased from 56% in 1935 to 89% by 1957 (46).

The Emerson Report had advanced several targets for the national public health system including one calling for complete coverage of the population by full-time LHDs (meaning those with full-time health officers) (14). However, other targets established in the Emerson Report also allow for some interesting insights into the capacity of the national public health system at this time. For example, the committee found that the nation had 64% of the public health personnel and 63% of financial resources needed to assure full coverage of the population (14).

Outside of these APHA-generated efforts, there were only scattered efforts to capture information on public health practice in a composite fashion. These include a follow-up to Chapin's 1914 examination of state health departments performed by Ferrell in 1929 (48) and Mountin's authoritative report (33) on federal, state, and local public health activities in 1950. More extensive information on state health agencies became available later through the establishment by ASTHO of a national Public Health Reporting System in 1970 through the Public Health Foundation (PHF). Although useful in terms of expenditures and programs for the official state health agencies, until the 1990s, these reports had very little information on the public health activities of LHDs. Information on state-level environmental protection, substance abuse, and mental health services was also incomplete if these services were the responsibility of agencies other than

the official state health agency. An effort to capture all core function-related expenditures of states through these various state agencies was piloted in 1996 after an earlier effort to identify core function-related expenditures of official state health agencies was completed in 1994 (42).

Information on local public health activities became increasingly available after 1987 through the efforts of PHF, CDC, and NACCHO. PHF has attempted to enhance information reported by state health agencies about local public health activities in its reporting system and also in its 1994 study of core function-related expenditures in six states (42). However, the most extensive information on local public health activities has been provided by recent profiles of LHD by NACCHO (35, 37), and of state-local systems by CDC (11).

Lessons from 80 Years of Measurement

During the 60-year period from 1925–1985, an increasing body of information was being assembled on the structure of public health practice (LHDs, expenditures, health officers, boards of health, state-local relationship, size and type of jurisdiction, agency staff, professional disciplines of staff, organization, structure, etc). At the same time, information on services provided to the community was increasingly available for the basic six, as well as chronic disease prevention, medical care services, and a variety of optional and optimal services. Even with such information on the inputs and outputs of public health practice, the links between inputs and outputs were not clear, and their relationship to an effective governmental presence were even less so. Further, this information base was largely generated and used within the governmental public health sector at the state and local level, with little impact on national policy or on nongovernmental stakeholders in the health system.

Efforts during the post-IOM report period have also failed to be comprehensive; as a result, we have neither a clear nor a complete picture of the status of public health practice at the end of the twentieth century. The NACCHO profiles provide considerable information on LHD characteristics, especially with respect to structure and services (inputs and outputs), and allow for a current estimate of full-time coverage. While there is no nationally agreed upon tool or instrument to asses whether LHDs are effectively carrying out the core functions (processes/practices), inferences from the NACCHO profiles, together with the practice performance studies stimulated by CDC, suggest that the current level of public health practice performance is 50–70% of what would be considered "fully" effective, and that fewer than 40% of the population in the United States is served by a LHD effectively addressing public health's core functions within its jurisdiction (56).

The various evaluations performed in the two eras described here are not readily comparable, and the standard of practice has no doubt changed over the past 75 years. Meaningful comparisons between the findings of the committee on Administrative Practice's evaluation in the mid-1940s and those from the early 1990s are not possible because of differences in the methods and measures. The earlier studies largely examined inputs and out-puts (services) whereas later efforts emphasized processes/practices (functions). These different approaches are illustrated in Table 1, which compares key measures from the Evaluation Schedule with 20 core function-related measures used in several studies completed in the 1990s.

These tracings are far from complete, but several common themes emerge. The first is that measurement for the sake of measurement has never been the purpose of these activities; the intent has consistently been to gather information that would be useful for improvement of local public health practice. The earliest available instruments, including the Appraisal Form and Evaluation Schedule, placed considerable emphasis on results, although generally the results of specific services rather than broader functions. In this light, they examined whether things were being done right rather than measuring whether the right things were being done.

In both periods, it has been easier to measure aspects of the public heath system than to develop consensus as to what these measurements tell us about the effectiveness of public health practice.

It was Chapin's epoch-making study of state health departments in 1914 that was mainly instrumental in directing attention to the practical advantages of expressing the extensive details of health surveys in terms of simplified numerical scores or grades; which would be combined into a single total score. This proposal of expressing public health activity and achievements in terms of numerical scores precipitated heated debate in the early meetings of the Committee on Administrative Practice . . . On the one side was the fear of scientific unsoundness in attempting to place weighted values on the separate measures and practices followed in a public health program. Opposed to this was the feeling that the promotion of public health require some means of ready visualization of degrees of achievement in order to create understanding and interest on the part of both the public and professional groups (6).

Where the Appraisal Form of the 1920s and 1930s placed emphasis on health department effort such as "number of visits" and "number of inspections," the Evaluation Schedule of the 1940s and 1950s focused on the resulting health protection of the community as a whole, recognizing contributions in efforts from all sources—private practitioners, voluntary agencies, and others—as well as from the health department. This information was quite useful for the local jurisdictions that voluntarily participated in these assessments. Participation was far from universal, however, so that the aggregated information could not adequately characterize the national effort. When efforts were undertaken to assess the national public health system, it was simpler to measure basic structural aspects such as number of LHDs and full-time coverage than either services or functions that were not well-defined.

In the current period, the preference for counting inputs and outputs (services) has inhibited efforts to gain national consensus on surveillance strategies and methods to assess progress toward Objective 8.14, which focuses on core function-related performance. Seven years after this important national health objective was unveiled, there are still no nationally agreed upon methods and tools for its measurement. Therefore, only limited information is available as to how close the nation is to its achievement.

Examples of Performance Measures from Evaluation Schedule[a] (1947)	**Consolidated Panel of Core-Function Related Performance Measures[b] (1995)**
Hospital beds: percentage in approved hospitals	***Assessment***
Practicing physicians: population per physician	For the jurisdiction severed by your local health department, is there a community needs assessment process that systematically describes the prevailing health status in the community?
Practicing dentists: population per dentist	In the past three years in your jurisdiction, has the local public health agency surveyed the population for behavioral risk factors?
Water: percentage of population in communities over 2500 served with approved water	For the jurisdiction served by your local health agency, are timely investigations of adverse health events, including communicable disease outbreaks and environmental health hazards, conducted on an ongoing basis?
Sewerage: percentage of population in communities over 2500 served with approved sewerage systems	Are the necessary laboratory services available to the local public health agency to support investigations of adverse health events and meet routine diagnostic and surveillance needs?
Water: percentage of rural school children served with approved water supplies	For the jurisdiction served by your local public health agency, has an analysis been completed of the determinants and contributing factors of priority health needs, adequacy of existing health resources, and the population groups most impacted?
Excreta disposal: percentage of rural school children served with approved means of excreta disposal	In the past three years in your jurisdictions, has the local public health agency conducted an analysis of age-specific participation in preventive and screening services?
Food: percentage of food-handlers reached by group instruction program	***Policy Development***
Food: percentage of restaurants and lunch counters with satisfactory facilities	For the jurisdiction served by your local public health agency, is there a network of support and communication relationships which includes health-related organizations, the media, and the general public?
Milk: percentage of bottled milk pasteurized	In the past year in your jurisdiction, has there been a formal attempt by the local public health agency at informing elected officials about the potential public health impact of decisions under their consideration?
Diphtheria: percentage of children under 2 years given immunizing agent	For the jurisdiction served by your local public health agency, has there been a prioritization of the community health needs which have been identified from a community needs assessment?
Smallpox: percentage of children under 2 years given immunizing agent	In the past three years in your jurisdiction, has the local public health agency implemented community health initiatives consistent with established priorities?
Whooping cough: percentage of children under 2 years given immunizing agent	
Tuberculosis: newly reported cases per death, 5-year period	
Tuberculosis: deaths per 100,00 population, 5-year period	

(Continued on next page)

Table 1 (Continued) Comparison of Public Health Practice Performance Measures Used in 1947 and 1995

Examples of Performance Measures from Evaluation Schedule[a] (1947)	Consolidated Panel of Core-Function Related Performance Measures[b] (1995)
Tuberculosis: percentage of cases reported by death certificate	For the jurisdiction served by your local public health agency, has a community health action plan been developed with community participation to address priority community health needs?
Syphilis: percentage of cases reported in primary, secondary, and early latent stage	During the past three years in your jurisdiction, has the local public health agency developed plans to allocate resources in a manner consistent with the community health action plan?
Syphilis: percentage of reported contacts examined	*Assurance*
Maternal: puerperal deaths per 1000 total births, 5-year rate	For the jurisdiction served by your local public health agency, have resources been deployed as necessary to address the priority health needs identified in the community health needs assessment?
Maternal: percentage of antepartum cases under medical supervision seen before sixth month	In the past three years in your jurisdiction, has the local public health agency conducted an organizational self-assessment?
Maternal: percentage of women delivered at home under postpartum nursing supervision	For the jurisdiction served by your local public health agency, are age-specific priority health needs effectively addressed through the provision of or linkage to appropriate services?
Maternal: percentage of births in hospital	
Infant: deaths under 1 year of age per 1000 live births, 5-year rate	In the past three years in your jurisdiction, has there been an instance in which the local public health agency has failed to implement a mandated program or service?
Infant: deaths from diarrhea and enteritis under 1 year per 1000 live births, 2-year rate	For the jurisdiction served by your local public health agency, have there been regular evaluations of the effect that public health services have on community health status?
Infant: percentage of infants under nursing supervision before 1 month	In the past three years in your jurisdiction, has the local public health agency used professionally recognized process and outcome measures to monitor programs and to redirect resources as appropriate?
School: percentage of elementary children with dental work neglected	
Accidents: deaths from motor accidents per 100,000 population, 5-year rate	For the jurisdiction served by your local public health agency, is the public regularly provided with information about current health status, health care needs, positive health behaviors, and health care policy issues?
Health department budget: cents per capita spend by health department	In the past year in your jurisdiction, has the local public health agency provided reports to the media on a regular basis?

Sources: [a]1947 Evaluation Schedule measures (5), pp. 53–54.

[b]1995 Consolidated core function-related measures (20), pp. 14–15.

As would be expected standards, when used before 1990, primarily related to inputs and outputs rather than to the processes necessary to carry out the public health core functions characterized in the IOM report. Standards, or performance expectations, for public health core functions developed after 1990 have proven to be useful for a variety of applications, including some efforts at practice surveillance vis-à-vis Objective 8.14 (56), agency self-assessment for capacity building (29–31), and the development of performance standards in state-local public health systems (54). Still, these standards appear to be in an early stage of development. Perfor-mance standards for other health organizations have become commonplace in recent decades (21), often involving the Joint Commis-sion on the Accreditation of Health Care Organizations (JCAHO). The establishment of a national accreditation or certification initiative for LHDs through either the national public health organizations or JCAHO has not been given serious consideration. Absent a federal initiative to support and fund core function activities of LHDs through block grants to states, a voluntary national accreditation program for LHDs may be the most realistic approach to promoting widespread adoption of practice standards related to the core functions (53).

The somewhat interchangeable use of the terms functions and services, particularly in the earlier period, is revealing in that it suggests that, at least as perceived initially, the prime function of local public health was to serve. The "basic six" were essentially six services, five clearly so (communicable disease, environmental sanitation, public

Table 2 Types of Measures Used in Activities Designed to Measure Public Health Practice

Activity	Inputs	Functions/ Processes	Outputs	Outcomes
Appraisal Forms (1920s and 1930)	×		×	
Evaluation Schedule (1940s)	×		×	
Public Health Reporting System (1970s thru 1990s)	×		×	
NACCHO Profiles (1990s)	×	×	×	
Practice Performance Measures (1990s)		×		
Comprehensive Performance Monitoring System for Public Health Practice	×	×	×	×

Source: Authors.

health lab services, maternal and child health, health education), whereas the sixth (vital statistics) reflected primarily the service elements of registering vital events. This confusion of services with functions is of more than passing interest in that measuring the performance of public health functions is essential to improve performance. If services are considered synonymous with functions, and services are measured, then the best that can be expected is that the performance of those services may be improved. Yet these may or may not be the right services in terms of community need and expectations. Operational definitions for the core functions (such as practice performance standards), to be measured along with inputs, outputs (including services), and outcomes, provide a more comprehensive framework for performance monitoring of the public health system (Table 2). This type of comprehensive performance monitoring activity requires a performance data base similar to the one proposed by Studnicki (50).

Revised LHD certification requirements in Illinois illustrate these issues. As part of an exten-

sive re-examination and restructuring of state-local public health activities, the framework for rules governing state certification of LHDs in Illinois was changed from one based on services provided to one based on carrying out public health's core functions within the community (54). Before 1993, to be certified by the state health department, Illinois LHDs had to meet program requirements for ten specific programs. After 1993, LHDs were required to meet performance expectations related to public health core functions. This requirement virtually changed the definition of a LHD from one based on its outputs to one based on its performance relative to its core functions (Table 3). Services that would result from each LHD's carrying out of its core functions would include three categories: those required by state public health laws (communicable disease control, food sanitation, sewage, water); those required by local laws or ordinances (variable from jurisdiction to jurisdiction) and those addressing priority community health needs established through a community needs assessment and planning process. Assessing programs and

Table 3 Requirements for Certification of Local Health Departments in Illinois Before and After July 1993	
Before July 1993, to Be Certified As a Local Health Department in Illinois, a Local Health Agency Must Carry Out the Following Programs:	**After July 1993, to Be Certified As a Local Health Department in Illinois, a Local Health Agency Must:**
Food sanitation	Assess health needs of the community
Potable water	Investigate health effects and hazards
Maternal health/family planning	
Child health	Advocate and build community support
Communicable disease control	
Private sewage	Develop policies and plans to address needs
Solid waste	
Nuisance control	Manage resources
Chronic disease	Implement programs
Administration	Evaluate and provide quality assurance
	Inform and educate the public

Source: Authors.

services alone, without examining performance of the processes that generate such services, leaves gaps in our understanding of LHD effectiveness vis-à-vis its core functions. Measuring inputs and outputs (i.e. services), without the core function-related processes, is similarly inadequate.

The preceding examination raises the interesting question as to whether the functions of public health have changed over this century. One possibility or suggestion is that it is not the functions that have changed but our ability to measure their performance; we now have a conceptual framework that allows for services to be distinguished from practices and new tools developed subsequent to the IOM report that can be used to measure different aspects of this framework.

An alternative or even additional explanation is that an understanding of the functions of

public health has matured over time. The development and expansion of the public health infrastructure in the Untied States advanced at a rapid pace between 1900 and 1950. It is conceivable that maturation of the functions of local public health was not possible until that infrastructure had been put into place. While the IOM core functions are often conceptualized as a linear process (assessment → policy development → assurance), it appears that the assurance function, at least in terms of emphasis, developed without commensurate maturation of the other core functions. The limited studies to date consistently identify higher performance on assurance-related practices rather than those related to either assessment or policy development (37, 44, 45, 55, 56). However, improved local public health performance through implementation of APEXPH and its

derivatives has been demonstrated (55). Greater promotion of these approaches will require new federal incentives to states and localities and greater commitment of the LHD community to performance improvement.

The lack of direct federal public health leadership throughout both periods, but most clearly before 1988, is also of interest. PHS involvement in public health practice measurement efforts can be traced back to the early days of the Committee on Municipal Health Department Practice, despite the lack of an effective public health presence in the federal government. Before the mid-1930s the Public Health Service was a unit of the US Treasury Department. After its placement in the Federal Security Agency and the succession of federal health agencies, there was some improvement. The PHS agency most closely identified with public health practice, CDC, was not created until 1946. Most of CDC's early emphasis was on categorical programs, although in the late 1980s its Public Health Practice Program Office catalyzed several national capacity-building initiatives. Notably missing even from the 1990 National Health Objectives (established in the early 1980s) was any allusion to local public health functions or to the extent of their availability across the United States. Although this omission was corrected with the year 2000 national health objectives, the lack of national policy and operational plans to measure and achieve that objective suggests a continuing lack of federal leadership. While PHS led the effort to develop a consensus vision for public health in the United States including a formulation of ten essential public health services, there has been little success in reaching consensus on a national practice surveillance system. In addition, the switch to the essential public health services framework from the public health practices may have slowed efforts to measure public health practice effectiveness (52). In an era of increasing political pressure against vast federal bureaucracies and in favor of returning decision-making to state and local governments, another federal government-inspired surveillance system faces formidable obstacles. Without strong federal leadership, the task might only be accomplished if the national practice organizations (especially ASTHO, NACCHO, and APHA) were to make it their priority. Amid other challenges to the public health system in the late 1990s, this is unlikely. APHA's leadership role from 1920 through the 1970s is noteworthy, although it appears to have diminished considerably since the days of Winslow and Emerson.

Efforts from both eras fail to link public health practice to health outcomes in the community. Before 1990, there was no real effort to do so. After 1990, only one study has attempted to relate LHD practice performance levels to some general community health status indicators (47). No clear links were found, but the study did not focus on health outcomes targeted by community needs assessments. It is now possible to perform such an examination where practice performance has been tracked over time, and where community needs assessments have led to interventions for high priority community health problems. Various levels of practice performance can now be related to changes in key outcome measures to identify the effectiveness of the various practices.

The increased interest in the broader aspects of public health performance monitoring is apparent in several initiatives developed since 1995. Many of these were stimulated by a 1994 CDC-sponsored Symposium on Mea-suring Public Health Practice, which examined the state of the art and spawned several important additional initiatives. In 1995, an IOM Committee on Using Performance Monitoring to Improve Community Health was established to broadly examine data needs for monitoring the performance of health services in relation to community health (20). In the same year, PHS funded a project to define information needs for a national public health infrastructure surveillance system that would collect information on inputs, processes, services, and outcomes of public health activities at all three governmental levels. Also in 1995, HRSA funded an evaluation of the training and education needs of the public health workforce to determine the size and composition of the professional public health workforce as well as its qualifications, staffing patterns, and distribution by public health core function. The longitudinal study funded by the Robert Wood Johnson Foundation tracking changes within the health systems of 12 metropolitan areas has added a component to specifically monitor changes in the public health activities within those sites. The findings and recommendations of these panels and studies will help define the public health system information needs for the next decade and beyond, as well as facilitate the use of information for community health improvement initiatives.

Conclusions

The history of measuring public health practice before the IOM report lacked a conceptual framework that viewed services as an output of the public health system's functions. As needs and conditions changed, appropriate public health responses in the form of services changed. An initial set of six basic services may have represented an appropriate product of a functioning public health system in the 1920s, at least for LHDs serving large urban populations. But to measure various aspects of those services as a means of assessing performance of the underlying functions is incomplete at best. Performance measurement in the public health system must be able to measure inputs, processes, outputs, and outcomes in ways that allow for changes in one to be linked one with another. Without such a comprehensive public health practice performance monitoring system, we will not be able to make the changes necessary to improve the results we seek. After 80 years of trial and error, the essential ingredients are in place. A conceptual framework, useful instruments, a national objective for the public health system, and the means of tracking progress over time are all in place. However, the commitment from the public health practice community and the national leadership to get the job done remains elusive. Although it may have taken 75 years to put the pieces in place, any further delay in establishing a comprehensive national system for public health practice will be costly. Ironically, it will now be much easier to measure that price in terms of the unrealized gains in health status that can be achieved through improved public health practice.

Literature Cited

1. American Public Health Association, Committee on Municipal Health Department Practice. 1922. *First Report*, Part 1. *Am. J. Public Health* 12(2):7–15

2. American Public Health Association, Committee on Municipal Health Department Practice. 1922. *First Report*, Part 2. *Am. J. Public Health* 12(2):138–47

3. American Public Health Association, Committee on Municipal Health Department Practice. 1926. *Fifth Report, Am. J. Public Health* 16(1):2–4 (Suppl. Abstr.)

4. American Public Health Association, Committee on Administrative Practice. 1926. Appraisal form for city health work. *Am. J. Public Health* 16(1):1–65 (Suppl.)

5. American Public Health Association, Committee on Administrative Practice. 1947. *Evaluation Schedule for Use in the Study and Appraisal of Community Health Programs.* New York: APHA

6. American Public Health Association. 1944. From health honor roll to national reporting area. *Am. J. Public Health* 34:1099–102 (editorial)

7. American Public Health Association. 1951. The local health department—services and responsibilities: an official statement of the American Public Health Association adopted November 1, 1950. *Am. J. Public Health* 41:302–7

8. Baker EL, Melton RJ, Stange PV, Fields ML, Koplan JP, et al. 1994. Health reform and the health of the public: forging community health partnerships. *JAMA* 272:1276–82

9. Berwick DM, 1995. From measuring to managing the improvement of prevention. *Am. J. Prev. Med.* 11(6):385–87

10. Brooks EF, Miller CA. 1987. Recent changes in selected local health departments: implications for their capacity to guarantee basic medical services. *Am. J. Prev. Med.* 3(3):134–41

11. Cent. Disease Control Prev., Public Health Practice Program Off., Div. Public health Systems. 1991. *Profile of state and territorial public health systems, 1990.* Atlanta, GA: CDC

12. Cent. Disease Control Prev., US Public Health Service. 1994. Public health core functions—Alabama, Maryland, Mississippi, New Jersey, South Carolina and Wisconsin. 1993. *MMWR* 43(1):13–15

13. DeFriese GH. Hetherington JS, Brooks, EF, Miller CA, Jain SC. et al. 1981. The program implications of administrative relationships between local health departments and state and local government. *Am. J. Public Health* 71(10):1109–15

14. Emerson H, Luginbuhl M. 1945. *Local Health Units for the Nation.* New York: Commonwealth Fund

15. Halverson WL. 1945. A twenty-five year review of the work of the committee on administrative practice. *Am. J. Public Health* 35(12):1253–59

16. Handler AS, Turnock BJ, Hall W, Potsic S, Munson J. et al. 1995. A strategy for measuring local public health practice. *Am. J. Prevn. Med.* 11(6):29–35 (Suppl.)

17. Hanlon JJ. 1973. Is there a future for local health departments. *Health Serv. Rep.* 88(10):898–901

18. Harrington HJ. 1978. *The Improvement Process: How America's Leading Companies Improve Quality.* New York: McGraw Hill

19. Institute of Medicine, Committee on the Future of Public Health. 1988. *The Future of Public Health.* Washington, DC: Natl. Acad. Press

20. Institute of Medicine, Committee on Using Performance Monitoring to Improve Community Health. 1996. *Using Performance Monitoring to Improve Community Health: Exploring the Issues.* Washington, DC: Natl. Acad. Press

21. Joint Commission on Accreditation of Healthcare Organizations. 1990. *Primer on Indicator Development and Application: Measuring Quality in Health Care.* Oakbrook Terrace, IL: JCAHO

22. Kaluzny AD, McLaughlin CP, Simpson K. 1992. Applying total management concepts to public health organizations. *Public Health Rep.* 107(3):257–64

23. Krantz FW. 1942. The present status of full-time local health organizations. *Public health Rep.* 57:194–96

24. Miller CA, Brooks EF, DeFriese GH, Gilbert B, Jain SC, Kavaler F. 1977. A survey of local public health departments and their directors. *Am. J. Public Health* 67(10):931–39

25. Miller CA, Gilbert B, Warren DG, Brooks EF, DeFriese GH. et al. 1977. Statutory authorizations for the work of local health departments. *Am. J. Public Health* 67(10):940–45

26. Miller CA, Moose MK, Kotch JB, Brown ML, Brainerd MP. 1981. Role of local health departments in the delivery of medical care. *Am J. Public Health* 71(1):15–29 (Suppl.)

27. Miller CA, Moore KS, Richards TB. 1993. The impact of critical events of the 1980s on core functions for a selected group of local health departments. *Public Health Rep.* 108(6):95–700

28. Miller CA, Moore KS, Richards TB, Kotelchuck M, Kaluzny AD. 1993. Longitudinal observations on a selected group of local health departments: a preliminary report. *J. Public Health Pol.* 14(1):34–50

29. Miller CA, Moore KS, Richards TB, Monk JD. 1994. A proposed method for assessing the performance of local public health functions and practices. *Am. J. Public Health* 84(11):1743–49

30. Miller CA, Moore KS, Richards TB, McKaig C. 1994. A screening survey to assess local public health performance. *Public Health Rep.* 109(5):659–64

31. Miller CA, Richards TB, Davis SM, McKaig CA, Koch GG. et al. 1995. Validation of a screening survey to assess local public health performance. *J. Public Health Manage Pract.* 1(1):63–69

32. Mountin JW. 1952. The health department's dilemma. *Public Health Rep.* 67(3):223–29

33. Mountin JW, Flook E. 1953. *Guide to Health Organization in the United States, 1951.* Public Health Serv. Publ. No. 196. Washington, DC:US GPO

34. Myers BA, Steinhardt BJ, Bruce J, Mosley ML, Cashman JW. 1968. The medical care activities of local health units. *Public Health Rep.* 83(9):757–69

35. National Association of County and City Health Officials. 1990. *National Profile of Local Health Departments.* Washington, DC: NACCHO

36. National Association of County and City Health Officials. 1994. *Blueprint for a Healthy Community: A Guide for Local Health Departments.* Washington DC: NACCHO

37. National Association of County and City Health Officials. 1995. *1992–1993 National Profile of Local Health Departments.* Washington, DC: NACCHO

38. National Association of County Health Officials, 1990. *An Assessment Protocol for Excellence in Public Health.* Washington, DC: NACCHO

39. Oberle MW, Baker EL. 1994. Healthy People 2000 and community health planning. *Annu. Rev. Public Health* 15:259–75

40. Pickett G. 1980. The future of health departments: the governmental presence. *Annu. Rev. Public Health* 1:297–321

41. Pratt M, McDonald S, Libbey P, Oberle M, Liang A. 1996. Local health departments in Washington State use APEX to assess capacity. *Public Health Rep.* 111:87–91

42. Public Health Foundation, 1995. Measuring state expenditures for core public health functions. *Am. J. Prev. Med.* 11(6):58–73 (Suppl.)

43. Rawlings ID. 1927. *The Rise and Fall of Disease in Illinois.* Springfield, IL: IL Dep. Public Health

44. Richards TB, Rogers JJ, Christenson GM, Miller CA, Gatewood DD, Taylor MS. 1995. Assessing public health practice: application of ten core function measures of community health in six states. *Am. J. Prev. Med.* 11(6):36–40 (Suppl.)

45. Richards TB, Rogers JJ, Christenson GM, Miller CA, Taylor MS, Cooper AD. 1995. Evaluating local public health performance at a community level on a statewide basis. *J. Public Health Manage. Pract.* 1(4):70–83

46. Sanders B. 1959. Local health departments: growth or illusion. *Public Health Rep.* 74(1):13–20

47. Schenk SE, Miller CA, Richards TB. 1995. Public health performance related to selected health status and risk measures. *Am. J. Prev. Med.* 11(6):55–57 (Suppl.)

48. Shonick W. 1995. *Government and Health Services: Government's Role in the Development of U.S. Health Services.* New York: Oxford Univ. Press

49. Studnicki J. 1995. Evaluating the performance of public health agencies: information needs. *Am. J. Prev. Med.* 11(6):74–80 (Suppl.)

50. Studnicki J, Steverson B, Blais HN, Goley E, Richards TB, Thornton JN. 1994. Analyzing organizational practices in local health departments. *Public Health Rep.* 109(4):485–90

51. Terris M, Kramer NA. 1949. Medical care activities of full-time health departments. *Am. J. Public Health* 39:1129–35

52. Turnock BJ, Handler AS. 1995. Evaluating the performance of local health agencies. II. The 10 public health practices vs the 10 public health services. (letter) *Am. J. Public Health* 85:1295–96

53. Turnock BJ, Handler AS. 1996. Is public health ready for reform? The case for accrediting local health departments. *J. Public Health Manage. Pract.* 2(3):41–45

54. Turnock BJ, Handler AS, Dyal WW, Christenson G, Vaughn EH, et al. 1994. Implementing and assessing organizational practices in local health departments. *Public Health Rep.* 109(4):478–84

55. Turnock BJ, Handler AS, Hall W. Lenihan DP, Vaughn EH. 1995. Capacity-building influences on Illinois local health departments. *J. Public Health Manage. Pract.* 1(3):50–58

56. Turnock BJ, Handler AS, Hall W. Potsic S, Nalluri R, Vaughn EH. 1994. Local health department effectiveness in addressing the core functions of public health. *Public Health Rep.* 109:653–58

57. Vaughan HF. 1972. Local health services in the United States: the story of CAP. *Am. J. Public Health* 62:95–108

58. US Public Health Service. 1990. *Healthy People 2000: National Health Promotion and Disease Prevention Objectives.* DHHS Publ. No. (PHS) 91–50212. Washington, DC: US GPO

59. Walker WW. 1939. The new appraisal form for local health work. *Am. J. Public Health* 29(5):490–500

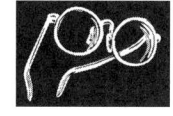 **Article Review Form at end of book.**

List the five issue areas that are "important" to local health departments (LHDs). Discuss the difficulties the LHDs faced in obtaining reimbursements from managed care organizations.

Assessing the Impact of Medicaid Managed Care on TB Activities in Local Health Departments

Liza C. Corso, Grace Gorenflo, Thomas B. Richards, Zachary Taylor, Carol K. Brown, and Patricia J. Gadow

Liza C. Corso, MPA, is Project Manager for the National Association of County and City Health Officials in Washington, D.C.
Grace Gorenflo, RN, MPH, is Associate Executive Director for the National Association of County and City Health Officials in Washington, D.C.
Thomas B. Richards, MD, is a Medical Officer with the Public Health Practice Program Office of the Centers for Disease Control and Prevention in Atlanta, Georgia.
Zachary Taylolr, MD, is Chief, Prevention Effectiveness Section, Research and Evaluation Branch, Division of Tuberculosis Elimination of the Centers for Disease Control and Prevention in Atlanta, Georgia.
Carol K. Brown, MS, is Director of Research and Development for the National Association of County and City Health Officials in Washington, D.C.
Patricia J. Gadow, MPH, is Director and Health Officer of the Madison Department of Public Health in Madison, Wisconsin, and Chairperson of the Tuberculosis Committee at the National Association of County and City Health Officials in Washington, D.C.

Three in-depth case studies were conducted to explore the impact of Medicaid managed care on local health department prevention activities. Tuberculosis (TB) was selected as a sentinel issue because TB includes both clinical treatment and population-based public health considerations (such as surveillance and contact tracing). Overall, study results indicated that there has been a minimal impact on TB prevention and control services, primarily because few TB patients are served by managed care. However, the sites offer many suggestions for areas to monitor, possible collaborative opportunities, and mechanisms to assure continued TB prevention and control.

The shift to managed care as a major method of health care delivery raises many questions about the effect it will have on public health activities. Knowledge of the working relationships and interactions between managed care organizations (MCOs) and local health departments (LHDs) can provide invaluable insights and advice for communities as MCOs provide more commercial health insurance and serve increasing numbers of Medicaid recipients.[1]

An issue of primary concern is the degree to which managed care will affect prevention activities. To examine this issue more closely, TB was selected as a potential sentinel marker for change because TB includes both clinical treatment and population-based considerations (such as surveillance and contact tracing).[2] Through their public health authority, state and local health departments have the ultimate responsibility for preventing and controlling TB. However, with the proliferation of MCOs, managed care may begin to provide some population-based services that have been traditionally provided by LHDs.

Methodology

In 1995, the National Association of County and City Health Officials (NACCHO), in collaboration with the Public Health

From *Journal of Public Health Management Practice,* November 1998 (Vol. 4, No. 6), pp. 62–68.

Practice Program Office (PHPPO), Centers for Disease Control and Prevention (CDC), and the Division of Tuberculosis Elimination at the National Center for HIV, STD, and TB Prevention (NCH-STP), CDC, established a work group to explore the impact of managed care on TB prevention and control. Under the guidance of this group, NACCHO identified three LHD jurisdictions where a state-based Medicaid managed care program existed and where the community TB incidence warranted an active TB prevention and control program. In addition, NACCHO identified the following five issues that were of particular importance to LHDs in TB prevention and control:

1. obtaining sustainable, long-range funding for clinical services and maintaining the essential resource base of TB control programs
2. maintaining the authority and leadership of LHDs in TB prevention and control strategies
3. improving the expertise of health care providers in treating and controlling TB
4. providing appropriate social services to TB patients
5. providing appropriate care to high-risk populations

In-depth case studies were conducted in three LHD jurisdictions: Metropolitan Nashville-Davidson County Health Department, Nashville, TN; St. Louis Department of Health and Hospitals, St. Louis, MO; and Palm Beach County Public Health Unit, West Palm Beach, FL. Before the site visit, NACCHO asked LHD staff at each site to complete a questionnaire that included 86 items about characteristics of the jurisdiction, TB prevention and control indicators, TB services provided by the LHD, the man-

aged care environment, and the five identified topics of special interest to LHDs. After NACCHO received the completed questionnaires, a team consisting of two NACCHO representatives and one CDC representative conducted a two-day site visit at each LHD during May and June of 1996. These visits included discussions with LHD staff; state personnel; and representatives from hospital, community-based organizations, and managed care. A detailed report on the case studies, including a copy of the questionnaire used, is available from NACCHO.[3]

Findings

The experiences of the three study sites indicate that the introduction of Medicaid managed care has had minimal impact on TB prevention and control activities thus far. A primary reason for this is that few of the traditional Medicaid population are at high risk for TB—with the exception of persons infected with human immunodeficiency virus (HIV) and refugees. These case studies do offer insight into new procedures or mechanisms that should be considered to assure continued TB prevention and control in a changing health care environment. The case studies also suggest opportunities for collaboration among LHDs, MCOs, state agencies, and others, and also may be considered for other prevention activities.

Characteristics of the Jurisdiction

The three study jurisdictions served populations ranging in size from 500,000 to 1 million. Each study site showed a decrease in the overall TB rate, and

an increase in the rate among high-risk populations from 1990 to 1995. Among those eligible for Medicaid, specific high-risk populations, such as those infected with HIV and refugees, represent increasing TB rates. Therefore, it is possible that MCOs will be treating more of these patients for TB in the future. Additionally, expanding eligibility for state Medicaid programs to populations such as the homeless could further increase the number of TB patients under the care of MCOs. See Table 1 for more information about the characteristics of the study sites.

The Managed Care Environment and TB

The three case study sites exist in somewhat varied managed care environments. Tennessee's Medicaid managed care program (TennCare) had been in place for two years at the time of the study and provides care for both the traditional Medicaid population as well as the uninsured and insurable. Missouri's program, Managed Care Plus (MC+), which had been in place for approximately six months at the time of the study, is being implemented in stages across the state, thus offering opportunity for changes and improvements within the system. In the first phase of the program, only the traditional Medicaid population was eligible: Aid to Families with Dependent Children (AFDC) recipients, pregnant women, children in poverty, children in state custody, and adults eligible under the refugee program. Florida's program (MediPass), which had been operating for about two years at the time of the site visit, also provides care to the traditional Medicaid eligible population

Table 1 Selected Characteristics for the Three Local Health Departments (LHDs)*

Characteristic	Metropolitan Nashville-Davidson County Health Department, Nashville, Tennessee	City of St. Louis, Missouri Department of Health and Hospitals, St. Louis, Missouri	HRS Palm Beach County Public Health Unit, West Palm Beach, Florida
Total population in jurisdiction served, 1995	529,892	369,000	962,802
Overall TB case rate per 100,000 population, 1995	14.9	10.8	13.5
Percent of cases known to be HIV seropositive, 1995	14.2%	10%	68%
Percent of TB cases among the foreign born, 1995	9.5%	10%	20%
Total LHD expenditures for TB control, 1995	$723,000	$339,000	$2,615,054
Total LHD staff, 1995	558	465	1095.5
Total LHD staff dedicated to TB control (FTEs), 1995	21.5	10.5	39
Medicaid Managed Care Program	TennCare	Managed Care Plus (MC+)	MediPass
HCFA Waiver	1115	1915(b)	1915(b)

*All data were provided by the study site local health departments.

through contracts with MCOs in the state. Unique to the Palm Beach County site is the fact that the LHD serves as a gatekeeper and provider for indigent health care and also operates a Medicaid HMO.

In comparing the three sites, we found that each LHD plays a different role in its managed care environment. The Nashville and St. Louis LHDs are moving toward a role that focuses less on providing primary care services and concentrates more fully on the core functions of public health, assessment, assurance, and policy development. On the other hand, the Palm Beach County LHD is retaining a strong foothold in providing primary care services and competes with the other HMOs in the community. Additionally, each LHD is experiencing different relationships with the MCOs, both formally and informally. The Nashville LHD has had formal contracts with several of the MCOs in its jurisdiction, but com-

munication and collaboration with them has been limited so far. The St. Louis LHD, which has been operating in a managed care environment for a much shorter time, has already extended invitations to MCOs for discussion. In that community, the MCO representatives appear very interested in establishing in-depth relationships with the LHD in the future, although they have been busy with enrollment and establishing a niche in the market. On the other hand, the Palm Beach County LHD is seen as a competitor by HMOs, which has limited its relationships with HMOs.

In each of the sites, various efforts are being made to promote TB prevention activities in the new managed care environment. For example the TennCare contracts with MCOs state that LHDs must obtain prior authorization before providing TB services to patients. However, recognizing the importance of providing prompt and immediate care, the Nashville LHD and the six MCOs

in the jurisdiction made informal agreements that no prior approval is necessary. On the other hand, the Missouri MC+ RFP included contract language stating the MC+ plan is responsible for reimbursing the LHD on a fee-for-service basis for TB-related screening, diagnosis, and treatment services provided to plan members. Florida also recently implemented legislation waiving the pre-authorization requirement for selected services, including TB. All of these provisions enhance the LHDs' ability to promptly identify and treat TB in managed care patients.

The Five Issue Areas

An analysis of each of the five issue areas that are important to LHDs indicates interesting trends and differences. Additionally, several opportunities for collaboration to improve TB control and prevention were noted. Examples include: establishing a TB task force to develop a strategic plan for TB prevention and control, including input from MCOs; developing patient treatment protocols and decision trees that MCOs could distribute to MCO providers; working together to ensure that provider profiles maintained by MCO administrators to monitor referrals from MCO primary care providers to "expensive" specialty care providers did not inhibit referral of TB patients to LHDs for evaluation and treatment[4]; and identifying data and establishing standards for evaluating the performance of MCOs in preventing and controlling TB. The five issue areas are described in detail below.

Funding for TB Control

To analyze changes in funding over the period studied, NACCHO examined changes in revenues from local, state, federal, and private sources from 1990 to 1995, as well as changes in reimbursement levels from MCOs and Medicaid (all figures were adjusted for inflation). Each of the sites indicated that expenditures increased for both the TB control program and the overall LHD from 1990 to 1995. However, because revenue generated by the TB program is inadequate, all sites indicated that funds are shifted from other services to cover TB program expenditures. Patient fees and third-party reimbursements (including reimbursements from Medicaid and MCOs) do not appear to be a large source of funding for any of the study site TB control programs.

Each site described difficulties in obtaining reimbursement from MCOs for TB services, regardless of legislative or contractual language. Barriers encountered most often were caused by different billing requirements among the MCOs, difficulty with identifying the MCO responsible for the patient at the time of treatment, or MCO denial of LHD claims. The fact that these problems continue to occur in the presence of language such as that found in the Missouri request for proposal (RFP) indicates this issue requires further scrutiny.

Reimbursement issues were further complicated by the fact that LHDs were able to obtain reimbursement for only a few TB-related services, often at relatively low rates. In general, the LHD is eligible for Medicaid reimbursement for TB testing, x-rays, laboratory tests, and clinic visits. Some of the more expensive services that LHDs provide, such as directly observed therapy, contact tracing, and social services, are not reimbursable.

The case studies suggested several collaborative opportunities to help sustain and improve LHD reimbursement for TB prevention and control, and thus maximize the available funding. Several examples of these collaborative opportunities include: revision of state Medicaid billing codes to facilitate billing LHD TB-related services; direct funding of TB program activities, including clinical management of patients with TB at adequate levels; and establishment of a universal coding and billing system for TB services that would be easy to access and utilize. MCOs, LHDs, and state agencies could also collaborate to develop compatible billings systems with access to updated information on patient enrollment.

Authority for TB Control

As a result of their governmental role and power, state departments and LHDs have the ultimate responsibility for TB prevention and control. During site visit discussions, MCO representatives clearly recognized that state and local public health agencies have responsibility for follow-up activities (such as surveillance and contact tracing), as well as the ultimate police authority to ensure that "difficult patients" comply with TB treatment (such as directly observed therapy for substance abusers).

TB is a legally reportable disease to public health agencies: contracts in each of the sites mention the state reporting requirements for TB. However, because each of the sites indicated that physicians were not a highly reliable source of reporting, several collaborative opportunities were suggested during site visit discussions. Examples include: developing model language to include in state Medicaid contracts with MCOs that might facilitate future TB surveillance and contact tracing; exploring the use of MCO administrative databases (such as claim records and pharmacy billing records) to evaluate whether all TB patients are being reported; and identifying out-of-state laboratories used by MCOs for TB laboratory testing so that public health agencies can follow up to ensure that all TB laboratory reports are received.

TB Expertise

LHD expertise in TB prevention and control activities was well recognized in each of the three case study sites, as evidenced by the number of consultations and referrals they each receive (this was true even before the advent of managed care). The TB program staff in each of the sites indicated that primary interaction with private providers was to provide advice and guidance about the testing, diagnosis, and treatment of TB. In addition, two of the three sites worked with community coalitions and TB task forces to improve provider expertise and better educate high-risk population groups.

Each site indicated that private provider knowledge about TB was varied; unfortunately, unless providers encounter TB patients relatively frequently in their practice, they may not be current on recommended procedures for TB testing, diagnosis, and treatment. LHD staff typically addressed provider education on an individual basis, sending guidelines and information to providers who asked questions or who were discovered to be treating a case improperly.

The onset of managed care provides several potential opportunities to collaborate on strengthening the expertise of private providers. Examples include: using coalitions or task forces to begin discussions with MCOs about collaborative opportunities; adding MCO representatives to task forces for TB prevention and control; developing jointly sponsored educational seminars targeted at MCO providers; working with state agencies or medical associations in requiring educational seminars that cover TB for provider licensure; and exploring the feasibility of using MCO databases and claims records as tools for evaluating whether providers are current on procedures for TB testing, diagnosis, referral, and treatment.

Social Services

In each of the study sites, social services for TB patients (such as transportation; interpreter services; assistance with housing, food, and clothing) over-whelmingly continue to be coordinated by the LHDs and by TB outreach workers

more specifically. Because the LHDs had limited resources, providing social services represented a significant challenge that could be quite time-consuming for the outreach workers.

Although MCO representatives acknowledged the importance of case management, none of the MCOs had active social service programs targeted at TB patients nor had any made provisions to reimburse LHDs for providing social services to MCO enrollees. Additionally, MCO representatives also expressed doubt as to whether MCOs would ever deliver social services to the same extent that many LHDs do. Therefore, if TB funding were to decrease and LHDs were to turn over some of the clinical activities to MCOs, it is very possible that the provision of social services to TB patients could be adversely affected.

The case studies suggested two collaborative opportunities related to social services. An initial step would be to clarify which social services could be offered by the LHD and which social services could be provided or reimbursed by MCOs. A subsequent area for collaboration would be to work together with the community to gather resources (such as clothing, food, housing, and transportation) from a wide variety of donors.

High-Risk Populations

Although the reported overall incidence of TB is on the decline, the disease is on the rise in many special, high-risk populations. The study sites reported an increase in the TB case rates among the foreign-born, the HIV and acquired immunodeficiency syndrome (AIDS) populations, and the homeless during the period of 1990 to 1995. Given that some pa-

tients among these populations are eligible for Medicaid (such as refugees and HIV/AIDS patients), MCOs possibly may be providing more care to these patients in the future. Additionally, some states may choose to expand the eligible population to include the uninsured and the uninsurable (for example, TennCare's coverage includes the homeless population), thus creating more responsibility for MCOs with respect to special populations.

If MCOs are to assume the responsibility for treating these special populations, they will have to learn the particular needs of these groups and ways to address them, perhaps by contracting with or referring cases to the LHD. Additionally, educational efforts regarding updated treatment and referral information could be offered to providers who are most likely to treat high-risk populations, such as providers who treat a high number of foreign-born individuals.

The case studies suggest several collaborative opportunities related to high-risk populations. Examples include: improved integration of TB services with HIV services; improved collaboration between refugee resettlement organizations and Medicaid agencies to minimize the time required to process paperwork and establish eligibility for enrollment in a Medicaid MCO; development of computerized systems to determine which individual is enrolled in which MCO plan (for example, this would assist a homeless individual who has been assigned to a MCO plan but has "lost" his or her MCO identification card); and improved collaboration between correctional facilities and LHDs to assure that individuals who are released from jail receive appropriate follow up (for example, to avoid having a TB skin test applied but not read or to treat an inmate released before the full course of therapy was completed).

Discussion

Overall, the LHDs that were studied appear to be well positioned to continue providing TB screening and treatment, and most individuals interviewed during the site visits felt that LHDs should retain these functions. However, if funding decreases and the LHD moves to a role that is primarily focused on assurance and monitoring, the LHD will have to closely oversee the MCO providers because it was often mentioned that these providers have varied expertise. If this becomes the case, MCO databases could be very useful for monitoring the performance of MCO providers (although the timely availability of this information for surveillance of TB cases may be difficult to accomplish). MCO representatives also indicated that TB quality assurance and outcome studies could be conducted.

Additionally, the relatively brief time that the new state-based Medicaid managed care systems have been in place and the patterns of eligibility for Medicaid managed care may be contributing factors to the relatively low level of interaction between LHDs and MCOs in TB prevention and control. The pool of individuals eligible for Medicaid managed care in 1995–1996 often did not include some groups at highest risk for TB (such as males). Consequently, LHD TB programs and Medicaid MCOs operated relatively independently. These findings may change in the future if, for example, state-based Medicaid managed care plan eligibility requirements are expanded to include a greater proportion of groups at high risk for TB.

Similarly, because LHD and MCO relationships may vary depending on the overall rate of TB locally, caution is needed in drawing conclusions about relationships between LHDs and MCOs based on the current study. If TB rates are in the intermediate to low range, and a community has several MCOs, then the number of TB cases seen by any single MCO may not be sufficient to justify that each MCO develop an independent, full-service TB program. In such a situation, it might be relatively advantageous for all MCOs within the community to contract with the LHD to provide whatever TB services are needed. Further research is needed on whether a LHD that elects to directly provide personal health services is viewed as a competitor by MCOs and private sector health care providers and what impact, if any, this might have on the ability of the LHD to collaborate with MCOs and others in developing an effective community TB prevention and control program.

Despite limitations, which are primarily related to the small study size, the study provides interesting information for other jurisdictions to consider. Although managed care appears to have a minimal impact thus far on TB prevention and control activities, the case studies offer many suggestions for areas to monitor, possible collaborative opportunities, and mechanisms to assure continued TB prevention and control. On the other hand, each of the study sites was encountering difficulties in several areas. MCO and LHD representatives in any of the sites had not yet met or discussed TB prevention and control at length. Many MCOs may not have had the time because they are concentrating on establishing a niche in the market and enrolling patients—or have identified other priority areas to address. Both MCO and LHD representatives agreed a discussion on TB prevention and control should occur in the future; they considered it beneficial to discuss issues such as provider education and expertise, social services, the provision of TB for special populations, and the development of compatible billing systems.

Clearly, there is much to explore about the impact that managed care is having and will continue to have on TB prevention and control. Further research should be conducted, including follow-up case studies of the sites highlighted in this report, studies of a larger number of communities, and studies of selected other public health conditions that may be sentinel markers for change. In the meantime, the case studies reported in this article provide a glimpse of issues at the local level and the challenges and opportunities for LHIDs, MCOs, and others.

References

1. National Association of County and City Health Officials. *Medicaid Managed Care: A Handbook for Public Health Agencies.* Washington, D.C.: National Association of County and City Health Officials, 1995.
2. Halverson, P. K., et al. Managed Care and the Public Health Challenge of TB. *Public Health Reports* 112 (1997): 22–28.
3. National Association of County and City Health Officials. *Tuberculosis Prevention and Control in a Changing Managed Care Environment: Challenges and Opportunities for Local Health Departments, Managed Care Organizations, and Others.* Washington, D.C.: National Association of County and City Health Officials, 1997.
4. Berenson, R. Profiling and Performance Measures. What are the Legal Issues? *Medical Care* 33, no. 1 (1995): JS53–JS59.

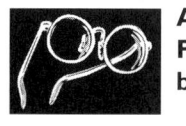

Article Review Form at end of book.

An estimated _____ would be needed to offset core public health productivity reductions associated with each 1 million in Medicaid funding losses. Discuss one of the three key steps for assessing the impact of Medicaid managed care on core public health responsibilities of Illinois local health departments.

Impact of Medicaid Resources on Core Public Health Responsibilities of Local Health Departments in Illinois

John R. Lumpkin, Laura B. Landrum, Angela Oldfield, Patti Kimmel, Michael C. Jones, Conny Mueller Moody, and Bernard J. Turnock

John R. Lumpkin, MD, MPH, is Director of the Illinois Department of Public Health in Springfield, Illinois.
Laura B. Landrum, MUPP, is Deputy Director of the Illinois Department of Public Health, Office of Epidemiology and Health Systems Development in Springfield, Illinois.
Angela Oldfield, MSW, is Chief, Division of Health Policy, for the Illinois Department of Public Health in Springfield, Illinois.
Patti Kimmell is Policy Section Administrator, Division of Health Policy, Office of Epidemiology and Health Systems Development, for the Illinois Department of Public Health in Springfield, Illinois.
Michael C. Jones, MS, is Senior Health Economist, Division of Health Policy,
Office of Epidemiology and Health Systems Development, of the Illinois Department of Public Health in Springfield, Illinois.
Conny Mueller Moody, MBA, is Policy Analyst, Division of Health Policy, Office of Epidemiology and Health Systems Development, for the Illinois Department of Public Health in Springfield, Illinois.
Bernard J. Turnock, MD, MPH, is Director and Clinical Professor of Community Health Sciences and Director of the Center for Public Health Practice at the School of Public Health, University of Illinois at Chicago.

With Illinois' plan to embark on a statewide Medicaid managed care program, the impact of Medicaid resources on core public health responsibilities of local health departments (LHDs) was assessed and found to be substantial. A reduction of $330,000 in core public health activities would likely accompany each $1 million in

Medicaid resources lost by these LHDs. Only by actively participating in the planning and implementation of these conversions can public health agencies maintain high productivity and efficiency in addressing core public health responsibilities in their communities.

Recently, managed health care delivery arrangements have proliferated both nationally and in Illinois. The growth of managed care is reflected in the increase in the variety and number of managed care delivery arrangements and by their market penetration. The potential of managed care to provide quality care and contain costs by managing utilization of services has been embraced by both employers purchasing health care benefits for their employees and by state governments seeking to contain burgeoning Medicaid costs. Applying managed care concepts to the delivery of care to the Medicaid population offers excellent opportunities to improve access to care and to seriously address the prevention of disease and injury in this population. However, such opportunities are not without potential ramifications for public health practice—as it now exists.

Although hope prevails for improving health care, there is concern about the ongoing role that public health agencies play in serving indigent populations. This concern has focused on the loss of Medicaid revenues that are now flowing to public health agencies that serve Medicaid clients when those clients transition into managed care arrangements, and on the possibility of losing public health capacity to continue performing essential public health responsibilities, including assurance of care to indigent populations.

This article describes a 1993 study that was commissioned by the Illinois Department of Public Health to determine the potential impact of Medicaid managed care on public health activities in Illinois. The resulting analysis, *Impact of Medicaid Resources on Public Health Activities of Illinois Local Health Departments*, employed a pragmatic approach of utilizing expert perceptions and available budget estimates in the absence of complete and comparable data. The study assumed that all primary care delivered by LHDs is "core" or essential public health activity—an assumption that is subject to debate. Although the research was conducted several years ago, when an Illinois Medicaid managed care waiver was under consideration by the Health Care Financing Administration (HCFA), the study continues to have significant value in illustrating the implications of a major, state-level policy change on local public health activities and on the health care delivery system. Those impacts are as follows:

- LHDs have become increasingly involved in providing direct clinical services to individuals who lack access to care, acting both as "providers of last resort" to those who lack access in the private marketplace and as "safety-net" providers at the request of various insurers such as Medicaid. The study focuses attention on the dilemma faced by LHDs as they struggle to maintain traditional public health and safety net capacities while revenue streams such as Medicaid reimbursement evaporate.

- The study argues that when LHD revenues diminish by $1, more than $1 in public health value is lost. By linking the funding for the provision of primary care and traditional, population-based public health services, LHDs have multiplied the beneficial health impacts that their program dollars deliver. For example, by offering "one-stop shopping," LHDs coordinate delivery of population-based and personal preventive care services at a common time and place, thereby improving their efficiency. In addition, by providing personal health services with clear community benefits, LHDs reach expanded populations and improve community health outcomes, enhancing their effectiveness. The study illustrates that linkages enable LHDs to magnify their available resources and improve the health of the communities they serve.

Finally, the study takes significant strides in examining relevant issues that have not been previously researched and lays the groundwork for future exploration through a model for analytical study of those issues until better quantitative data are available. Given the growing domination of the health care delivery system by managed care arrangements and the passage of the Balanced Budget Act of 1997—with its potential to expand Medicaid and cover more children who are currently uninsured—the implications of the study are even more significant today.

Introduction

Public health agencies, including LHDs serving populations of all sizes, have emerged as significant providers of personal health care services for low-income populations in the United States.[1] Some in the public health community fear that this expansion of personal health care services (including clinical, preventive, and primary care services) has occurred at the expense of the LHDs' ability to effectively carry out traditional responsibilities in the area of community-wide prevention.[2-4] Whether these changes reflect an increase, decrease, or steady state of output for core public health responsibilities depends, to a large extent, on how these responsibilities and activities are defined.

The term "core public health" (CPH) will be used here for those population-based and personal health services that are intended to:

- Prevent epidemics and the spread of disease.

- Protect against environmental hazards.

- Prevent injuries, both unintentional and intentional.

- Promote and encourage healthy behaviors.

- Respond to disasters/emergencies and assist communities in recovery.

- Assure the quality and accessibility of health services.

Among 10 essential public health services associated with these services is the duty "to link people to needed personal health services and assure the provision of health care when otherwise unavailable."[5] The provision of primary care and clinical preventive services to Medicaid recipients and other populations with limited access to health care services should be viewed as a CPH responsibility when its intent is to assure accessibility.

While resources to support the provision of personal health care services have increased from a variety of federal and state sources during the 1980s and 1990s, funding for population-based CPH activities has not kept pace. Nationally, expenditures for population-based CPH activities fell from 1.2 percent of all health expenditures in 1981 to 0.9 percent in 1993,[6] bolstering concerns that the nation's public health system is deteriorating.[7]

Core Public Health and Medicaid Managed Care Scenarios

The ever-increasing market penetration of managed care networks and the recent flurry of national and state health reform proposals signal even further changes in the financing and provision of health services in the United States. It is anticipated that a substantial portion of the personal health care and clinical preventive services now provided by public health agencies will shift to the private health sector to be provided under a variety of managed care arrangements.

This shift is likely to occur in one of three possible scenarios. Under one scenario, these changes would free up resources for expanded population-based CPH activities by LHDs. Under a second scenario, resources would follow clients to the private sector, resulting in a diminution of resources but no net reduction in either clinical services or population based efforts. Under a third scenario, the shift of services from public to private sectors would result in a decline in overall CPH efforts because Medicaid-reimbursable clinical service resources have enabled many LHDs to provide population-based CPH activities. These various scenarios are characterized by either an increase, decrease, or steady state of CPH output or productivity.

Increasingly in Illinois and elsewhere, LHDs have been encouraged to become Medicaid vendors and to expand their participation in various Medicaid–funded programs. LHDs have seized these opportunities both as a means to assure access for the low-income populations in their communities and as an attractive alternative to direct funding or grants. Illinois LHDs have responded by greatly increasing their participation and, at the same time, their dependency on Medicaid resources, especially since 1990. If Medicaid resources are now directly or indirectly enabling the provision of other CPH activities in Illinois, then the decision to enroll Medicaid recipients in private managed care systems in order to control the state's Medicaid costs could diminish public health productivity.

This effect could be offset by participation of LHDs in private managed care systems as providers of case management and primary care services, or by a provider "tax" on private managed care systems to support the local public health infrastructure. The latter option would recognize the contribution of LHDs' efforts to control infectious disease and abate environmental hazards and might include the provision that LHDs provide selected services like immunizations to managed care enrollees.

Will Medicaid Managed Care Impact Public Health Functions?

The intent of this study was to determine if—and to what extent—the loss of Medicaid resources would impact CPH activities in LHDs and the jurisdictions they serve when Medicaid recipients are enrolled in private managed care systems. Three basic questions were addressed:

1. Are Medicaid resources currently enabling other CPH activities of Illinois LHDs?

2. Would the loss of these Medicaid resources reduce the capabilities of Illinois LHDs to carry out their CPH responsibilities?

3. What additional resources may be needed to maintain the current level of CPH activities if Illinois LHDs lose these Medicaid revenues?

This study was commissioned by the Illinois Department

of Public Health (IDPH) in order to inform the budgetary, legislative, and implementation processes involved in the planned conversion to a Medicaid managed care model for Illinois (Illinois MediPlan Plus). The state agency responsible for the Medicaid program in Illinois is the Illinois Department of Public Aid (IDPA). Although previous examinations[8-14] have raised and clarified aspects of the possible impact of Medicaid managed care conversions on LHDs, none of the earlier studies quantified effects in terms of CPH output and resource requirements. This study utilized inputs from Illinois LHD administrators in order to describe and measure the effects that would occur with implementation of a statewide Medicaid managed care program.

Sources of Data and Input

Data and information used in this assessment were derived from both primary and secondary sources.[15-19] Eight Illinois LHDs participated in an in-depth analysis of their current budget and Medicaid revenues, the perceived impact of Medicaid revenue reductions on specific Medicaid-funded services and CPH activities, and their likely future roles under Illinois MediPlan Plus. These LHDs were selected to be generally representative of all 86 recognized LHDs in the state, including large LHDs from the Chicago metropolitan area, agencies serving both urban and rural populations in downstate Illinois, and small LHDs serving primarily rural populations. LHD administrators from these agencies completed a structured survey instrument that called for specific information and provided for both open- and closed-ended responses to queries. Detailed responses and comments from LHD administrators are included in the full report of this study.[20]

Using a brief structured survey form, 15 Illinois LHDs (including two of the eight agencies involved in the in-depth analysis) participated in a less extensive examination of their current budgets and the likely effects of Medicaid revenue reductions within their agencies. These agencies also supplied information on the proportion of their current budgets supporting Medicaid services and CPH activities. They also estimated what cuts in Medicaid services and CPH activities would likely accompany Medicaid funding reductions and identified which CPH responsibilities would suffer most heavily from these reductions.

Data on various IDPA and IDPH program and service expenditures also were examined. Finally, information from states where Medicaid managed care programs have already been implemented was collected through structured telephone interviews of key informants.

Key Steps for Assessing the Impact of Medicaid Managed Care on Core Public Health Responsibilities of Illinois LHDs

1. Identify Medicaid revenues that are "at risk of loss"
   - Determine level of total resources for LHDs
   - Determine sources of total resources for LHDs
   - Identify Medicaid-related resources of LHDs
   - Identify Medicaid resources "at risk" per waiver
2. Assess *potential* impact of lost Medicaid revenues on CPH output and forecast resource requirements to maintain current CPH output levels:
   - Determine current LHD CPH output (expenditures)
   - Estimate CPH output reductions associated with loss of "at-risk" Medicaid revenues
   - Estimate resources needed to compensate for CPH output reduction for each CPH function
3. Based on likely future roles for LHDs, forecast *actual* resource requirements to maintain current CPH output levels

Steps for Impact Assessment

The framework for this impact assessment (see the Box, "Key Steps for Assessing the Impact of Medicaid Managed Care on Core Public Health Responsibilities of Illinois LHDs") involved the following three key steps:

1. Identify Medicaid revenues that are "at risk of loss" to Illinois LHDs as a result of the conversion to a Medicaid managed care model and examine the relationship of these revenues to other resources available to LHDs.

2. Assess the potential impact on CPH output if all Medicaid revenues that are "at risk" are lost by Illinois LHDs and forecast resource requirements necessary to maintain current CPH output levels.

3. Based on the likely future roles for LHDs within new Medicaid managed care networks, forecast actual impact and resource requirements necessary to maintain current CPH output levels.

Table 1

Table 1 Medicaid Resources "at Risk of Loss," by Illinois LHDs with Medicaid Managed Care Conversion (1994).

	$ Million	% of LHD Total $
Estimated total 1994 resources for Illinois LHDs*	310.0	100
Estimated percent of LHD resources from selected sources**		
Local resources (taxes and fees)	170.5	55
Federal funds	21.7	7
IDPH local health protection grant	9.3	3
Other state categorical funds	65.1	21
Medicaid funds (total)	43.4	14
Identify selected Medicaid-related revenues***		
Medical services: Healthy Kids, FQHC and MD services ("at risk" per waiver)	13.0	4
Medical services plus public aid case management	32.9	11
Medical services plus public aid and public health case management	43.7	14
Medical services plus PA and PH case management plus PH family planning and lead services	50.1	16

*Based on a comparison of 1990 and 1994 agency budgets for 20 Illinois LHDs.[18–20]

**Estimates derived from various sources.[18–20]

***Based on 1994 expenditures reported by IDPA and IDPH,[15,17] with percents based on estimated total expenditures of $310 million.

Key findings related to each of these steps are described in the following sections.

Medicaid Revenues "at Risk of Loss"

Total LHD expenditures from all sources have risen to more than $300 million in Illinois. The recent rapid budget growth for Illinois LHDs has been largely due to increased Medicaid and Medicaid-related revenues, such as IDPA and IDPH Healthy Moms/Healthy Kids (HM/HK) funding. HM/HK programs provide case management and related services to Medicaid recipients from Medicaid resources as well as to non-Medicaid recipients from state funding through contracts extended from the state agencies to LHDs. LHDs and other vendors of medical services provided directly to Medicaid recipients are reimbursed separately by the Illinois Department of Public Aid in addition to these case management contracts.

It is not uncommon for 15 to 25 percent of LHD budgets to depend on Illinois' Medicaid program for medical, case management, mental health, and substance abuse services; the average for the 21 Illinois LHDs examined in this study was 14 percent. Virtually all Illinois LHDs now provide Medicaid early periodic screening, diagnosis, and treatment (EPSDT/ Healthy Kids) and HM/HK case management services. Medical service reimbursements alone account for only about 4 percent of total LHD resources, but these revenues are linked closely with HM/HK funds from IDPA and IDPH and with other health programs such as family planning and lead screening. These funding streams together comprise about one-sixth of the total revenues for Illinois LHDs (see Table 1).

As a result of initial decisions for Illinois MediPlan Plus to fold in medical services but not case management services, a total of $13 million in Medicaid resources was at immediate risk of loss by Illinois LHDs. These funds represented various direct medical services previously funded through EPSDT/ Healthy Kids, federally qualified health center (FQHC) encounters, and physician services. Nonetheless, LHDs participating in this study feared that case management resources provided through HM/ HK also would be lost as managed care approaches were expanded in Illinois. Seven of the eight LHDs participating in the in-depth examination perceived the loss of resources for these services as likely to have a very significant, negative impact on their agencies and their role in the community.

Potential Impact of Lost Medicaid Revenues on CPH Output

The loss of $13 million would not necessarily reduce CPH activity because these services would still be available to Medicaid recipients through other providers. However, Illinois LHDs participating in this study projected a reduction in CPH output that would be greater (by $4.3 million) than the value of the services they perceived would be lost. This net reduction in CPH output exceeds the value of direct effects that are associated with redeployment of staff from other CPH activities to provide direct services that would no longer be reimbursed by Medicaid. LHDs estimated that they would likely continue to provide 10 to 20 percent of the previous levels of medical services for Medicaid recipients, even without reimbursement as part of their safety-net responsibilities. This level of nonreimbursed service provision would take place through redeployment of staff who would be taken away from other CPH activities—at a cost of $2 million in CPH output.

Due to the integrated nature of the health services offered by LHDs, additional impacts also were expected in other areas of the agencies and would account for the remaining $2.3 million in CPH output reduction. LHDs reported that the loss of funding for medical services would result in numerous missed opportunities for immunizations, WIC and lead screenings, family planning contacts, counseling, and education. With an actual loss of $13 million in Medicaid revenues creating a net reduction of $4.3 million in CPH output, an estimated $330,000 would be needed to offset CPH productivity reductions associated with each $1 million in Medicaid funding losses (see Table 2).*

As reported by Illinois LHDs, core public health responsibilities that would be most negatively impacted include preventing epidemic/disease spread, promoting/assuring healthy behaviors, and assuring the quality and accessibility of care in the community. By proportionately

*Tables not included in this publication.

weighing the responses of Illinois LHDs, the $4.3 million total reduction in CPH output would require $3.2 million in additional funding to offset the productivity losses for these three core duties. An additional $1.1 million would be needed to offset reductions in efforts to prevent injuries, protect against environmental hazards, and respond to disasters (see Table 3).*

Likely Impact on CPH Output

There is no consensus view among Illinois LHDs as to likely future relationships between LHDs and managed care networks. While most LHDs foresee themselves continuing to provide at least some medical services within one or more managed care networks, LHDs perceive their future role to be less central to the health needs of Medicaid recipients than they currently are. LHDs also see a need to continue to offer some services to those populations that will fall between the cracks of the managed care networks.

The resulting actual impact—assuming some continued provision of Medicaid reimbursable medical services by Illinois LHDs—is estimated at $2.2 million. The assumptions for continued provision of medical services both in Chicago and downstate are noted in Table 3. Of this impact, $1.6 million would be needed to maintain CPH capabilities and output for preventing epidemics and spread of disease, promoting healthy behaviors, and assuring the quality and accessibility of health services. An additional $600,000 would be needed to offset reductions in efforts to prevent injuries, protect against environmental hazards, and respond to disasters.

In sum, the range of possible impacts and resource requirements to maintain current CPH output is forecast at $2.2 million to $4.3 million, with the lower figure considered more likely because actual Medicaid losses to LHDs will probably be $6.5 million to $7 million, rather than the entire $13 million that is at risk.

Implications and Limitations

The intent of this study was to determine the extent to which Medicaid will enable CPH activities in LHDs as a basis for forecasting the impact of reduced Medicaid resources on these LHDs when Medicaid recipients are enrolled in private managed care systems. Illinois LHDs have provided clear but somewhat disconcerting answers to each of the three central questions examined in this assessment:

1. Medicaid resources are now enabling CPH activities primarily through facilitating access to populations at greatest risk of health problems and poor health status, thereby increasing CPH productivity at any given funding level.

2. The integrated nature of LHD programs, through the provision of complementary health and social support services, means that reduced medical services will decrease the productivity of public health prevention efforts directed toward these and other low-income populations.

3. The loss of Medicaid reimbursement to Illinois LHDs for medical services likely would be $6.7 million to $13 million and would result in the need for $2.2 million to

$4.3 million in additional funding in order to maintain the current level of CPH output from Illinois LHDs.

These conclusions support the argument that the productivity of CPH efforts is increased when these services are colocated. Fragmentation of CPH activities may require additional resources in order to maintain overall levels of CPH output for the community. The possibility of reduced public health services to the community should be considered, especially where Medicaid managed care models are driven by pressures to reduce public outlays for health services. Otherwise, community health status may become a casualty of Medicaid managed care conversions.

Any attempt to quantify the likely effects of conversion to a Medicaid managed care model will encounter both methodological obstacles and varying local circumstances. While there have been a number of reports raising the specter of diminished public health productivity, there has been scant effort to quantify the potential effects, let alone the actual effects. This study is a small step in that direction because it uses the perceptions and estimates of LHD administrators to identify effects to these agencies that go beyond the loss of Medicaid revenues. Illinois LHDs predicted that the CPH output of their agencies would decline more than can be accounted for by the movement of Medicaid resources to other providers in the community.

The quantification of this differential effect may not be viewed as great at only $330,000 for each $1 million in lost Medicaid revenues, especially when only $13 million in funding is at imme-

diate risk. However, given the extent of Medicaid funding within Illinois LHDs (14 percent) and the likelihood that additional services will be rolled into managed care arrangements in the future, the eventual impacts could be staggering. If the entire $43.4 million in Medicaid revenues to Illinois LHDs were to be displaced, an additional $14.5 million would be needed statewide just to maintain the current level of CPH output. That additional need is 150 percent more than the basic public health protection grant that is extended to certified LHDs for CPH activities.

While perceptions of Illinois LHD administrators were used to quantify possible effects, the actual funding and CPH output may be greater or less than described here. While most components used in this model were treated conservatively (for example, so that they would serve to understate the actual effects), it was apparent that Illinois LHDs misunderstood, or were extremely skeptical of, which services were included in Illinois MediPlan Plus. All eight LHDs participating in the in-depth portion of the study perceived that Medicaid-funded case management resources would be lost to their agencies with the managed care conversion. This belief was prevalent despite widespread dissemination of the waiver application proposal and repeated statements to the contrary by state agency officials. It is possible that this widely held perception could have prompted administrators to overestimate the conversion's impact on CPH output. However, the conservative handling of other variables used in this model may have resulted in underestimates of CPH output impacts.

The reliability and accuracy of LHD self-reporting have been demonstrated in studies of public health practice performance by investigators at the University of North Carolina and University of Illinois-Chicago Schools of Public Health.[21-24] These studies suggest that LHD administrators' perceptions and estimates of impact on CPH output can provide the basis for designing more definitive impact evaluations, which can be used to better quantify primary and secondary effects. Unfortunately, CPH responsibilities do not easily lend themselves to quantification and measurement. Instruments based on 10 public health practices[21-24] that implement the three core functions of public health described in the Institute of Medicine report[7] (assessment, policy development, and assurance) or based on 10 essential public health services[5] could be applied in a before-and-after format for this purpose. In view of the many different forms that Medicaid managed care models can assume—with some services included and others "carved out"—the diversity of community providers and networking arrangements in urban, suburban, and rural settings as well as the primacy of some conversion objectives over others (cost control vs. health status improvement), it is clear that more definitive impact evaluations will need to be both tailored and flexible.

The questions and issues addressed in this study are being examined in other parts of the country as well. A review of the national experience with LHD participation in Medicaid managed care systems bolsters the findings in this study that the major effects on LHDs of Medicaid managed care arrangements include both primary and secondary impacts.[8-14,20] Primary impacts are apparent in the reduction of specific services and staff, and the redeployment of existing staff to maintain safety-net levels of service provision even without Medicaid reimbursement. Secondary effects include erosion of the critical mass needed to provide an effective safety net, loss of the capability for direct provision of services with community benefit, and reduction of the synergistic effect that integrated programs and services have one on the others.

Nationwide, state and local public health agencies will have to continue to grapple with the impact of Medicaid managed care on their ability to carry out core functions. This poses a stern leadership test for these agencies that often may be exacerbated by inter- and intra-agency politics and barriers. Statewide public health organizations found that the Illinois MediPlan Plus program failed to adequately delineate functional roles and reimbursement mechanisms for LHDs. In response, these statewide organizations sought to include LHDs in the program on an "any willing provider basis." This situation highlights how critically important it is for the entire public health community to become involved in the policy-making process to ensure the integration of public health approaches with those of managed care. In this light, it is critically important for the entire public health community at the state and local level to be very involved in the policy-creating process in order to assure the integration of public health approaches with the managed care model. Such issues will continue to challenge the Illinois' public health community.

References

1. Shonick, W. *Governmental Health Services: Government's Role in the Development of U.S. Health Services 1930–1980.* New York, NY: Oxford University Press, 1995.
2. Lipman, J. The Impact of Health Care Reform on Local Health Departments. *Journal of Public Health Management and Practice* 1 (1995):viii–ix.
3. Pearson, T. A., et al. Who Will Provide Preventive Services? The Changing Relationships between Medical Care Systems and Public Health Agencies in Health Care Reform. *Journal of Public Health Management and Practice* 1 (1995):16–27.
4. Saunders, S. E., et al. Maternal and Child Health and Health Care Reform. *Journal of Public Health Management and Practice* 1 (1995): 78–85.
5. Baker, E. L., et al. Health Reform and the Health of the Public: Forging Community Health Partnerships. *JAMA* 272 (1994): 1,276–1,282.
6. Lee, P. R. Reinventing Public Health. *JAMA* 270 (1993): 2,760.
7. National Academy of Science, Institute of Medicine. *The Future of Public Health.* Washington, D.C.: National Academy Press, 1988.
8. Association of State and Territorial Health Officials. *The Impact of Medicaid Managed Care on Public Health Systems in Arizona: A Case Study of Public Health and the Arizona Health Care Cost Containment System.* Washington, D.C: ASTHO, May 1993.
9. Greenberg, E. L., and Atchison, C. G. The Impact of Medicaid Managed Care on the Public Health System in Arizona: Case Study. *Journal of Public Health Management and Practice* 1 (1995): 7–15.
10. Miline, T. Public Health in A Reformed Health Care System. Annual Conference of Idaho Association of District Boards of Health. Sun Valley, ID: May 19, 1993.
11. National Association of County Health Officials. *Managed Care, Medicaid and the Public Health System.* July 1993.
12. National Association of County Health Officials. *Medicaid Managed Care Arrangements and Local Health Departments.* 1994.
13. Papin, T. Current Issues and Future Trends in County Government Involvement in Managed Care. NACO Annual Meeting. Chicago: July 17, 1993.
14. Peck, M., and Hubbert, E. D. *Changing the Rules: Medicaid Managed Care and MCH in U.S. Cities.* City MatCH: University of Nebraska Medical Center: July 1994.
15. Illinois Department of Public Aid. *FY-1994 Medicaid Payments to Illinois Local Health Departments.* September 1994.
16. Illinois Department of Public Health. *Core Public Health Functions Expenditures Pilot Data.* Submitted to Public Health Foundation. Springfield, IL: May 1994.
17. Illinois Department of Public Health Data. *FY-94 and FY-95 Contract and Expenditure Data for Healthy Moms/Healthy Kids Case Management Services (from both IDPA and IDPH), Family Planning Services, Lead Screening Services, and Local Health Protection Grant Services.* 1994.
18. Project Health, Systems Development Committee, Finance Subcommittee. *Budget Development Survey for Local Health Departments.* Springfield, IL: May–September 1991.
19. Project Health, Public Health Systems Committee, Organizational Subcommittee. *Preliminary Assessment of Selected Organizational Characteristics of Illinois Local Health Departments.* Springfield, IL: January 1992.
20. Illinois Department of Public Health. *Impact of Medicaid Resources on Public Health Activities of Local Health Departments in Illinois.* Springfield, Illinois: October 1994.
21. Miller, C. A., et al. A Proposed Method of Assessing the Performance of Local Public Health Functions and Practices. *American Journal of Public Health* 84 (1994): 1,743–1,749.
22. Miller, C. A., et al. Validation of a Screening Survey To Assess Local Public Health Performance. *Journal of Public Health Management and Practice* 1 (1995): 63–71.
23. Turnock, B. J., et al. Local Health Department Effectiveness in Addressing the Core Functions of Public Health. *Public Health Reports* 109 (1994): 653–658.
24. Turnock, B. J., et al. Capacity Building Influences on Illinois Local Health Departments. *Journal of Public Health Management and Practice* 1(3) (1995): 50–58.

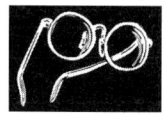

Article Review Form at end of book.

What is "community empowerment?" Compare the role mass media outlets play in community-based intervention programs with the role of community organizations.

Community-Based Approaches for the Prevention of Alcohol, Tobacco, and Other Drug Use

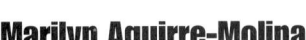

Marilyn Aguirre-Molina

Robert Wood Johnson Foundation, College Road East, Princeton, New Jersey

D. M. Gorman

Center of Alcohol Studies, Rutgers—The State University of New Jersey

Abstract

This paper summarizes what is known about community-based approaches for the prevention of ATOD problems and how the current practices in the field reflect these approaches. The first section of the chapter provides a brief summary of events early in this century when community-based approaches were central to addressing alcohol and other public health problems. The second section contains an overview of current research and empirical findings that yield consensus as to what conceptually and in practice constitutes a comprehensive, community-based prevention program for the prevention of ATOD problems.

The third section reviews the literature of existing programs to assess the extent to which they include the salient elements and employ interventions determined to be fundamental to comprehensive community-based prevention programs. The final section discusses some of the challenges that confront researchers and practioners when developing prevention initiatives and programs in high-risk environments.

Introduction

Research findings demonstrate that the risk of using alcohol, tobacco, or other drugs (ATOD) increases disproportionately with the number of risk factors present in a community. For example, adolescent alcohol and other drug-related problems appear to be linked with poor family management practices, low family bonding and conflict, neighborhood deterioration, economic deprivation, and inner-city schools (21, 49). Other environmental factors have been identified as contributing to these risks. They include, for example, the easy access and availability of alcohol and tobacco in a community (70, 81, 103, 111), pricing and taxes on alcohol and tobacco (17, 103), as well as marketing and promotional activities targeted by the alcohol and tobacco industries to consumer groups such as young people, communities of color, and women (4, 34, 37, 47, 72, 88, 90). These research findings have led to an understanding of the complex etiology underlying the use of alcohol and other drugs.

This current understanding of the combined effects of environmental and social conditions on ATOD risks has resulted in an emphasis on interventions that extend beyond single-focused education programs targeting individual behavior to include comprehensive, community-based approaches. Such approaches attempt not only to influence the individual but also to incorporate the participation of the general community and its institutions to address the environmental and social factors that contribute to ATOD problems (60, 68, 79, 108, 112, 117). These approaches are characterized by systematic applications of integrated and sustained prevention strategies that are guided by public health theory and practice (8, 55, 76, 113).

Comprehensive, community-based approaches have emerged as the most viable way of reducing the risk of alcohol and other drug use (17, 21, 32, 33). As such, these prevention strategies have received substantial support from both the public and private sectors in the form of federal grants (e.g. Center for Substance Abuse Prevention-Community Partnership Program), foundation support (e.g. The Robert Wood Johnson Foundation-Fighting Back Program), and the adoption of these approaches by the voluntary sector (e.g. 4-H, the Junior League). This support is based on the observation that community-based approaches hold a great deal of promise because they endeavor to address the social context and environmental conditions that contribute to and sustain ATOD problems in a community (48, 56, 60).

Early Community-Based Efforts

Focus on the community as a unit of intervention is not a new phenomenon nor a unique approach to addressing problems that affect substantial numbers in a population. This focus has been at the core of public health practice in the United States since the 1800s,

as the country struggled to bring under control the morbidity and mortality produced by infectious diseases and environmental conditions (58, 93, 94, 96). In like manner, community-focused action for alcohol problems has a long-standing history dating back to the 1830s and the advent of the temperance movement, when diverse constituent and citizen groups organized to address problems at the local level, where they were most directly and personally experienced (63). Although the temperance movement has been characterized by some as a failure because of the ultimate repeal of the 18th Amendment to the Constitution (which prohibited the "manufacture, sale and transportation of intoxicating liquors"), it nevertheless represents one of the most successful grass-roots, community-driven social movements in United States history. As Goldberg states, the movement's "leaders not only converted their proposals into law but achieved polity-member status" (39, p. 19).

Once again, the community is the locus of intervention as the ATOD field and grass-roots groups struggle with the public health problems posed by alcohol, tobacco, and illicit drug use. The current focus on community-based interventions for addressing ATOD problems has many parallels with early public health practice and community action. For example, then, as now, the specific mechanisms of disease were not fully understood, as is the case with the etiology of alcohol, tobacco, and other drug use today. Nevertheless, during both periods it is evident that collective action against the disease-producing agent and attention to the individual and environment

(physical, social, and economic) have the greatest potential for yielding positive public health outcomes.

However, certain features distinguish current community-based action for ATOD problems from earlier efforts. For example, unlike the movements of the 1940s, 1950s, and 1960s when primary emphasis was placed on building a treatment system for alcoholics and the drug addicted, present-day community-based action for alcohol and other drug problems includes a distinct focus on prevention, the adoption of the public health model, and the use of public policy for change (92). Additionally, tobacco is prominent on the list of drugs in need of intervention. There has also been a shift away from reliance on professional change agents to the active participation of a diverse cadre of community members taking over the functions of initiating and mobilizing support for social change (10, 11). Prominent among these change agents are youth and parents, members of the faith community, local officials (elected and appointed), the business sector, and other concerned citizens.

Elsewhere, Room (92) provides an informative account of the events of the 1960s and 1970s that resulted in what he describes as the "new alcohol problems perspective" from which present-day community-based action programs for alcohol and other drugs have evolved. Additionally, Mosher & Jernigan (76), in their 1989 review of alcohol policy, provide a detailed overview and analysis of the alcohol policy movement at the core of today's public health action for the prevention of alcohol-related problems.

Community-Based Prevention

A review of the current literature reveals that community-based programs with the greatest promise for positive prevention outcomes rely heavily on the principles and models of community action for social change (11, 73) and place a high value on *community empowerment;* both concepts have their origins in the tradition of *community development* (5, 22). Programs are comprehensive and recognize the importance of social policy, use the tools of *public health practice,* and draw on the best available *research knowledge* to guide the interventions. Below we briefly review issues related to the comprehensiveness of programs, community empowerment, community development, and public health practice. Different types of intervention programs tend to draw upon different bodies of theory and research knowledge; for example, some draw upon studies of individual-level risk factors such as deficiencies in social skills, whereas others draw upon research pertaining to environmental factors such as drug availability. In the section discussing specific ATOD prevention interventions, we describe the underlying theory and research upon which these are based.

Comprehensive

A comprehensive community-based intervention targets multiple systems and employs multiple strategies (8). The targeting of multiple systems assures the identification of and attention to all factors within the environment that contribute to community risks (55). Equally important, targeting multiple systems enables

the recruitment and participation of sectors and constituencies within a community that have an important and vital role in addressing ATOD problems. These sectors and constituencies include youth and families, the media, community organizations, and local institutions such as schools, the business sector, the faith community, government, and law enforcement.

Most prominent among the promising strategies employed at the community level are a combination of community organization (75), coalition development (13), media advocacy (118), and advocacy for public policies that influence the availability and marketing of alcohol and other drugs (25, 57, 86, 103). Embedded in an advocacy strategy for public policies is the understanding that individual behavior is shaped by the environment, which in turn is shaped by public policy. By making changes in public policy that affect the social, legal, and economic environments in which people make health decisions, there exists the opportunity for making the greatest progress.

Community Empowerment

Wallerstein & Bernstein (119, 120) provide thorough reviews of the concept of empowerment and its application in a number of community settings for varied health outcomes. They define community empowerment as ". . . a social-action process in which individuals and groups act to gain mastery over their lives in the context of changing their social and political environment" (120). The most effective community-based prevention programs are designed with the understanding that sustained change is achieved by individuals and communities

that attain personal and community empowerment. This empowerment enables them to become active players (subjects) in the processes of community change vs passive recipients (objects) of prevention programs and services (73, 112, 120). It is in this domain where prevention specialists such as researchers, service providers, and health educators may encounter the greatest challenge. Many specialists approach communities as empowered experts with a ready constructed prevention model and assumptions, and thus find it difficult to hear community voices or learn ways to become part of a process that promotes social responsibility and social justice. The potential for conflict is increased when the community is ethnically, racially, or economically different from that of the specialist. Hill and colleagues (50) found that ". . . the barriers to the success of community-level prevention programs may lie more in overcoming the paternalism (by the expert) that arises as these programs actually unfold" (50, p. 86).

Community Development

Community development is the process of communities becoming invested in the identification and reinforcement of those aspects of everyday life, culture, and political activity that are conducive to health. Community development should be the ultimate goal of prevention strategies because it enables individuals and communities to increase their control over the determinants of health by securing the tools (resources, skills, authority, etc) needed to change their environment (1). These efforts are needed to change the social, political, and economic systems that contribute to neighborhood deterioration and community disorganization (see final section for details).

Public Health Model

Program interventions that are structured on the principles of the public health model take into consideration the host, agent, and environment, and focus on the interaction of this triad for the spread of alcohol and other drug-related problems. This analytic framework has moved the ATOD field away from the traditional focus on individual behavior as the primary domain of intervention to include an assessment of the drug's availability, accessibility, marketing, and the contribution of environmental structures within which these problems occur. Following Holder (53), we use the public health model to review existing community-based programs for the prevention of ATOD use and related problems.

In assessing state-of-the-art ATOD community-based prevention efforts in the United States, the following section reviews the available literature on existing community-based prevention programs. This assessment is guided by an attempt to answer the following questions: (*a*) Are the majority of the programs identified in the literature as comprehensive community-based ATOD prevention programs accurately classified, given that such programs improve their potential for success by employing multi-system/multi-strategy interventions? (*b*) Have these programs moved beyond a primary focus on individual behavior change to include environmental and public policy changes that facilitate and enhance individual behavior change? (*c*) Are the principles of community action, development,

participation, and empowerment evident to the processes and interventions described? (*d*) Are these programs guided by public health theory and the best available research? The review of the literature represents a preliminary step toward answering these questions so that we might better understand the strengths and limits of the processes currently under way in the field of prevention.

Community-Based Intervention Programs

As noted above, we use the three elements of the traditional public health model—the host, the agent, and the environment—to structure our review of community-based ATOD interventions. Of course, some programs are designed to affect more than one of the components of the public health model. For this review, a judgment has been made concerning the primary focus of the program. It should be noted that the review is restricted to programs targeted specifically at preventing drug use. Thus, it does not include programs that have a broader focus (such as preventing cardiovascular disease) and includes some types of drug use (typically cigarette smoking) among the many risk factors they target. Shea & Basch (100, 101) have reviewed these studies in detail. It also means that programs intended to reduce or stop drug use among established heavy users, such as the Community Intervention Trial for Smoking Cessation (110), are not included in the review.

Despite the attention given to community-based ATOD interventions, there are few well-designed studies reporting program effects on behavioral outcomes rather

than on attitudes or knowledge. Gorman & Speer (44) conducted a detailed review of community interventions designed to prevent alcohol use and alcohol-related problems. They identified just eight studies that reported program effects on behavior and used controlled evaluation or time-series analysis to assess program impact. Most of these studies were concerned with changing the behavior of individuals rather than with influencing alcohol availability or changing the environment in which host and agent are brought together and interact. The primary focus of the present review is not methodological issues such as study design and techniques of data analysis. Such issues are discussed in detail by others (19, 54, 66, 78).

Strategies Designed to Change Host

Strategies designed to change the behavior of individuals have relied principally upon educational programs, mainly in the form of mass media interventions or community-based skills training for adolescents. Mass media programs typically target specific types of drug (i.e. alcohol or tobacco or illicit substances such as marijuana or crack cocaine). Community-based skills training programs typically target the so-called gateway substances, alcohol, tobacco, and marijuana.

Mass Media Interventions

Mass media campaigns have been widely used in the United States as part of the "war on drugs." Examples are the Just Say No campaign of the early 1980s and the succession of public service announcements (PSAs) mounted by the Partnership for a Drug-Free

America since the late 1980s. As Wallack (116) observes, these campaigns are premised on the idea that ATOD use results from lack of information and focus primarily on individual behavior and personal responsibility. Advocates of this approach claim that its effectiveness can be inferred from national survey data showing a decline in drug use and in attitudes favorable to drug use since the campaigns have been in operation (87). However, there are a number of reasons why causality cannot be inferred from the association suggested by these data. For example, such an inference represents an example of the so-called ecological fallacy—meaning that changes occurring at one level of analysis (in this case, individual reports of drug use) cannot be inferred as resulting from changes occurring at another level of analysis (in this case, society-wide media campaigns) (35). Beyond such methodological issues, it has been suggested that the Partner-ship campaign might actually do more harm than good since it focuses attention exclusively on individual-level factors, thereby undermining potential support for initiatives that target the socioeconomic and political factors contributing to ATOD use (116).

Reviews and empirical studies from the 1980s consistently showed that broad-based mass media interventions, by themselves, had little impact on use of alcoholic beverages and cigarettes (30, 31, 77). Consequently, it has been suggested that mass media interventions be used primarily to supplement other approaches such as school-based and community-based programs. This supplementary approach has been most fully developed in the prevention of cigarette smoking among youth (30), but has also been used in community-based initiatives designed to prevent alcohol problems (14, 36, 38).

In addition to a shift toward a supplementary approach, Flay & Sobel (31) recommended more formative research into mechanisms and processes through which media interventions work, so that messages can be more appropriately targeted at their intended audiences. Some laboratory-based research has been conducted in this area (20). Obviously, from a public health perspective, the goal of this approach is to refine media messages such that salient information reaches the largest possible number of the target high-risk audience. In one of the few evaluations of such use of mass media, Barber et al (6) assessed the effectiveness of a 30-second televised PSA designed on the principals of behavioral self-control training and targeted at heavy drinkers in North Queensland, Australia. Some subjects in the evaluation were sent a letter one week before advertisements were screened alerting them to the commencement of the campaign (it was hypothesized that forewarning the audience would enhance the effects of mass media interventions). In an evaluation involving 96 subjects, alcohol consumption was found to be significantly lower at post-test among subjects who were sent the letter and viewed the PSA compared with those who only received the letter or viewed the PSA or who got no intervention. The effects of the program were specific to alcohol use, as might be expected from such a narrowly focused clinically oriented approach. There were no effects on participants' perceptions of the dangers associated with alcohol use or attitudes toward social policies designed to control alcohol use and availability.

The key to such a targeted approach is to refine media messages such that high-quality information reaches the largest possible number of the appropriate target audience whose behavior the intervention is intended to change. This falls within what Wallack (115) refers to as the *personal-individual* approach to health promotion. In contrast, the *social-political* approach emphasizes changing the way in which a community thinks about the broader issues related to drug use and related problem, e.g. the marketing strategies of the liquor industry and laws regulating the sale of alcoholic beverages (see below).

Community-Based Skills Training

Community-based skills training programs typically use curricula that are employed in school-based ATOD prevention programs. Opinion concerning the effectiveness of school-based social and resistance skills training curricula varies. Advocates claim that they are effective in preventing drug use among adolescents (9, 26, 84), whereas others maintain that their impact has been overstated (18, 35, 40, 42, 43, 67).

A number of community-based prevention programs are centered on the use of social influence curricula (e.g. 98, 109, 119). The best known of these programs is the Midwestern Prevention Project (MPP), a six-year longitudinal study targeted at youth in Kansas City and Indianapolis (59, 82, 83). The MPP consists of five components, introduced sequentially: a mass media component (comprised of television, radio, and print media events); a school-based social skills training curriculum; a parent program (oriented around six homework assignments); community organization involving training of city leaders in the planning and implementation of prevention efforts; and a health policy change component designed to initiate change in local ordinances regulating the availability of alcohol and tobacco products. Influences operating within the school (notably peer group pressure) were considered the most proximal in the sequence leading to drug use initiation, and therefore the school-based curriculum and mass media component were introduced first in the intervention sites, followed by the other three components at 6- to 12-month intervals. The school, family, and media components were concerned essentially with *demand* reduction, whereas the community organizing and policy change components were considered *supply* reduction strategies (82).

Pentz and associates (83) reported one-year follow-up data from more than 5000 students in the Kansas City site following the implementation of the school, family, and media components. Prevalence rates for cigarette, alcohol, and marijuana use were significantly lower among those who had taken part in the program than among controls. Johnson and colleagues, in a three-year follow-up study of a subsample of 1607 subjects from the Kansas City site, described two additional components: a parent organization program concerned with reviewing school prevention policy and training parents in communication skills, and initial training of community leaders in an attempt to establish a prevention task force. Significantly fewer subjects were using cigarettes and marijuana at fol-

low-up among those who had received the program than among control subjects (25 vs 31% in the case of cigarettes, and 12 vs 20% in the case of marijuana). However, there were no differences between groups in terms of alcohol use.

One of the main weaknesses of the MPP is that allocation to study conditions was, for the most part, not random, and only limited data pertaining to initial equivalence have been reported (35). Of the 42 schools involved in the study in Kansas City, only 8 were randomly assigned to study conditions; the other 34 were allocated on administrator flexibility, with 20 rescheduling their existing activities and being assigned to the intervention group and 14 not rescheduling and being assigned to the comparison group. Also, although conceived as a comprehensive multicomponent intervention, only limited aspects of the MPP have been evaluated to date. Published accounts from the Kansas City evaluation give few details on the level of participation in the parenting program, while two other components—the mass media program and the community organization efforts—appear to have been implemented in both the intervention and control communities, which makes it impossible to assess their impact on outcome variables (59). In the Indianapolis site, participation in the parenting program was also not experimentally controlled, and the sample of self-selected participants differed in many crucial respects (e.g. socioeconomic status, ethnicity, and reported cigarette and alcohol use) from nonparticipants (91). Those who took part in the parenting program generally engaged in the least demanding activity (namely, the homework sessions), with participation in

more demanding activities (e.g. skills training and community meetings) limited to about one in five of the participants.

A methodologically more sophisticated community-based study that builds upon a school-based program was recently started in 24 public school districts located in six counties in northeastern Minnesota (85). Fourteen of the school districts have been randomly allocated to the intervention condition (Project Northland) and ten to the control condition. The intervention program employed in this project has three components: a parent program (oriented around four activity books for students to work on at home with their parents/guardians), a peer-led school-based resistance skills training program, and a community program built around task forces comprised of representatives from various community organizations. The goal of the latter is to develop strategies to reduce the access of adolescents to alcohol. These strategies fall into four broad areas: education of alcohol merchants; enforcement of existing laws on alcohol sales; development of new local ordinances regulating sales; and development of school policies concerning alcohol use. Community organizers are responsible for the formation of the task force in each community.

Strategies Designed to Change the Agent

Community-based drug prevention programs can do little to change the agent per se: They cannot reduce the production and manufacture of drugs such as alcohol, tobacco, marijuana, and cocaine. However, they can influence drug availability and access.

In recent years, field trials of illegal sales have documented the ease of availability of tobacco products to minors (16). This technique has also been employed in pretest-post-test trials to evaluate the impact of preventive treasures (2, 3, 29). The outcome measure in these studies has been sales by merchants, and little is known about the effects of these efforts on use of tobacco products (2, 29). Interventions used in these studies employ one of two strategies, education of merchants and enforcement of laws. Research shows that educational approaches produce only short-term change in merchants' behavior, and that enforcement is necessary to achieve sustained reduction in availability (3, 29). However, one study (29) found that judges frequently dismissed citations against merchants for selling to minors, and observed that a successful enforcement effort could be undermined by judicial leniency. This finding suggests that interventions need to have an impact upon other institutions within a community if they are to have a sustained effect.

To date, very few studies report using field trials of merchant behavior to assess the extent of illegal sales of alcohol to minors (80, 89), and just two report employing this approach to assess the effectiveness of community prevention initiatives in reducing such sales and hence underage drinking, Project Northland (85) (see above) and Communities Mobilizing for Change on Alcohol (112) (see below).

Strategies Designed to Change the Environment

It is increasingly recognized that it is not sufficient to simply inoculate young people against the social pressures to use drugs, as is the case with many programs that target the individual without taking into consideration the enormous contribution of the social environments (51). Similarly, programs designed to limit access and availability must work through a range of institutions within a community if they are to have a sustained effect. The most comprehensive prevention programs in this area now draw upon conceptual models that emphasize the social and environmental determinants of behavior rather than individual and intrapsychic processes (e.g. 52, 112). Before discussing these broad-based initiatives, programs that target specific community agencies and organizations are discussed.

Community Organizations

Sociologists argue that the social organization of communities depends to considerable extent on the viability of its institutions (27, 121), ranging from government agencies like schools and social service departments to small private businesses such as the corner grocery store. In socially disorganized communities, institutions are typically nonexistent or function in a manner that is detrimental to local residents. Such communities are also vulnerable to the emergence of drug use, crime and delinquency, and violence (104). Conversely, communities characterized by high citizen participation in formal and informal organizations and with well-established local networks that foster meaningful social ties between individuals are more resilient to such problems and better able to respond to external pressures toward increased availability of drugs. The efforts of many community-based organizations are designed to restore local control and accountability of neighborhood institutions. Much of this effort has focused on the role of law enforcement agencies, although in recent years attempts have also been made to control the sale practices of local retail outlets for tobacco products and alcoholic beverages (see above).

Law enforcement Community policing represents an excellent example of the attempt to rebuild communities through restructuring the role and functions of key institutions (27). In many urban minority communities, the main function of the police is to control local residents rather than to serve them. The tactics used in such areas differ markedly from those employed in white middle-class communities (17), and there is little evidence to suggest that they have much impact on the illicit drug markets (64). Community policing is intended to reduce the estrangement of the police from those they are supposed to serve, emphasizing as it does a commitment to problem-solving, (two-way channels of communication between the police and citizens, responsiveness to community demands, neighborhood outreach and ministrations, and community self-help (95, 104). Drug use prevention frequently becomes the focus of community policing in urban neighborhoods since the sale and use of drugs are prominent among problems confronting residents of these areas.

Although there has been considerable rhetoric surrounding community policing, there have been relatively few systematic and methodologically sound evaluations of specific programs. Data from the few available studies show that community policing has the greatest impact upon residents' assessment of police performance, rather than on drug availability and related social disorder (69, 95, 105). As with other types of community-based programs, community policing as implemented often only loosely adheres to the key philosophies and principles underlying the approach (95). Police may have little enthusiasm for engaging in the activities required by community policing, and community participation is frequently hard to secure. This is especially true in socioeconomically and racially diverse neighborhoods, in which community policing can serve the needs of some members of the community (typically white, middle-class) at the expense of others (46, 95, 105).

Despite these problems and limited empirical support, community policing is likely to remain a popular drug prevention strategy given its appeal across the political spectrum: Conservatives like it because it is tough on those who sell drugs within neighborhoods and emphasizes the need for self-help, while liberals find its focus on community involvement and problem-solving attractive (41). Thus, it represents a politically expedient approach to the prevention of illicit drug use, although its capability to engage residents of those communities most affected by this problem has yet to be demonstrated (106).

Local media As noted above, the mass media can be used to influence the way in-which a community thinks about the broader issues related to ATOD use and related problems. Radio, television, and print media can provide people with the skills and information necessary to change the social and environmental factors that influence their health, rather than simply providing skills and

knowledge intended to change personal behavior (115, 116). The goal of such media advocacy is to empower people such that they become active participants in the decision-making processes shaping the social and political context in which individual-level decisions about behavior are made. The behavior and health of the community, not the individual, is the central concern. Wallack and colleagues (118) discuss the principles underlying this approach to health promotion, and present a number of case studies illustrating the effective use of this strategy. The issues addressed in these case studies include the location of billboards advertising alcohol close to schools, the promotion and sale of alcohol at a large amusement park, a loophole in one state's law concerning alcohol-impaired driving, and the targeted marketing of malt liquor to African Americans.

Broad-Based Community Change

To date, the two most comprehensive, community-based drug prevention-programs have both focused on alcohol. Communities Mobilizing for Change on Alcohol (CMCA) is an 18-community trial designed to assess the effectiveness of a community mobilization strategy in reducing the availability of alcohol to those under 21 years of age and the level of alcohol use and alcohol-related health and social problems among this age group (112). The program is designed to accomplish these goals through change in community policies and practices concerning alcohol use, as opposed to simply changing "the behavior of an aggregate of individuals in the community" (112, p. 80). The project does not involve a set of pre-established program components

for implementation in participating communities. Rather, the intervention entails a standardized process of community activation and mobilization, with communities free to implement whichever strategies and approaches they consider most appropriate in dealing with the problems they face. In line with this emphasis on community autonomy, the role of the research team is to help shape local policies and practices and not to try to directly control them. The research design of the CMCA is eloquent, involving both a randomized community trial and time-series analysis with multiple sources of data (e.g. school-survey, merchant survey, field trial of alcohol purchase attempts).

The Prevention Research Center (PRC) Project entails a more formal invention than the CMCA Project, but is similar in its emphasis upon community-level processes (52). The intervention is intended to reduce the number of accidents and fatalities resulting from alcohol use, and is designed in accordance with a clearly articulated theoretical model in which the community is conceived of as a system involving the interaction of the individual and the social, economic, and physical environment. Alcohol-related accidents and fatalities are considered outputs of this system. The key factors operating within a community to produce these outputs are the level and pattern of alcohol consumption, the level of alcohol sales, the availability and marketing of alcohol, access to alcohol, community norms governing use, the enforcement of laws, community education, the level of risk-related activities (e.g. driving or using heavy machinery), and general background influences (e.g. the use of private automobiles compared to public transport).

The PRC intervention has five components: (*a*) community mobilization through the development of organizations and coalitions and increased public awareness; (*b*) training bar staff and management in responsible service practices; (*c*) community, parent, and retailer education aimed at reducing underage drinking; (*d*) increased effectiveness of DUI enforcement (both actual and as perceived by community residents); and (*e*) improved implementation of local ordinances governing youth accessibility to alcohol. The program is structured to ensure that an ongoing process of information sharing is established between the project staff and community representatives. The program has been implemented in two communities in California and one in South Carolina, each with a matched comparison community. A range of measures are being used to assess the intervention, including surveys, monitoring DUI arrest data and media accounts, and analysis of outlet densities and changes in policies.

Intervening in High-Risk Communities

Despite some large-scale funding initiatives (e.g. the Center for Substance Abuse Prevention-Community Partnership Program), relatively little empirical research is available from which to assess the impact of community-based initiatives in areas most adversely affected by alcohol, tobacco, and other drugs. Although no community is immune from the adverse consequences of ATOD use, the markets for the most potent but inexpensive drugs tend to concentrate in poor, urban neighborhoods. This is true not only of

illicit drug markets such as those in crack cocaine (24), but also the sale of tobacco products and alcohol (71, 102). Not surprisingly, although there has been some decline nationally in illicit drug use by adolescents since the mid-1980s (at least until the past year or two), evidence suggests that rates remain high among low-income, inner-city youth (7, 74). Consequently, many social and public health problems associated with drug use also concentrate in disadvantaged, urban communities (23, 45, 99, 114). As Kandel & Davies (62) observe, such findings suggest that drug use is becoming one further dimension of the increasing polarization evident in the United States between the economically advantaged and disadvantaged.

In communities beset by intense economic deprivation, social dislocation, and the ready availability of inexpensive drugs, the environmental factors sustaining drug use are immensely compelling, and agent-level biological and psychological risk factors (e.g. low self-esteem, poor decision-making skills) are probably of only minimal importance in explaining elevated levels of risk. Interventions that target only agent-level risk factors are likely to have minimal impact in terms of reducing ATOD use and ATOD-related problems. The need to target multiple systems, to build and develop community institutions, and to empower community members is especially acute in such settings.

Neighborhood and community social organization is crucial in mediating the impact of broader environmental influences (such as social deprivation and inequality) on ATOD use and ATOD-related problems.

Socioeconomic Environment
(e.g. economic inequalities)

Community/Neighborhood
(e.g. disorganization)

Family
(e.g. conflict)

School
(e.g. peers)

Agent
(e.g. ATOD use)

Figure 1 Hypothesized causal chain from socioeconomic factors through community and inter-personal influences to individual behavior.

Neighborhood and community factors have an especially profound impact upon risk factors such as family management practices and the formation and activities of youth peer groups (28, 97). In turn, family management practices and peer group affiliations interact in influencing individual-level factors such as self-esteem, self-efficacy, and decision-making skills as well as in facilitating or discouraging children's drift into later high-risk activities such as engaging in antisocial acts (12, 61). This suggests a causal chain of the type depicted in Figure 1. Again, intervening at the lower end of this causal chain (i.e. only with the agent) is likely to prove ineffective.

Research suggests that those environmental factors that elevate the risk of drug use among the residents of impoverished urban neighborhoods (high rates of unemployment, inadequate social services, high incidence of teenage pregnancy and crime) might also mitigate against the development of community-based action. For example, Klitzner et al (65) in their study of parent-led drug prevention initiatives found that membership was comprised predominantly of white middle- and upper-class females, with "low income, minority, and high-risk youth . . . largely unreached by the programs." Research in crime prevention also indicates that collective citizen action is less likely to arise in low-income, urban neighborhoods (104). However, against this, recent research shows evidence of effective community participation in prevention efforts in low-income neighborhoods beset by drug problems (69, 107). Confrontational tactics (such as marches) were most frequently used by groups in these neighborhoods, and the existing organizational capacity of the community was important in stimulating antidrug activism. One of the main challenges of future research is to find ways to engage those individuals and groups involved in prevention efforts within their communities, rather than imposing top-down prevention models and programs considered suitable by outside experts.

Conclusions

We began by presenting a brief overview of historical events showing how community-based approaches have been central to addressing issues related to alcohol use and other public health problems in the United States. We then reviewed current research indicating what conceptually and in practice constitutes a comprehensive, community-based prevention program to avert public health problems. The third section of the chapter reviewed major community-based prevention programs and initiatives in the ATOD field to assess the extent to which these include the salient elements and employ in-terventions determined to be fundamental to comprehensive community-based prevention programs. While it is evident from this review that there are numerous such interventions currently in progress in the field of ATOD prevention, it is also clear that the majority of these fall short of what has been described as comprehensive community-based programs. Although nearly all prevention initiatives are now conceptually driven, the focus of most of these remains to reduce demand for drugs through changing the attitudes and behavior of individuals. Programs that are truly comprehensive and attempt to change environmental-level as well as agent-level risk factors, and that empower and build community capacity for change, remain the exception. Most prevention initiatives come in the form of standardized packages and curricula devised by experts from outside the community, with minimal community participation in their design and delivery and little attention to the unique factors that contribute to ATOD problems within the target community. Not surprisingly, it has proved difficult to generate community involvement in such programs (e.g. 109). These problems are especially acute in high-risk communities—an issue addressed in the final section of this chapter.

The two most comprehensive community-based drug prevention programs described in this review both focus on alcohol (52, 112). Both draw upon the public health model in emphasizing the social and environmental determinants of alcohol use, and both attempt to foster community involvement in the design and implementation of their interventions. To date, evaluation data from these studies have yet to be reported.

Finally, it is important to note some of the factors that impede the design and implementation of comprehensive community-based ATOD prevention programs. First, such programs are difficult and complicated to set in motion and guide to completion; supervising and orchestrating the implementation of the diverse elements required of comprehensive programs is an extremely demanding enterprise (compared, for example, with delivering a tailor-made, single-focus program). Second, and related to the first issue, such activities are extremely difficult to evaluate. Expertise in methods and data analysis techniques other than those associated with traditional randomized experiments (e.g. time-series analysis) is required of the investigator. Third, when programs are truly based on the principals of community action and development, they are likely to encounter obstacles posed by the political and economic interests that are threatened by empowered communities. Fourth, to a considerable extent, the field of ATOD research is still conceptually grounded in models that attribute drug use to individual biological, psychological, and psychosocial factors such as personality traits, low self-esteem, inadequate coping skills, and peer pressure. Consequently, it is these factors that we set out to alleviate when trying to prevent drug use. Finally, an equally important deterrent to moving toward truly comprehensive community-based prevention programs is the fact that experts in the field of ATOD use (i.e. researchers, service providers, and health educators) frequently do not know how to work effectively with communities toward the empowerment and social justice that are essential for community change and the prevention of alcohol-, tobacco-, and drug-related problems. The latter requires a new way of conceiving of the community as an active partner in prevention. As case studies and accounts in the press indicate, residents of high-risk communities beset by drug problems do, of their own accord, develop and implement initiatives designed to limit the availability of alcohol, tobacco, and other drugs (97, 107, 118), and in the future prevention experts should make more effort to build upon such neighborhood-based movements.

Literature Cited

1. Aguirre-Molina M, Parra PA. 1995. Latino youth and families as active participants in planning change. In *Understanding Latino Families—Scholarship, Policy and Practice*, ed. R. Zambrana, pp. 130–53. Thousand Oaks, CA: Sage
2. Altman DG, Rasenick-Douss L, Forster V, Tye JB. 1991. Sustained effects of an educational program to reduce sales of cigarettes to minors. *Am. J. Public Health* 81:891–93
3. Altman DG, School C, Basil M, 1991. Alcohol and cigarette advertising on billboards. *Health Ed. Res.* 6:487–90
4. Altman D, Carol J, Chalkley C, Cherner J, DiFranza J. et al. 1992. Report of the Tobacco Policy Research Study Group on access to tobacco products in the United States. *Tobacco Control* 1(Suppl.): S45–S51
5. Bailey A. 1980 Community development theory and practice. *Commun Forum* 6:1–4
6. Barber, JG, Bradshaw R, Walsh, C. 1989. Reducing alcohol consumption through television advertising. *J. Consult. Clin. Psychol.* 57:613–18

7. Barr KEM, Farrell MP, Barnes GM, Welte JW. 1993. Race, class, and gender differences in substance abuse: evidence of middle-class/underclass polarization among black males. *Soc. Probl.* 40:314–27
8. Benard B. 1990. An overview of community-based prevention. In *Prevention Research Findings: 1988*, ed. KH Rey, CL Faegre, P Lowery, pp. 126–47. Rockville, MD: OSAP Prev. Monogr. 3
9. Botvin G. 1990. Substance abuse prevention: theory, practice and effectiveness. See Ref. 110a, pp. 461–519
10. Braithwaite RL, Lythcott N. 1989. Community empowerment as a strategy for health promotion for black and other minority populations. *JAMA* 261:282–83
11. Brown ER. 1991. Community action for health promotion: a strategy to empower individuals and communities. *Int. J. Health Serv.* 21:441–56
12. Brown BB, Mounts N, Lamborn SD, Steinberg L. 1993. Parenting practices and peer group affiliation in adolescence. *Child Dev.* 64:467–82
13. Butterfoss FD, Goodman RM, Wandersman A. 1993. Community coalitions for prevention and health promotion. *Health Ed. Res.* 8:315–30
14. Casswell S, Ransom R. Gilmore L. 1990. Evaluation of a mass-media campaign for the primary prevention of alcohol-related problems. *Health Prom. Int.* 5:9–17
15. Cent. Dis. Control. 1989. *Reducing the Health Consequences of Smoking: 25 Years of Progress. A Report to the Surgeon General*. Washington, DC: CDC
16. Cent. Dis. Control. 1993. Minors' access to tobacco—Missouri. 1992, and Texas, 1993, *Morbid, Mortal, Wkly. Rep.* 42: 125–28
17. Chambliss WJ. 1994. Policing the ghetto underclass: the politics of law and law enforcement. *Soc. Probl.* 41:177–94
18. Cleary PD, Hitchcock JL, Semmer N, Flinchbaugh LJ. Pinney JM. 1988. Adolescent smoking: research and health policy. *Milbank, Q.* 66:137–71
19. Collins LM, Seitz LA. 1994. *Advances in Data Analysis for Prevention Intervention Research (NIDA Res. Monogr. 142)*. Rockville, MD: Nail. Inst. Drug Abuse

19a. Davis RC, Lurigo AJ, Rosenbaum DP, eds. 1993. *Drugs and the Community: Involving Community Residents in Combatting the Sale of Illegal Drugs*. Springfield, IL: Charles C. Thomas
20. Donohew L, Lorch. E, Palmgreen P. 1991. Sensation seeking and targeting of televised anti-drug PSAs. In *Persuasive Communication and Drug Abuse Prevention*, ed. L Donohew, HE Sypher, WJ Bukoslki, pp. 209–26. Hillsdale, NJ: Lawrence Erlbaum
21. Dryfoos JG. 1993. Preventing substance abuse: rethinking strategies. *Am. J. Public Health.* 83:793–95
22. Dubey SN. 1970. Community action programs and citizen participation: issues and confusion. *Soc. Work.* 15:76–84
23. Dunlap E. 1992. The impact of drugs on family life and kin networks in the inner-city African-American single-parent household. In *Drugs, Crime and Social Isolation: Barriers to Urban Opportunity*, ed. AV Harrell, GE Peterson, pp. 181–207. Washington, DC: Urban Inst. Press
24. Dunlap E, Johnson BD. 1992. The setting for the crack era: macro forces, micro consequences (1960–1992). *J. Psychoact. Drugs* 24:307–21
25. Edwards G, Anderson P, Babor T. Casswell S, Ferrence R, et al. 1995. *Alcohol Policy and the Public Good*. New York: Oxford Univ. Press/WHO
26. Ellickson, PL. 1995. Schools. In *Handbook on Drug Abuse Prevention: A Comprehensive Strategy to Prevent the Abuse of Alcohol and Other Drugs*. ed. RH Coombs, D Ziedonis, pp. 93–120. Boston. MA: Allyn & Bacon
27. Etzioni A. 1993. *The Spirit of Community: The Reinvention of American Society*. New York: Simon & Schuster
28. Fagan J. 1993. The political economy of drug dealing among urban gangs. See Ref. 19a. pp. 19–54
29. Feighery E, Altman DG, Shaffer G. 1991. The effects of combining education and enforcement to reduce tobacco sales to minors: a study of four northern California communities. *JAMA* 266: 3168–71

30. Flay BR. 1986. Mass media linkages with school-based programs for drug abuse prevention. *J. School Health* 56: 402–6

31. Flay BR, Sobel JL. 1983. The role of mass media in preventing adolescent substance abuse. In *Preventing Adolescent Drug Abuse: Intervention Strategies.* ed. TJ Glynn, CG Leukefeld, JP Ludford pp. 5–35. Washington. DC: US GPO. NIDA Res. Monogr. 47

32. Florin P, Chavis D. 1990. Community development and substance abuse prevention. In *National Training System Trainer Resource Manual.* Rockville, MD: Off. Subst. Abuse Prev.

33. Florin P, Wandersman A. 1990. An introduction to citizen participation, voluntary organizations and community development: Insights for empowerment through research. *Am J. Comm. Psychol.* 18:41–54

34. Gerbner G. 1990. Stories that hurt: tobacco, alcohol and other drugs in the mass media. See Ref. 90. pp. 53–127

35. Gerstein DR, Green LW. 1993. *Preventing Drug Abuse: What do we Know?* Washington, DC: Natl. Acad. Press

35a. Giesbrecht N, Conley P, Denniston RW, Gliksman L, Holder HD, et al. eds. 1990. *Research, Action, and Community: Experiences in the Prevention of Alcohol and Other Drug Problems.* Washington, DC: OSAP Prev. Monogr. 4

36. Giesbrecht N, Pranovi P, Wood L. 1990. Impediments to changing local drinking practices: lessons from a prevention project. See Ref. 35a. pp. 161–82

37. Gitlin T. 1990. On drugs and mass media in America's consumer society. See Ref. 90. pp. 31–52

38. Gliksman, L. Douglas RR, Thomson M, Moffatt K, Smythe C, Caverson R. 1990. Promoting municipal alcohol policies: an evaluation of a campaign. *Contemp. Drug probl.* 17:391–420

39. Goldberg RA. 1991. *Grassroots Resistance—Social Movements in Twentieth Century America.* Belmont, CA: Wadsworth

40. Gorman DM. 1992. Using theory and basic research to target primary prevention programs: recent developments and future prospects. *Alcohol Alcohol.* 27: 583–94

41. Gorman DM. 1993, "War on drugs" continues in United States under new leadership. *Br. Med. J.* 307:369–71

42. Gorman DM. 1995. Are school-based resistance skills training programs effective in preventing alcohol misuse? *J. Alcohol Drug Ed.* 41:74–98

43. Gorman DM. 1995. Do school-based social skills training programs prevent alcohol use among young people. *Addict. Res.* In press

44. Gorman DM, Speer PW. 1995. Preventing alcohol abuse and alcohol-related problems through community interventions: a review of evaluation studies. *Psychol. Health* 10:1–38

45. Greenberg M, Schneider D. 1994. Violence in American cities: Young black males is the answer, but what was the question? *Soc. Sci. Med.* 39:179–87

46. Greene JR. McLaughlin E. 1993. Facilitating communities through police work: drug problem solving and neighborhood involvement in Philadelphia. See Ref. 19a. pp. 141–61

47. Grube JW, Wallack L 1994. Television beer advertising and drinking knowledge, beliefs and intentions among schoolchildren. *Am. J. Public Health* 84:254–59

48. Hansen WB, Graham JW. 1991. Preventing alcohol, marijuana, and cigarette use among adolescents: peer pressure resistance training versus establishing conservative norms. *Prev. Med.* 20:414–30

49. Hawkins JD, Lishner D, Catalano R. 1992. Risk and protective factors for alcohol and other drug problems in adolescence and early adulthood: implications for substance abuse prevention. *Psychol. Bull.* 112:64–105

50. Hill H, Piper D, Moberg DP. 1995. "Us planning prevention for them": the social construct of community prevention for youth. *Int. Q. Health Ed.* 15:65–89

51. Holder HD. 1992. Undertaking a community prevention trial to reduce alcohol problems: translating theoretical models into action. See Ref. 54, pp. 227–43

52. Holder HD. 1993. Prevention of alcohol-related accidents in the community. *Addiction* 88:1003–12

53. Holder HD. 1994. Public health approaches to the reduction of alcohol problems. *Subst. Abuse* 15:123–38

54. Holder HD, Howard JM. 1992. *Community Prevention Trials for Alcohol Problems: Methodological Issues.* Westport, CT: Praeger

55. Holder HD, Wallack L. 1986. Contemporary perspectives for preventing alcohol problems: an empirically derived model. *J. Public Health Pol.* 7:324–39

56. Howard-Pitney B. 1990. Community development is alive and well in community health promotion. *Comp. Psychol.* Summer, 4–5

57. Hu T, Sung HY, Keeler T. 1995. Reducing cigarette consumption in California: tobacco taxes vs. an antismoking media campaign. *Am. J. Public Health* 85:1218–22

58. Institute of Medicine. 1988. *The Future of Public Health.* Washington. DC. Natl. Acad. Press

59. Johnson CA, Pentz MA, Weber MD, Dwyer JH, Baer N, et al. 1990. Relative effectiveness of comprehensive community programming for drug abuse prevention with high-risk and low-risk adolescents. *J. Consult. Clin. Psychol.* 58: 447–56

60. Kaftarian SJ, Hansen WB. 1994. Improving methodologies for the evaluation of community-based substance abuse prevention programs. *J. Comp. Psychol.* 22:3–5 (OSAP Spec. Issue)

61. Kandel DB, Andrews K. 1987. Processes of adolescent socialization by parents and peers. *Int. J. Addict.* 22:319–42

61. Kandel DB, Davies M. 1991. Decline in the use of illicit drugs by high school students in New York State: a comparison with national data. *Am J. Public Health* 81:1064–67

63. Keer KA. 1985. *Organized for Prohibition: A New History of the Anti-Saloon League.* New Haven, CT: Yale Univ. Press

64. Kleiman MAR, Smith KD. 1990. State and local drug enforcement: in search of a strategy. See Ref. 110a, pp. 69–108

65. Klitzner M, Bamberger E. Gruenewald PJ. 1990. The assessment of parent-led prevention programs: a national descriptive study *J. Drug Ed.* 20:111–25

66. Koepsell TD, Wagner EH, Cheadle AC, Patrick DL, Martin DC, et al. 1992. Selected methodological issues in evaluating community-based

health promotion and disease prevention programs. *Annu. Rev. Public Health* 13:31–57

67. Kozlowski LT, Coambs RB, Ferrence RG, Adlaf EM. 1989. Preventing smoking and other drug use: Let the buyers beware and the interventions be apt. *Can. J. Public Health* 80:452–56

68. Lorion RP. 1991. Prevention research. In *DHHS Drug Abuse and Drug Abuse Research.* Trienn. Rep. Congr. Sec., 3rd, Washington, DC: DHHS, GPO

69. Lurigio AJ, Davis RC. 1992. Taking the war on drugs to the streets: the perceptual impact of four neighborhood drug programs. *Crime Delinq.* 38:522–38

70. Lynch BS, Bonnie R.J. 1994. *Growing Up Tobacco Free: Preventing Nicotine Addiction in Children and Youths.* Washington, DC: Natl. Acad. Press

71. Marriot M. 1993. For minority youths, 40 ounces of trouble. *NY Times,* April 16:Al, B3

72. Maxwell B, Jacobson M. 1989. *Marketing Disease to Hispanics.* Washington, DC: Cent. Sci. Public Interest

73. McLeroy KR, Bibeau D, Streckler A, Glanz K. 1988. An ecological perspective on health promotion programs. *Health Ed Q.* 15:351–77

74. McNagny SE, Parker RM. 1992. High prevalence of recent cocaine use and the unreliability of patient self-report in an inner-city walk-in clinic. *JAMA* 267:1106–8

75. Minkler M. 1991. Improving health through community organization. In *Health Behavior and Health Education—Theory, Research and Practice,* ed. K Glanz, FM Lewis, BK Rimer, pp. 257–87. San Francisco. CA: Jossey-Bass

76. Mosher JF, Jernigan DH. 1989. New directions in alcohol policy. *Annu. Rev. Public Health* 10:245–79

77. Moskowitz JM. 1989. The primary prevention of alcohol problems: a critical review of the research literature. *J. Stud. Alcohol* 50:54–88

78. Murray DM, Rooney BL, Hannan PJ, Peterson AV, Ary DV, et al. 1994. Intraclass correlation among common measures of adolescent smoking: estimates, correlates, and application in smoking prevention estimates. *Am J. Epidemiol.* 140:1038–50

79. National Cancer Institute. 1991. *Strategies to Control Tobacco Use in the United States: A Blueprint for Public Health Action in the 1990's.* Bethesda, MD: NIH. Smok. Tob. Control Monogr. 1.

80. O'Leary D, Gorman DM, Speer PM. 1994. The. sale of alcoholic beverages to minors. *Public Health Rep.* 109:816–18

81. O'Malley P, Wagenaar A. 1991. The effects of minimum drinking age laws on alcohol use, related behaviors, and traffic crash involvement among American youth, 1976–1987. *J. Stud. Alcohol* 52:478–91

82. Pentz MA. 1993. Comparative effects of community-based drug abuse prevention. In *Addictive Behaviors Across the Life Span: Prevention, Treatment, and Policy Issues.* ed. JS Baer, GA Marlatt, RJ McMahon, pp. 69–87. Newbury Park, CA: Sage

83. Pentz MA, Dwyer JH, MacKinnon DP, Flay BR, Hansen WB. et al. 1989. A multicommunity trial for primary prevention of adolescent drug abuse: effects on drug use prevalence. *JAMA* 261: 3259–66

84. Perry CL, Kelder SH. 1992. Models of effective prevention. *J. Adolesc. Health* 13:355–63

85. Perry CL, Williams CL, Forster JL, Wolfson M, Wagenaar AC, et al. 1993. Background, conceptualization and design of a community-wide research program on adolescent alcohol use: Project Northland. *Health Ed Res.* 8:125–36

86. Peterson DE, Zeger SL, Remington PL, Anderson HA. 1992. The effects of state cigarette tax increases on cigarette sales, 1955 to 1988. *Am. J. Public Health* 82:94–96

87. Pisani RG. 1995. Advertising industry. In *Handbook of Drug Abuse Prevention,* ed. RH Coombs, D Ziedonis, pp. 217–48. Boston, MA: Allyn & Bacon

88. Pollay RW, Lee JS, Carter-Whitney D. 1995. Separate but not equal—racial segmentation in cigarette advertising. In *Gender, Race and Class in Media,* ed. G Dines, JM Humez. pp. 109–11. Thousand Oaks, CA: Sage

89. Preusser DF, Williams AF. 1992. Sales of alcohol to underage purchasers in three New York counties and Washington, D.C. *J Public Health Pol.* 13:306–17

90. Resnick H, Gardner SE, Lorion RP, Marcus CE. eds. 1990. *Youth and Drugs: Society's Mixed Messages.* Rockville. MD: OSAP Prev. Monogr. 6

91. Rohrbach LA, Hodgson CS, Broder BI, Montgomery SB, Flay BR, et al. 1994. Parental participation in drug abuse prevention: results from the Midwestern Prevention Project. *J. Res. Adolesc.* 4:295–317

92. Room R. 1990. Community action and alcohol problems: the demonstration project as an unstable mixture. See Ref. 35a, pp. 1–21

93. Rosen G. 1958. *A History of Public Health.* New York. MD Publ.

94. Rosen G. 1975. *Preventive Medicine in the United States 1900–1975.* New York: Sci. Hist. Publ.

95. Rosenbaum DP, Lurigio AJ. 1994. An inside look at community policing reform: definitions, organizational changes, and evaluation findings. *Crime Delinq.* 40:299–314

96. Rossi PH. 1965. *Community.* New York: Free Press

97. Sampson RJ. 1992. Family management and child development: insights from social disorganization theory. In *Facts, Framework, and Forecast: Advances in Criminological Theory,* ed. J McCord, 3:63–93. New Brunswick. NJ: Transaction

98. Schinke SP, Orlandi MA, Cole KC. 1992. Boys & Girls Clubs in public housing developments: prevention services for youth at risk. *J. Comp. Psychol.* 20:118–28. OSAP Spec. Issue

99. Selik RM, Chu SY, Buehler JW. 1993. HIV infection as leading cause of death among young adults in US cities and states. *JAMA* 269:2991–94

100. Shea S, Basch CE. 1990. A review of five major community-based cardiovascular disease prevention programs. Part 1: Rationale, design, and theoretical framework. *Am. J. Health Promot.* 4:203–13

101. Shea S, Basch CE. 1990. A review of five major community-based cardiovascular disease prevention programs. Part II: Intervention strategies, evaluation methods, and results. *Am. J. Health Promot.* 4:279–87

102. Sims C. 1992. Community groups attack the industry's rich franchise at the corner store. *NY Times*, Nov. 29, Sect. 3:1, 6

103. Single E. 1994. The impact of social and regulatory policy on drinking behavior. In *The Development of Alcohol Problems: Exploring the Biopsychosocial Matrix of Risk*, pp. 205–48. Rockville. MD: NIAAA. Res. Monogr. 26

104. Skogan WG. 1990. *Disorder and Decline: Crime and the Spiral of Decay in American Neighborhoods.* Berkeley: Univ. Calif. Press

105. Skogan WG. 1994. The impact of community policing on neighborhood residents: a cross-site analysis. In *The Challenge of Community Policing: Testing the Promise*, ed. DP Rosenbaum. pp. 167–81. Thousand Oaks, CA: Sage

106. Skogan WG, Annan S. 1993. Drug enforcement in public housing. See Ref. 19a. pp. 162–74

107. Skogan WG, Lurigio AJ. 1992. The correlates of community antidrug activism. *Crime Delinq.* 38:510–21

108. Stokols D, 1992. Establishing and maintaining healthy environments: toward a social ecology of health promotion. *Am. Psychol.* 47:6–22

109. St. Pierre TL, Kaltreider DL, Mark MM, Aikin KJ. 1992. Drug prevention in a community setting: a longitudinal study of the relative effectiveness of a three-year primary prevention program in Boys & Girls Clubs across the nation. *Am. J. Comp. Psychol.* 20:673–706

110. The COMMIT Research Group. 1995. Community Intervention Trial for Smoking Cessation (COMMMIT): 1. Cohort results from a four-year community intervention. *Am. J. Publ. Health* 85: 183–92

110a. Tonry M, Wilson JQ, eds. 1990. *Drugs and Crime.* Chicago: Univ. Chicago Press

111. Toomey L, Jones-Webb R, Wagenaar A. 1993. Recent research on alcohol beverage control policy: a review of the literature. *Annu. Rev. Addict. Res. Treat.* 3:279–92

112. Wagenaar AC, Murray DM, Wolfson M, Forster JL, Finnegan JR. 1994. Communities Mobilizing for Change on Alcohol: design of a randomized community trial. *J. Comp. Psychol.* 22:79–101. OSAP Spec. Issue.

113. Wagenaar AC, Perry CL. 1994. Community strategies for the reduction of youth drinking: theory and application. *J. Res. Adolesc.* 4:319–45

114. Wallace R. 1990. Urban decertification, public health and public disorder. "Planned shrinkage," violent death, substance abuse and AIDS in the Bronx. *Soc. Sci. Med.* 31:801–13

115. Wallack L 1990. Two approaches to health promotion in the mass media. *World Health Forum* 11: 143–54

116. Wallack L. 1994. Media advocacy: a strategy for empowering people and communities. *J. Public Health Pol.* 15: 420–36

117. Wallack L, Corbett K. 1990. Illicit drug, tobacco, and alcohol use among youth: trends and promising approaches in prevention. See Ref. 90, pp. 5–29

118. Wallack L, Dorfman L, Jernigan D, Themba M. 1993. *Media Advocacy and Public Health: Power for Prevention.* Newbury Park, CA: Sage

119. Wallerstein N, Bernstein E. 1998. Empowerment education: Friere's ideas adapted to health education. *Health Ed Q.* 15:379–94

120. Wallerstein N, Bernstein E. 1994. Introduction to community empowerment, participatory education, and health. *Health Ed Q.* 21:141–48

121. Wilson WJ. 1987. *The Truly Disadvantaged: The Inner City, the Underclass, and Public Policy.* Chicago: Univ. Chicago Press

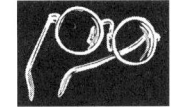 **Article Review Form at end of book.**

About half of all smokers die in middle age, resulting in a loss of
_____ of potential life. What does the study show regarding
gender and smoking?

The Use of Prevalence Data to Unite the Community in Prevention Programs

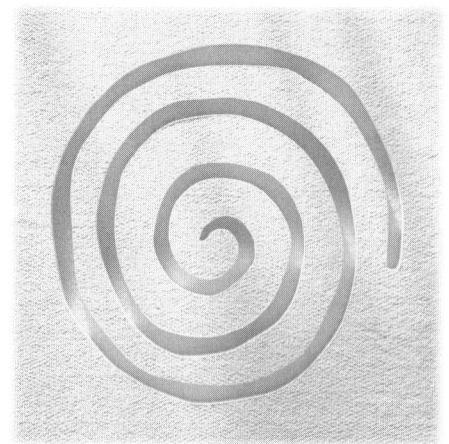

Bernard J. Healey

Bernard J. Healey, PhD, is an Assistant Professor of the Graduate Program in Health Care Administration at Kings College, Wilkes Barre, Pennsylvania.

This study examined the prevalence of cigarette smoking in a three-county area of northeastern Pennsylvania. More than 14,000 questionnaires have been returned, and results reveal that 5,411 children have experimented with cigarettes and 2,962 of those children continue smoking today. Cigarette experimentation begins as early as age 5 in northeastern Pennsylvania, with the highest number of children (19.8%) experimenting by age 12. This experimentation occurs less frequently among females in the lower grades and more frequently among females in the later years of high school. The results of this study were used to unite the health community of northeastern Pennsylvania in a number of prevention initiatives.

The Centers for Disease Control and Prevention (CDC) attributes approximately 10 million deaths to cigarette smoking since the first Surgeon General's report on smoking and health was published in 1964.[1] Cigarette smoking remains the largest single preventable cause of premature mortality in this country. In fact, the CDC expects tobacco use to become the single greatest risk factor for death and disability in the world by the year 2020.

In conjunction with the alarming mortality associated with cigarette smoking, the Department of Health and Human Services (DHHS) has called teen smoking a national public health crisis and contends that the crisis is worsening.[2] Studies have shown that more than 80 percent of these young tobacco users began their addictive habit before they were 18 years old.

The CDC reports that the prevalence of smoking cigarettes for adults in the United States was 27.7 percent for males and 22.5 percent for females in 1994.[3] The prevalence for smoking for children under age 18 was 29.8 percent for males and 31 percent for females in that same year. The CDC reports that the prevalence of smoking cigarettes for adults in Pennsylvania is 24 percent for both males and females.[3] In 1994, the prevalence in Pennsylvania for children grades 9 to 12 was 31 percent for boys and 32 percent for girls. Very little information is available on a national level regarding the prevalence of smoking among elementary and middle-school children.

One of the major long-term effects is found in the increased number of cigarettes smoked and the continued smoking as a child grows older. The Institute of

Medicine found that nicotine addiction develops in the first few years of cigarette use and that the earlier a child smokes, the more likely he or she will become addicted.[4] The majority of young people who smoke on a daily basis confirm that they want to quit smoking but are unable to do so. Nicotine in tobacco causes and sustains addiction.[4] There is evidence that manufacturers deliberately design their products to provide the consumer with a pharmacologically addictive dose of nicotine to continue the consumer's need for the product.

Despite many studies, society still underestimates the dangers presented by adolescent smoking. About half of all smokers die in middle age, resulting in the loss of at least 20–25 years of potential life.[5] It is well documented in the literature that nicotine addiction begins very early in life and most likely has occurred prior to high school graduation for most individuals who use tobacco. Health problems associated with smoking are a function of duration (years) and intensity (amount). Most people could be prevented from becoming addicted if they could be kept tobacco-free during their childhood years.

In the long term, the reduction in the number of children smoking seems to be the most effective way to reduce the nation's leading cause of preventable death in older Americans and perhaps to reduce the development of other high-risk health behaviors. The CDC in 1994 reported that adolescents began cigarette smoking as a result of social influences, promotional efforts by tobacco producers, social pressure, and curiosity.[5] But once

the habit is established, it becomes the norm.

One study found that most young people do not actively seek to start smoking but are pushed into the habit by friends, older brothers and sisters, and others.[6] A report in 1994 by the Surgeon General, *"Preventing Tobacco Use Among Young People,"* reveals that the onset of tobacco use is influenced by sociodemographic, environmental, behavioral, and personal factors.[2] Furthermore, the earlier one begins to smoke, the more likely one is to be a smoker as an adult.

The Institute of Medicine believes that the entire community, especially community leaders, must become involved if prevention efforts are to be successful.[4] In order for community leaders to become involved in problem solving, they must first become aware of the nature of the problem under consideration. Gregg believes that the starting point in a successful prevention program is descriptive epidemiology,[7] which allows the problem under investigation to be better understood.[6] Dever argues that in order to understand the health needs of a population, a health status assessment is of paramount importance.[8]

The purpose of this study was to describe the use of tobacco by children in northeastern Pennsylvania and to use the survey results to unite the community in prevention initiatives to reduce the experimentation with cigarettes. In order to accomplish these goals, the following study questions were developed and answered by this study.

1. What is the prevalence of cigarette use by children under 18 years of age in northeastern Pennsylvania?

2. Is there a gender difference in age of first cigarette experimentation, continuation of the smoking habit after first experimentation, and mean number of cigarettes smoked each day?

3. Can the results of a large community health survey be utilized to generate support and resources to implement prevention programs in the community?

Methods
Study Population
The sample chosen for this study included six school districts in northeastern Pennsylvania that were representative of school districts in this part of the state and included urban and rural students as well as public and private schools. A letter was sent to 15 randomly chosen school superintendents requesting permission to survey all students in grades 4–12. To protect their privacy, students were allowed to complete the survey anonymously, but their participation was mandatory. Homeroom teachers administered the questionnaire during the last class period.

Instrument
The instrument used in this study was a two-page questionnaire consisting of 19 questions about tobacco, alcohol, and marijuana use. A review of the literature was utilized to establish face validity of the instrument. Three health experts then evaluated the questionnaire to assess the instrument's content validity. The questionnaire was field tested on several students in grades 4–12 in a school district not utilized in this study.

Results

The final response for this study was 15,227 returned questionnaires. There were responses from all six school districts representing private, public, and rural school districts in northeastern Pennsylvania. These questionnaires were then evaluated for accuracy and entered into a computer utilizing a statistical software program provided by the CDC. There were 774 questionnaires containing unrealistic responses that were not entered into the computer. Therefore, the total number of questionnaires analyzed was 14,523.

What is the prevalence of cigarette use by children under 18 years of age in northeastern Pennsylvania?

In the six school districts surveyed, the frequency of experimentation with smoking cigarettes ranged from a low of 31.5 percent to a high of 41.4 percent, with an average of 37.3 percent having tried cigarettes. Of those children who had tried cigarettes, the numbers of children who continue to smoke ranged from 38.7 percent to 67.2 percent, with the average being 54 percent. More than 80 percent of these children had no desire to quit smoking. There were 5,411 children who had tried cigarettes and 54 percent of them (2,962) were still smoking. In the fourth grade, 8.1 percent of the students had tried cigarettes, and 36.5 percent of those fourth graders who had tried smoking cigarettes were still smoking. The number of individuals who tried smoking cigarettes increased for each year until it reached 63.9 percent in the 12th grade, and the number of those who tried cigarettes and continued to smoke also in-

Table 1 Age of First Attempt at Using Cigarettes: Children Grades 4 to 12, Northeastern Pennsylvania, December, 1996

Age	Males		Females	
	N	%	N	%
5	41	1.8	19	0.7
6	58	3.7	32	1.9
7	106	7.7	43	3.4
8	178	14.4	107	7.3
9	217	22.6	176	13.8
10	369	36.5	270	23.6
11	344	49.4	358	36.7
12	500	68.2	568	57.4
13	386	82.8	530	76.7
14	239	91.8	329	88.7
15	132	96.7	187	95.5
16	60	99.0	94	99.0
17	23	99.8	24	99.9
18	4	100.0	4	100.0
Totals	2,661		2,750	

N = 5411; Male: mean age 11.2, Female: mean age 11.9.

creased each year until it peaked at 60.8 percent in the 12th grade (see Table 1).

This study found that in northeastern Pennsylvania, first experimentation with cigarettes begins as early as age 5 (1.3 percent), with the highest number of students (19.8 percent) having their first cigarette at age 12. The incidence of new smoking dropped off dramatically as children enter the later years of adolescence. By age 16, new cigarette experimentation dropped off in a dramatic way (see Table 2).

Is there a gender difference in age of first cigarette experimentation and continuation of the smoking habit after first experimentation and the mean number of cigarettes smoked each day?

This study included 7,168 males and 7,356 females between the ages of 10 and 19. There were

2,661 males and 2,750 females in this study that experimented with cigarettes, 44.7 percent of the male experimenters and 52.3 percent of the female experimenters continued to smoke.

The mean number of cigarettes smoked each day was 5.9 for males and 5.0 for female respondents. The number of cigarettes smoked each day rose from 2.0 for males and 1.1 for females in fourth grade to 8.0 for males and 7.0 for females in 12th grade (see Table 3).

This experimentation occurred less frequently for females in the lower grades and more frequently for females in the later years of high school. The mean age for cigarette experimentation was 11.2 for males and 11.9 for females. The greatest escalation in cigarette experimentation occurred at age 12 for males and

Table 2 — Number of Children Who Have and Have Not Experimented with Cigarettes, Northeastern Pennsylvania, December, 1996

Grade	N	Tried	Percent	Did Not	Percent
4	1,561	126	8.0	1,435	92.0
5	1,666	190	11.4	1,476	88.6
6	1,829	301	16.5	1,528	83.5
7	1,796	566	31.5	1,230	68.5
8	1,783	764	42.8	1,019	57.2
9	1,634	887	54.3	747	45.7
10	1,511	848	56.1	663	43.9
11	1,411	878	62.2	533	37.8
12	1,332	851	63.9	481	36.1
Total	14,523	5,411	37.3	9,112	62.7

Table 3 — Mean Number of Cigarettes Smoked Each Day by Grade and Gender, Northeastern Pennsylvania, December, 1996

Grade	Male	Female
4	2.0	1.1
5	1.5	1.0
6	2.5	2.1
7	3.4	3.3
8	3.7	3.7
9	6.1	4.9
10	6.2	6.0
11	8.0	6.1
12	8.0	7.0

females. Although females started smoking at a slightly older age than males, a higher percentage of females continued to smoke (see Table 4).

Can the results of a large-community survey be utilized to generate support and resources to implement prevention programs in the community?

The results of this study were utilized to unite the health care community in several initiatives aimed at reducing the prevalence of children using cigarettes in northeastern Pennsylvania. The first initiative was a three-day conference held at King's College in April 1997 for student leaders, health professionals, and local teachers. This conference brought together national experts on nicotine addiction who shared prevention strategies with conference participants. All costs associated with this conference were paid by local health care facilities.

The second community prevention initiative resulting from this study will be a week-long, three-credit undergraduate college course titled "Leadership in Health Education." The course will be offered at King's College to 20 advanced-placement student leaders from 14 school districts in northeastern Pennsylvania. This course will prepare student leaders to develop and implement tobacco prevention programs in their respective school districts. The tuition for this college course will be paid by local health care facilities.

Local health care facilities paid all costs associated with this survey and a future survey to measure the effectiveness of initiatives to reduce children smoking, the three-day conference, and the college training program. The survey of smoking prevalence in northeastern Pennsylvania was the catalyst that brought the health care community together in a united effort to reduce the number of children smoking in the community.

Discussion

The CDC recognizes that the duration and intensity of tobacco use are important causes of early mortality and the loss of years of potential life among the users of these products.[5] The results of this study demonstrate that children in northeastern Pennsylvania begin using cigarettes at a very early age and that most of these children continue to smoke as they grow older. The majority of the smokers use an increasing number of cigarettes each year, and the majority do not want to quit smoking. The Institute of Medicine reports that most addicted individuals cannot quit their habit.[4] This study demonstrates the need for and the value of the development of community surveillance systems for the prevalence of high-risk health behaviors.

Table 4	A Comparison of the Number of Children That Experiment with Cigarettes and the Number That Continue to Smoke by Grade Level and Gender, Northeastern Pennsylvania, December, 1996							
	Male				**Female**			
	Experiment		Continued		Experiment		Continue	
Grade	N	%	N	%	N	%	N	%
4	75	9.9	28	37.3	51	6.3	18	35.3
5	101	12.0	52	51.4	89	10.8	32	36.0
6	179	19.8	58	32.4	122	13.2	45	37.2
7	285	32.6	128	44.9	281	30.5	138	49.1
8	397	43.9	217	54.8	367	41.8	195	53.1
9	446	54.3	262	59.0	441	54.3	279	63.3
10	381	50.5	206	54.1	467	61.8	283	60.7
11	408	59.0	234	57.4	470	65.3	267	56.8
12	388	63.0	224	57.7	462	64.6	292	63.2
Total	2,660		1,409		2,750		1,399	

Based on the results of this study, the following recommendations are made:

1. Educational programs that are developed to reduce cigarette experimentation by children need to begin in the very early elementary grades and continue through high school.

2. The CDC reports that the prevalence of smoking cigarettes for children under 18 was 29.8 percent for males and 31 percent for females.[3] In 1994, the prevalence of smoking in northeastern Pennsylvania among children in grades 9–12 was 31 percent for males and 32 percent for females. This study found the prevalence of cigarette use by the children of northeastern Pennsylvania to be higher than both state and national averages. Therefore, greater resources are needed to change cigarette experimentation in this community.

This study demonstrates that local surveillance data about high-risk health behaviors can be used to attract community attention and resources for local prevention efforts. Other communities need to complete similar studies and collaborate with local health care institutions to develop and implement community preventive health initiatives.

A follow-up study of the same school districts needs to be completed in a few years to evaluate the success or failure of the various prevention initiatives.

References

1. Centers for Disease Control and Prevention. World No-Tobacco Day—May 31, 1997. *Morbidity and Mortality Weekly Report 46*, no. 2 (1997): 433.
2. U.S. Department of Health and Human Services, *Preventing Tobacco Use Among Young People: A Report of the Surgeon General.* Atlanta, GA: U.S. Department of Health and Human Services, Public Health Service, Centers for Disease Control and Prevention. National Center for Chronic Disease Prevention and Health Promotion, Office on Smoking and Health, 1994.
3. Centers for Disease Control and Prevention. Surveillance for Selected Tobacco-Use Behaviors—United States, 1990–1994. *Morbidity and Mortality Weekly Report 43*, no. SS U.S. (1994):1–6.
4. Institute of Medicine. *Growing Up Tobacco Free: Preventing Nicotine Addiction in Children and Youths.* Washington D.C.: National Academy Press, 1994.
5. Centers for Disease Control and Prevention. CDC Surveillance Summaries. *Morbidity and Mortality Weekly Report 43*, no. SS-3 (1994): 1–6.
6. Skutchfield, D., and Keck, C. W. *Principles of Public Health Practice.* Albany, New York: Delmar Publications, 1997.
7. Gregg, M. *Field Epidemiology.* New York: Oxford University Press, 1996.
8. Dever, G. E. *Improving Outcomes in Public Health Practice: Strategy and Methods.* Gaithersburg, MD: Aspen Publishers, Inc. 1997.

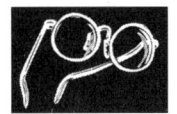 **Article Review Form at end of book.**

How does Citrin define *community*? Citrin states that, by following this path, public health will become the next significant societal enterprise to be converted into a commodity. Describe the "path."

Topics for Our Times:

Public Health— Community or Commodity? Reflections on *Healthy Communities*

Toby Citrin

*School of Public Health
University of Michigan
Ann Arbor*

I recently read the new Institute of Medicine report, *Healthy Communities*.[1] As a member of the earlier Institute of Medicine committee that authored *The Future of Public Health*,[2] I was anxious to see how a group of current public health leaders assessed the relevance of the earlier report to the current environment. I was gratified, informed, and disturbed by what I read.

The gratification came from the vote of confidence given by the authors to the earlier report, now almost 10 years old. The authors feel that *The Future of Public Health* is still the authoritative source for identifying the essential mission and core functions of public health and for establishing the vocabulary and basic framework for describing and assessing the effectiveness of our public health system.

The *Healthy Communities* report is also informative. It identifies two areas in which events since the initial report present opportunities and threats to public health, and it provides insight, advice, and real-world examples for addressing these challenges. The central portion of the report is divided into a description of the advantages of partnering with communities and their organizations and a description of the opportunities and challenges presented by the rapid advance of managed care. The report calls on public health agencies to partner with community-based organizations and urges the agencies to work out a set of relationships with managed care organizations that will strengthen the capacity of both systems to advance the public's health. The report could just as well have been titled *Healthy Partnerships*, since it iden-

tifies the current priority task for public health as creating effective partnerships with community-based organizations and with managed care systems.

It is this parallelism between partnering with community and partnering with managed care that caused my third reaction to the report: a disturbing feeling that the main point has been missed. By stating that public health's current agenda is to create productive relationships with communities and with managed care, the report overlooks the fundamental difference between these two features of the current American health scene, avoids discussion of the inherent tension between them, and fails to identify public health as an expression of community and not simply a potential partner with community.

Community is a concept based on the notion that society cannot exist and progress without

"Topics for Our Times: Public Health—Community or Commodity? Reflections on *Healthy Communities*." From *American Journal of Public Health*, March 1998 (Vol. 88, No. 3), pp. 351–352. Reprinted by permission from the American Public Health Association.

a set of mutual relationships expressing the obligations of individuals to each other and to the groups of which they are a part. Community-based organizations (e.g., community health centers, church-related health and social services organizations) are the embodiment of this concept, expressing the community's desire to organize into groups and associations to carry out projects and programs promoting the community's well-being. Fairness, equity, justice, caring, and concern are the values that guide communities and community-based organizations.

For many decades, public health leaders and scholars have identified the fundamental links between public health, the communitarian ethic, and principles of social justice. Winslow's classic definition of public health includes, as a component of public health's mission, "the development of the social machinery which will ensure to every individual in the community a standard of living adequate for the maintenance of health." [3] *The Future of Public Health,* in its articulation of the mission of public health, made it clear that public health is a societal function aimed at advancing the health of the total population. More recently, Turnock, in *Public Health: What It Is and How It Works,* [4] called attention to the relationship of public health with principles of social justice, as well as the sharp contrast between those principles and the principles of the marketplace: "In the case of public health, the goal of extending the potential benefits of the physical and behavioral sciences to all groups in the society, especially when the burden of disease and ill-health within that society is unequally

distributed, is largely based on principles of social justice." [4]

Public health practitioners, teachers, and students who have worked closely with community-based organizations have been gratified by the way in which these organizations and their members quickly come to understand that public health expresses their own experience-driven insights into the causes of health and disease and provides a vehicle for expressing their desire to work together to better their communities. For example, representatives of the 7 consortia that make up the Community-Based Public Health initiative, sponsored by the WK Kellogg Foundation, have defined their common vision of public health as follows:

The Community lies at the heart of public health. . . . Success with public health policies and programs depends upon the extent to which they reflect the community's values and priorities.

Public health, broadly defined, embraces virtually all of the community's priorities, and provides an organizing framework for the development of programs to address them. Public health encompasses the physical, mental, social, economic and spiritual health of the community. Public health recognizes that jobs, decent housing, the elimination of poverty, an end to racism, and economic justice, are all necessary ingredients to a comprehensive public health strategy.[5]

Managed care offers a sharp contrast to this vision of public health as an expression of community. Managed care is not a manifestation of community but a manifestation of the marketplace, driven by economic forces that call for slowing down the rate of increase in health care costs. The rapidity of its growth is a func-

tion of tightening budgets and competitive forces.

Managed care organizations, in contrast with community-based organizations, are driven not by shared values or mutual obligations but rather by the economics of producing a quality product at the lowest price that secures a maximum investment return and continued growth. While public health is concerned about the health status of the entire population, particularly those who are most vulnerable, managed care organizations are concerned about the retention of their current subscribers and their ability to add new subscribers. These fundamental differences between public health and managed care are exacerbated when one considers for-profit rather than nonprofit organizations, the former being even more exclusively oriented toward maximum growth and profit. The continuing pace of conversion of major nonprofit providers to for-profit status thus accentuates the contrast between the public and private health sectors.

The critical question for public health today is not whether it can engage in an effective partnership with both community-based organizations and managed care systems. The critical question is whether public health will be converted into yet another component of the marketplace or whether it will take a firm and clearly articulated stand as an expression of the community. As a partner with community and managed care organizations, public health simply bargains for roles and for funding along with managed care organizations and asks for the community's advice and support. A significant portion of the *Healthy*

Communities report is devoted to this kind of role allocation. Such a view of public health as representing a set of services and functions to be divided up between public and private entities suggests that public health should follow the path of medicine, once seen as a mission-driven, value-laden profession but increasingly spoken of as just another "commodity." By following this path, public health will become the next significant societal enterprise to be converted into a commodity.

If, on the other hand, public health recognizes its inherent role as an expression of society's desire to work together for the common good, its relationship to managed care will not be as a partner but as a representative of the community, to ensure that the resources and authority provided to the managed care system are used in ways that improve the health of the public as a whole in a cost-effective manner. Seen as an expression of community, public health, together with community residents and their organizations, identifies the root causes of health and disease and develops policies and programs that promote community health. This view has public health leaders advocating for social justice as instruments of the community rather than simply being partners with the community. Also, this view has public health working to ameliorate those social, economic, and environmental conditions that are responsible for illness and not simply running programs to control communicable disease, provide health education, and fill gaps in delivering health care services. And, under this conception of public health, the relationship between public health agencies and community-based organizations is not limited to one advising the other or the two splitting functions or program elements; rather, it is a much deeper relationship involving the sharing of the very ethical and social principles on which communities and, at its base, public health itself are founded.

Some might criticize this description of public health's role as overly idealistic and as likely to result in public health's losing the necessary fiscal resources on which the survival of public health agencies is dependent. I would take the contrary view. If public health becomes converted into a commodity—a set of services that can be performed by any efficient health care organization for a price—then the existing public health system is doomed to further diminution and possible extinction, as mission-driven public health organizations are replaced by government contracts, awarded to the lowest "responsible" public or private bidder. If public health agencies are converted into nothing more than service providers under contract communities will view them not as community advocates but as yet another of the corporate-controlled systems that sell goods and earn profits.

If, however, public health reaffirms its societal mission as an expression of community, then public health will have earned the respect and trust of the community; and that respect and trust will result in the community's becoming a strong advocate for public health. Indeed, while the *Healthy Communities* report correctly states that public health cannot alone save the health of communities, it ought to make clear that communities are essential to the future of public health.

As any student of American political history knows, our society's romance with individualism or communitarianism, with the free market or economic regulation, with libertarianism or social justice, goes through continuing swings and never remains constant. When the current wave of market-dominated politics shifts inevitably into a period in which America rediscovers principles of social justice and communal responsibility, and in which government again is entrusted with the task of expressing the notion of community, promoting the public's welfare, and—in the words of the earlier Institute of Medicine report—"assuring conditions for people to be healthy," where will public health be found? It will be found, it is hoped, staunchly embedded in the community, not as a commodity provided to the community, not only as a partner with the community, but as an intrinsic component of the community. We must all work toward the realization of this vision of public health's future as we move through the difficult challenges of the present.

References

1. Institute of Medicine. *Healthy Communities.* Washington, DC: National Academy Press; 1996.
2. Institute of Medicine. *The Future of Public Health.* Washington, DC: National Academy Press; 1988
3. Winslow CEA. The untilled field of public health. *Mod. Med.* March 1920:183.
4. Turnock B. *Public Health: What It Is and How It Works.* Aspen; 1997.
5. National Policy Task Force of the Community-Based Public Health Project; 1996.

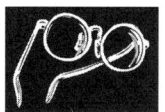 **Article Review Form at end of book.**

If done correctly, a community health needs assessment will identify
_____. Differentiate between the coalition-building process and
the collaboration-building process.

Community Assessment:

A Model "How-To" Based on Two Communities' Experience

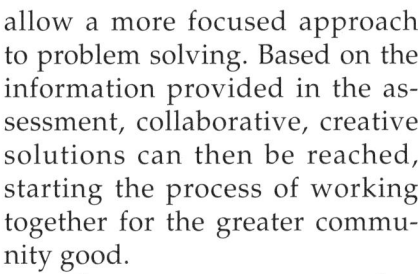

Virginia M. Pearson

If done correctly, a community health needs assessment is a systematic method for identifying the unmet human needs of particular populations at risk within a defined community or geographic area. It is a way to broaden a population's understanding of the concept of "health" beyond the medical/illness definitions to include all the many social and environmental areas that also impact an individual's sense of well-being.

A needs assessment requires the approval and encouragement of top management of the sponsoring organization(s). Ideally, this would come from the health care organization's board of directors and executives. These individuals, then, become the steering committee, receiving regular reports, approving staff time for the process, and providing final approval of the assessment document and resulting next steps.

Populations at risk, or vulnerable populations, are defined as those groups that are in need, whether that need stems from lack of finances, lack of human contact, or lack of ancillary services; in other words, "need" comes in a variety of forms and is not limited to economics.

The defined community may be a given primary or secondary service area(s), a specific geographic area, i.e., the entire town or an area within a given radius of a health care organization, or it may include an area that a health care organization is looking at for outreach services. No matter how it is defined, it must be broad enough to include the most vulnerable and undeserved populations.

The overall goal of a needs assessment is to provide baseline information that is factual and acceptable to a variety of health and health-related providers. This will prevent some of the duplication of efforts that occurs in many communities and will

allow a more focused approach to problem solving. Based on the information provided in the assessment, collaborative, creative solutions can then be reached, starting the process of working together for the greater community good.

There are many approaches being used in various communities. Most of them are similar in nature. The uniqueness of each community is what shapes each report's results and makes it different from those obtained in other areas.

To be most successful, a needs assessment should be viewed, from the start, as an ongoing process, one that is reviewed and updated on a regular basis. All of the interaction and creative planning that is started with the community should be integrated as part of a facility's regular marketing and planning cycles. The needs assessment process itself should be redone every three to five years. This not only provides updated informa-

Reprinted with permission from *The ASHCMPR Resource Collection.*

tion, but is also a way of measuring the impact of the work done based on the previous assessment.

The needs assessment information-gathering process is often seen as having three steps:

Step I. Community Overview

Community overview is a quantitative look at the defined community. It includes demographic, public health, economic and education profiles, and trends for the community and helps to identify those at-risk populations in the defined community and where they are located. This information can be gathered from such sources as the U.S. Census, local Chamber of Commerce, community health authority, a state's almanac, etc. Depending on internal resources, this work can be done by an organization's internal planning staff or an outside consultant, or by using a student intern from a local university.

Step II. Community Interviews

Community interviews can be accomplished through a number of methods, utilizing one or more of the following: one-on-one interviews, small focus groups, and mail or phone surveys. During this interviewing process, community residents have the opportunity to (1) validate the information contained in Step I through their own experiences, (2) provide information about the needs of vulnerable populations, and (3) create a network and interact with social service providers, community leaders, and the vulnerable populations to collaboratively address the priority needs identified in the community.

This step usually utilizes a team or task force composed of staff members from the sponsoring organization(s). Ideally, this group should represent a cross-section of the facility(s) including a variety of skills, male and female, ethnic and age mixed. The individuals should be chosen for their skills (or willingness to acquire these skills) in discovering and examining relevant written records (especially if they are to be integrally involved in all three steps), their ability to learn from community residents, willingness to listen carefully during interviews and also the informal conversations that surround those interviews, their awareness and sensitivity in making observations, and using common sense in analyzing written and spoken information. Task force members will be required to devote more individual hours to the assessment than will the other groups, and they will also require training in proper interviewing skills.

Individuals who should be included in the community interview process should include:

- Community key informants because of their official positions or professional experience have knowledge about the entire community, i.e., the mayor, religious leaders, etc.

- Provider key informants provide health and social services, i.e., physicians, social workers, etc.

- Community advocates are advocates for vulnerable populations and are trusted and respected by those populations. They are involved in addition to, not because of, the other work they do, i.e., leaders of community action

organizations, United Way, or church volunteers.

- Vulnerable or at-risk populations directly feel the effects of needs and benefit the most from any possible solutions, i.e., the elderly, teenage parents, etc.

Step III. The Report

In this step, the information gathered in steps I and II are assessed and a report is drafted pending approvals from those authorizing the assessment. The final report should include an executive summary, introduction, overview of the community (step I), summary of the methodology used for the report (step II), basic findings (step III), and possible recommendations for future planning and action.

Note: This is merely the first phase of a multiphase, ongoing process. Following this three-step process provides the information that sets the stage for the coalition-collaboration-partnership building phase. This phase will determine if the end result will have real impact toward improving the community, or merely providing a report to sit on the shelf. At least two types of partnerships can be formed in this phase. Each has positive and negative aspects. One is no better than another. One may be more appropriate for a given need than another. Both types may be used for different needs in a given community. The type of partnership will be shaped by the community, the need, and the comfort level of the organizers.

- In a coalition building process, any individual or organization that is interested can participate. This process takes longer because of the need to build trust levels and handle "turf" issues. But the result is a community-led project, with the assessment's sponsor(s) willing to give up control. If the assessment sponsor(s) discontinues its support, the project will most likely continue.

- In a collaboration building process, the assessment's sponsor(s) picks its partners. The project belongs to the sponsor(s) and, if for some reason, the sponsor(s) discontinues support, the project will most likely cease.

These partnerships, then, are given the responsibility for determining what needs will be addressed, action plans, funding sources (grants or other), review of the results, and communications to the appropriate publics.

Ten Rules for Conducting a Community Health Needs Assessment

Rule #1

Don't get bogged down in all the rules. It is better to get started and make any needed adjustments along the way rather than wait for divine inspiration or perfection.

Rule #2

For greatest impact, make sure the needs assessment has the support of top management. In addition to the CEO, the board of directors should, if possible, be active participants in the decision, with project updates provided on a regular basis.

Rule #3

You cannot and should not do an assessment alone. Choosing a project leader is critical. This should be an individual who (a) can devote long hours to the project, (b) has leadership and team-building skills and can get past territorial issues, and (c) has the ability to assess all the information and put it into report form. For greatest visibility in the community, and in the interest of time, two to three task forces should be identified to coordinate the data gathering, interviewing, and communications.

Rule #4

Getting the process defined and in place is one of the toughest parts, but critical to the success of the assessment.

- All task force members must have a clear understanding of the importance of the project to the health care organization(s). This message should be clearly presented by the CEO.

- All task force members must have a clear understanding of just what an assessment is and what the expected results will be. This should come from the project leader.

- Task force members should begin early in the process with a session designed to set down a purpose statement and objectives for the assessment.

- Confidentiality must be promised to all respondents and then held as a sacred trust by all task force members.

- Respondents need to be assured that they will receive feedback about the assessment's results in executive summary or some other form.

Rule #5

It is important to run a "tight ship" or the process will get off schedule. A timeline and future meetings should be determined early. Most community needs assessments can be accomplished in a six- to eight-month time-frame. While this is an aggressive schedule, it can be done.

It also helps to insure that the momentum that builds during the Assessment is not lost by stringing out the process. Both task force members and top management need to be clear about the time commitment from the beginning.

A typical schedule allows for about two months of preparation and training, two months to conduct the interviews, and about two months to assess the information and draft the report.

Most interviews and small (4–10 people) focus groups will last about two hours including travel time.

Rule #6

You will never be able to interview everyone who wants to be included in the process, so don't drive yourself crazy trying to make everyone happy. When putting together the initial list, don't hold back. It is better to have too many names than not enough. And duplicates can always be deleted. The goal is to create a list that presents a good cross-representation of the community and its many populations.

Rule #7

Open-ended questions yield the best information. By keeping the questions short, top-of-mind answers are received. And these answers tend to be most important to the respondents. This type of question is also harder to analyze and this should be taken into consideration when determining how to question respondents.

Rule #8

Do not raise community expectations that *all* of the identified needs will be met, or that one (or even all) of the community's organizations has all the answers and enough resources. The assessment is simply an information-gathering part of what should be a greater project. The second phase should consist of forming partnerships in the community to identify creative and appropriate solutions to address the needs. This is an on-going process, and the assessment should be redone every three to five years.

Rule #9

Share the results. Information is a powerful tool and it is only as good as the number of organizations and individuals who have access to it—and make use of it in their planning efforts. Keeping the results for one organization will serve to create suspicion on the part of the community, especially with the individuals who gave you their time and observations. Partnerships and progress will not occur in a vacuum.

Rule #10

See Rule #1.

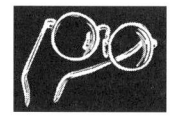 **Article Review Form at end of book.**

WiseGuide Wrap-Up

- Following the Institute of Medicine's 1988 report, efforts began to focus on performance related to public health departments "core functions." Since then, efforts have been made to improve health practices to reach targeted 2000 goals.

- The five issue areas important to LHDs are funding for TB control, authority for TB control, TB expertise, social services, and high-risk populations.

- The switch to a Medicaid managed care system will cause some reduction in medical and social support services from LHDs. This will decrease the productivity of public health prevention efforts directed toward low-income populations.

- Mass media intervention programs typically target specific types of drugs. Community cases skills training programs typically target the so-called gateway substances.

- Teen smoking has been called a national smoking crisis that is worsening, due to the alarming mortality rates associated with smoking.

- Community-based organizations express the community's desire to organize into groups and associations to carry out projects and programs promoting the community's well-being. Fairness equity, justice, caring, and concern are the values that guide communities and these organizations.

- The overall goal of a needs assessment is to provide baseline information that is factual and acceptable to a variety of health and health-related providers.

R.E.A.L. Sites

This list provides a print preview of typical **Coursewise** R.E.A.L. sites. (There are over 100 such sites at the **Courselinks**™ site.) The danger in printing URLs is that web sites can change overnight. As we went to press, these sites were functional using the URLs provided. If you come across one that isn't please let us know via email to: webmaster@coursewise.com. Use your Passport to access the most current list of R.E.A.L. sites at the **Courselinks** site.

Site name: Community Health Needs Assessment/Managing Change

URL: http://wchd.neobright.net/wc_community_assessment.html

Why is it R.E.A.L.? This site is from the Wayne County Combined General Health District. It provides links to numerous community health projects, both national and international.

Key topics: needs assessment, health policy, data analysis

Try this: Select *Community Focused/Population Based Activities*. Select *Four Case Studies in Community Transformation*. Review the Orlando, Florida, project. Orlando has mounted one of the most comprehensive, inclusive, full-bore efforts to be found in any large city.

···

Site name: Community Profiler

URL: http://207.87.15.154/commpro/

Why is it R.E.A.L.? This profiler will allow you to generate rates of health-related behaviors and conditions in your community, or any other community in the United States. You can see rates for such indicators as average height and weight, cigarette smoking, alcohol consumption, visits to doctors, and income. You can also view comparisons among all communities in a state.

Key topics: community profile

Try this: Complete the process for your community.

···

Hospital/Health Care–Based Programming

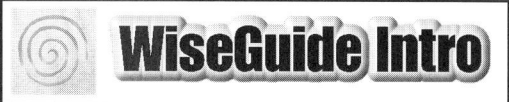

Hospitals and health care systems historically have been known as places of healing, a last resort in the effort to regain one's health. In present day, that emphasis has shifted from one of healing the ill to maintaining health and preventing illness. Many factors have influenced this shift—most notably, changes in insurance, a movement toward managed care, and Medicare/Medicaid reimbursement.

In this section, we will examine several hospital/health care–based programs. The review will include Medicaid issues, health initiatives used to boost prevention and revenues, managed care initiatives, and health-promoting hospitals.

Alina Salganicoff (Kaiser Commission) and Suzanne F. Delbanco (University of California, Berkeley) address "Medicaid and Managed Care: Meeting the Reproductive Health Care Needs of Low-Income Women." This article explores the implications for Medicaid recipients, physicians, and the agencies themselves as the current system is switched to a managed care system.

Healthcare Demand and Disease Management's "Community Health Initiative Uses Casefinding, Intervention to Boost Prevention and Revenues" discusses the results of a program that was initially designed to prevent disease, diabetes in particular. The Winchester Hospital's Clinical Health Initiative has not only resulted in earlier diagnoses but has also translated into significant risk pool savings, and more revenue for both the hospital and local physician practices.

Shirley Gordon (Gordon and Gordon Associates) presents "Removing Barriers and Improving Choices: A Case Study in Reproductive Health Services and Managed Care." This article recommends public policy strategies to overcome and prevent multiple barriers that were identified in a New York–based study in 1995. The study focused on access to reproductive health services in managed care settings.

Juergen Pelikan, Hubert Lobnig, and Karl Krajic, all from the World Health Organization (WHO), present "Health-Promoting Hospitals." The article discusses the health-promoting hospital concept, which was started in 1988 by a group at the WHO regional office. Since then, several directives have been issued, and many hospitals, especially in Europe, have become health-promoting hospitals. The goals, objectives, and strategies, of such hospitals are discussed.

Reading 25. List two of the three responsibilities state agencies will have to address by moving to a managed care system. Discuss the challenges Medicaid beneficiaries face with a move to a managed care system.

Reading 26. One of the prevention program's unforeseen benefits was the increase in _____. What kind of effect did this prevention program have on the hospital's physicians and patients?

Reading 27. FAIR recommends five priority strategies to reduce and prevent barriers to reproductive health care for managed care enrollees. List three. How does lack of adequate information about reproductive health care coverage affect appropriate care?

Reading 28. A health-promoting hospital promotes patients' health by continuously _____, thus reducing the risks involved in hospital stays and interventions. A health-promoting hospital is a "healthy organization." Explain.

List two of the three responsibilities state agencies will have to address by moving to a managed care system. Discuss the challenges Medicaid beneficiaries face with a move to a managed care system.

Medicaid and Managed Care:

Meeting the Reproductive Health Needs of Low-Income Women

Alina Salganicoff and Suzanne F. Delbanco

Alina Salganicoff, PhD, is Associate Director of the Kaiser Commission on Medicaid and the Uninsured and a Senior Program Officer of the Henry J. Kaiser Family Foundation in its Washington, D.C. office.

Suzanne Delbanco, MPP, MPH, was a program consultant for the Kaiser Family Foundation in Menlo Park, California. She is currently completing a PhD at the Goldman School of Public Policy at the University of California, Berkeley.

State Medicaid programs have increasingly turned to managed care with hopes of controlling spending while improving access to care. The move to managed care has significant implications for the provision of reproductive health services—family planning, abortion, sterilization, sexually transmitted diseases, and maternity care. However, the delivery of reproductive health services in a Medicaid managed care environment is wrought with many difficulties. The complexity inherent in Medicaid policy, the changing world of managed care, and the health and social needs of the Medicaid population are compounded by the sensitive nature of reproductive health needs.

Mirroring trends in the private sector, state Medicaid programs have increasingly turned to managed care with hopes of controlling spending while improving access to care. Today, nearly half, or more than 15 million Medicaid beneficiaries are enrolled in managed care.[1] The move to managed care has particularly significant implications for the provision of reproductive health services such as family planning, abortion, sterilization, treatment of sexually transmitted diseases (STD), and maternity care.

Providing reproductive care through Medicaid managed care arrangements poses challenges for beneficiaries, health care providers, health plans, and state agencies alike. Navigating the complexities inherent in the Medicaid program is no small feat. These include confusing and arcane eligibility policies, administrative hurdles, limited provider availability, and notoriously slow and low payment rates. In recent years, a new layer of intricacy has been placed on this flawed but vitally important safety net program—managed care. Medicaid beneficiaries are now commonly faced with learning how to use a new system of care and developing relationships with a new set of providers.

These changes do not affect beneficiaries alone. Providers, particularly those who have traditionally cared for the poor, are faced with a new range of activities. In part, these include competing for patients, negotiating contracts, and establishing or joining networks. State agencies are now charged with a new set of responsibilities, including assuring that plan networks are adequate and include the providers that best meet the complex health and social needs of Medicaid beneficiaries. State agencies also must take extra precautions to ensure that beneficiaries are protected from the many incentives in managed care to provide less care. Compounding these difficulties is the sensitive nature of reproductive health care, which adds the challenges of confronting societal preconceptions and taboos in the health care environment.

This article provides a brief overview of the reproductive health care needs of low-income women, discusses Medicaid's role in financing reproductive health services, and reviews trends in managed care for the Medicaid population. It also raises considerations for program administrators and policymakers that are integral to assuring that managed care best serves the reproductive health care needs of low-income women.

Reproductive Health Care Needs of Low-Income Women

Specifying the reproductive health care needs of low-income women is not simple. There is no standard definition of reproductive health care, and information about the specific health concerns of different income groups is not readily available. For the purposes of this discussion, reproductive health services are defined to include: routine gynecologic examinations; contraceptive counseling, services, and supplies; STD and human immunodeficiency virus (HIV) counseling, diagnosis, and treatment; screening for cancers of the reproductive system, including cervical and breast cancers; infertility services; abortion counseling and services; and pregnancy-related care.[2] To varying degrees, state Medicaid

programs cover most of these services.

To qualify for Medicaid, an individual must meet Medicaid's income criteria and be pregnant and low income, eligible for welfare assistance* (usually women with young children in their peak childbearing years), disabled and eligible for Supplemental Security Income (SSI), or over age 65. Because of this eligibility policy, the adult Medicaid population is overwhelmingly comprised of low-income women. Nearly three-quarters (71%) of the non-older adults that Medicaid covers are women, and of these women, 81 percent are between the ages of 18 and 44.[3]

While women enrolled in Medicaid have reproductive health needs and problems similar to those of their privately insured counterparts, many of those experienced by low-income women are compounded by poverty, low-educational attainment, and lack of access to timely and appropriate health care. As a result of these and other factors, low-income women experience a disproportionately greater incidence of unintended pregnancy, STDs, poor birth outcomes, and shorter survival times for cervical and breast cancer.

Unplanned pregnancy—while a problem among all groups of sexually active women of reproductive age—is especially prevalent among low-income women. Among poor women surveyed in the 1995 National

*The new welfare law eliminated the automatic link between cash assistance under Aid to Families with Dependent Children (AFDC) with a new block grant to states called Temporary Assistance for Needy Families (TANF). The new law requires states to use the AFDC eligibility criteria of July 1996 (before the law changed) to determine Medicaid eligibility for families with children.

Survey of Family Growth, 61 percent classified their pregnancies as unintended, compared with 41 percent of women whose incomes exceeded 200 percent of the poverty level.[4] Contraceptive use also varies with income. Low-income women are less likely than women with higher incomes to use contraception and more likely to have more difficulty using contraceptives regularly and correctly.[5] As a result, low-income women are more likely to get pregnant even when they report using contraception.[6]

While no data are available on the specific relationship between income and the incidence of STDs, information is available on STD rates by race and ethnicity. In the United States, race and ethnicity have been found to be risk markers that correlate with other basic determinants of health status such as poverty and access to health care. Women from some minority racial and ethnic groups have higher rates of STD and HIV infection than nonminority women.[7]

Similarly, although all sexually active women are at risk for cervical cancer, this preventable cancer is more commonly found in poor women.[8] While poor women are less likely to get breast cancer than are women with higher incomes,[9] women who are on Medicaid or are uninsured were found to have more advanced breast cancer at the time of diagnosis and have worse survival rates than privately insured women.[10] Cancer prevention efforts, including Pap smears, breast exams, and mammograms, are encouraged for all women, but those who are poor do not receive these screenings at recommended rates or at rates comparable to their higher income counterparts.[11]

Medicaid's Role in Reproductive Care

Medicaid, the jointly financed state-federal health care program for the poor, plays a key role in covering reproductive health care for low-income women. To participate in Medicaid, a state must agree to provide beneficiaries with a mandatory set of benefits, which include: inpatient and outpatient hospital care; physician, midwife, and certified nurse practitioner services; laboratory and X-ray services; and family planning services. A state also can provide optional services such as prescription drugs, screening, and preventive care. Medicaid covers a broad range of reproductive care, including family planning services and supplies (reimbursed at a 90% federal match), STD screening and treatment, prenatal care and delivery, and sterilization (only for individuals who are 21 years and over, mentally competent, and voluntarily give informed consent). Infertility treatment is defined as a family planning service under Medicaid, though the extent to which women on Medicaid can use this service is unknown. Federal funds can be used for abortions sought by Medicaid beneficiaries only in cases of life endangerment, rape, or incest. A state can use it own funds to pay for medically necessary abortions, but only 17 states currently do this to varying degrees.[12]

Because of their poor health status and greater health care needs, women on Medicaid seek health care more often each year than their low-income, privately insured and uninsured counterparts.[13] Low-income women on Medicaid or other public insurance are also more likely than women with private insurance to have made a gynecologic visit in the last year.[6] This can be attributed to the fact that women eligible for Medicaid include those who are pregnant or in their peak reproductive years. Where women get reproductive care also differs by insurance type. Compared with women who have private insurance, women who are covered by Medicaid or are uninsured are also more likely than those with private insurance to have obtained gynecologic care in a clinic-based setting than from a private doctor's office or health maintenance organization (HMO).[6]

Several indicators—such as the use of family planning services, pregnancy-related care, and preventive screenings—shed light on Medicaid's important role covering reproductive health care. Medicaid is the largest single source of public funding for family planning services, financing 46 percent of all public spending on contraceptive services.[14] For example, in 1995, Medicaid provided family planning services to 2.5 million Medicaid beneficiaries on a fee-for-service basis at a cost of $500 million (representing less than 1% of total Medicaid spending).[15] Because most services under full- and partial-risk managed care arrangements are paid for on a capitated basis, it is unknown on a national level what share of Medicaid spending went to family planning services for women enrolled in managed care.

One of Medicaid's most significant roles is financing pregnancy-related care. As a result of federal and state expansions of eligibility for pregnant women in the late 1980s and early 1990s, Medicaid has become a dominant payer for births. Medicaid pays for approximately 40 percent of all births in the United States, and more than half of all births in Georgia, Louisiana, Mississippi, New Mexico, and West Virginia.[17] Today, states are required to extend eligibility to all pregnant women with incomes below 133 percent of the poverty level and can opt to expand coverage to women with incomes up to 185 percent of poverty. Some states have used a variety of mechanisms to broaden eligibility beyond the federal ceiling. Section 1115 Research and Demonstration Waivers allow states to expand eligibility beyond federal requirements, while the Section 1902(r)(2) option allows states to use the more liberal income and assets test to determine Medicaid eligibility for children and pregnant women. Thirty-four states have extended eligibility to pregnant women who are beyond the federal floor of 133 percent of poverty.

Medicaid also plays a critical role for low-income women by covering preventive screening for cervical and breast cancer. Women with Medicaid coverage or private coverage are more likely than uninsured women to receive these services. In a survey of low-income people in five states, about 60 percent of women with Medicaid or private coverage had a Pap smear in the past year, compared with about 40 percent of uninsured women. Similarly, while about half of low-income women between the ages of 50 and 64 with Medicaid or private coverage had a mammogram in the past year, only one quarter of uninsured women reported having had one.[17]

As discussed previously, federal funding of most Medicaid abortions is prohibited by law; two-thirds of states do not provide any Medicaid funding for abortions. Because most poor women must pay for abortions out of their own pockets, an estimated one in five

Medicaid-eligible women who had second-trimester abortions would have had first-trimester abortions if the lack of public funds had not delayed raising sufficient money to pay for the procedure.[18] As a result of this policy and other factors, low-income women with unplanned pregnancies are less likely to have an abortion than their higher-income counterparts.[19] If they do have an abortion, they are more likely than their higher-income counterparts to have a higher risk, more expensive second-trimester abortion.

Despite Medicaid's important role, the low-income women it covers often experience difficulty gaining access to the reproductive health care services they need. From preconception counseling to postpartum care, cancer screening, and treatment, low-income women—including those with Medicaid coverage—do not receive recommended levels of services. The key question is whether the shift to Medicaid managed care improves or exacerbates this situation.

Medicaid Managed Care and Reproductive Health

Medicaid's use of managed care has grown explosively in the past decade. In 1987, an estimated 1.8 million Medicaid beneficiaries were enrolled in managed care arrangements. By 1997, enrollment had reached an estimated 15.3 million, about 48 percent of the Medicaid population. Although there are no precise estimates of the composition of the Medicaid managed care population, almost 90 percent of $9.9 billion in federal and state Medicaid payments to managed care orga-

nizations (MCOs) is estimated to be on behalf of children and their families (usually their mothers).[20]

Under Medicaid, managed care includes a wide array of arrangements designed to control costs and improve access. These arrangements usually follow one of three general models: primary care case management (PCCM); full-risk plans, such as HMOs; and limited-risk, prepaid health plans (PHPs). About one-third of Medicaid managed care enrollees are enrolled in PCCM arrangements, which identify a specific provider as the patient's gatekeeper and reimburse that provider on a fee-for-service basis.

Although states have always been able to allow beneficiaries to enroll in managed care voluntarily, they could not require beneficiaries to enroll in managed care plans until recently without a waiver from the Health Care Financing Administration (HCFA). Today, most states that mandate managed care enrollment are using either Section 1915(b) (freedom of choice) or Section 1115 (research and demonstration) waivers to waive the freedom of choice of provider provisions of the Social Security Act. As of March 1997, 40 states and the District of Columbia were operating nearly 100 1915(b) managed care waiver programs; and 18 states had received HCFA approval for Section 1115 waivers. As a result of the enactment of the Balanced Budget Act (BBA) of 1997, states can now require managed care enrollment for all Medicaid beneficiaries—except children with special needs, dually eligible Medicaid/Medicare beneficiaries, and American Indians—under the new Section 1932 of the Social Security Act. This means that states no longer need to obtain waivers to man-

date enrollment in managed care for most Medicaid beneficiaries.

In the mid-1980s, the freedom of choice legislation was enacted to protect access to timely and confidential family planning services for Medicaid beneficiaries in managed care, and to protect family planning providers without managed care contracts who otherwise would have lost a large base of patients.[21] These provisions are referred to as the family planning "freedom of choice" provisions. Thus, even if a beneficiary is enrolled in managed care, she can seek family planning services out-of-plan.

The type of waiver under which a state operates its mandatory managed care plan has implications for access to reproductive health care, particularly for family planning services. With Section 1915(b) waivers, states must allow all women in managed care plans to use their family planning provider of choice, even if family planning services are included in the plan's capitated rate. In contrast, states with Section 1115 waivers may request federal permission to require women to seek all family planning services from their plans, although few states have actually applied to waive these freedom of choice provisions. Because many states are opting to continue to operate their waiver program after passage of the BBA, the distinctions between the types of waiver programs are still relevant today for women in Medicaid managed care. The BBA is silent on family planning provider freedom of choice, which effectively maintains the ability of managed care enrollees to go outside their plans to obtain family planning services from the providers of their choice.

If a state supports Medicaid managed care beneficiaries' freedom of choice of family planning provider, it is incumbent on both plans and state Medicaid programs to provide information to members about their right to obtain family planning services directly from providers of their choosing. Most state agencies classify the following as family planning: contraceptive counseling, patient education, related examinations and treatment; laboratory tests for STDs, HIV, and pregnancy; Pap smears; and contraceptive devices. However, a number of reproductive services—including hysterectomies, breast exams, maternity care, abortion services, and treatment for STDs—are generally excluded from most state definitions of family planning services for the purposes of the freedom of choice exemption.[22]

Some states have also used Section 1115 waiver authority to expand Medicaid coverage for a limited range of family planning services for women who otherwise would be ineligible for Medicaid assistance. Eight states have expanded coverage to an estimated 35,000 women who would not qualify for assistance because they are either no longer pregnant and do not meet Aid to Families with Dependent Children (AFDC) eligibility, or because they lost Medicaid coverage for other reasons.[23] The goal of these limited-scope Section 1115 waiver programs is to decrease unwanted and mistimed pregnancies by increasing access to family planning services. These waivers must demonstrate federal budget neutrality, which is assessed by comparing estimated savings from averted births and costs during the first year of life to the costs of expanded family planning services. Of the states that have been granted waivers,

two require that women receiving family planning benefits enroll in an MCO. However, most states allow full freedom of choice of provider and pay for provider services on a fee-for-service basis.

One of the other key functions of Medicaid is financing prenatal care. Many states have used 1915(b) waivers to enroll pregnant women in managed care with the goal of increasing coordination and integration of care, providing unique community education and other specialized, nonmedical social and preventive services, and controlling spending.[24] Despite managed care's potential for innovation, most prior evaluations have not found that managed care improves access to prenatal care, the adequacy of care, or birth outcomes for the women enrolled in Medicaid managed care.[25–27]

Specific Issues in Delivering Reproductive Health Services

Much has been written about the challenges and opportunities managed care poses as an approach for the delivery of care to the low-income population. In general, the evidence is mixed because managed care does not appear to significantly improve access over fee-for-service arrangements, nor does it consistently appear to restrict access or worsen health outcomes.[28] Studies suggest that access and quality vary tremendously with type of plan and provider. Regardless of whether one views the growth of managed care as a positive or negative trend, managed care for the Medicaid population is rapidly becoming the dominant approach for the delivery of care to low-income women. Health care providers, adminis-

trators, and others concerned about access to reproductive health care services for women must consider other issues as they work to assure that low-income women have access to care.

Access and Availability of Care

All women, regardless of socioeconomic status or Medicaid eligibility, benefit from having the broadest possible range of reproductive health services. The Medicaid managed care contracting process can be used to ensure that coverage is comprehensive and that beneficiaries are able to seek reproductive health care from sources with which they are comfortable. Medicaid beneficiaries enrolled in managed care plans remain entitled to the full spectrum of Medicaid benefits even if the services are not included in the state's contract with the MCO. However, if specific reproductive health services are not included explicitly in a managed care contract—or are not discussed with the beneficiary by her primary care provider—the beneficiary may not know she is entitled to them.

States have flexibility in determining which benefits and service plans are included in their contracts. They also have the authority to identify which providers must be included as members of managed care networks, though most states give plans considerable discretion over the composition of their networks. In a landmark study of Medicaid managed care contracts, Rosenbaum and colleagues found broad variation among states in the specificity of reproductive health services that were covered.[29] Their study found that while a majority of states specified maternity care, enhanced prenatal services, and family planning services, only a handful specifically mentioned in their contracts coverage of intrauterine devices (IUDs), Depo-Provera, and Norplant. Similarly, only a fraction of states specifically identified infertility and other gynecological services in their contracts. Unless these benefits are specified in the contract, the plan or the network is not required to provide them, even though the beneficiary is still entitled to receive them from Medicaid-qualified providers outside of the plan.

Since Roe v. Wade in 1973, there have been legislative efforts to permit individuals and some medical facilities to refuse to provide services to which they have moral, ethical, or religious objections, such as abortion. "Conscience clauses" have reemerged with the growth of managed care, and their impact has expanded with the rapid rate of new affiliations between payers and providers of care, both religious and secular. Given that Medicaid recipients are already restricted in where they can seek care because of their insurance status, further limitations on the services their managed care plans provide can create serious barriers to care. The BBA allows Medicaid managed care plans, not just individuals, to refuse to "provide, reimburse for, or provide coverage of, any counseling or referral service to which it has a moral or religious objection." Plans that implement this option are required to alert beneficiaries of this denial. Ideally, these beneficiaries will continue to have alternative sources—such as freestanding family planning clinics—from which to seek care within the Medicaid system. But choices may be particularly limited in rural areas where there

may be only one provider of reproductive health services. Because women still have legal entitlement to these services under Medicaid, it will be critical that states ensure that women are informed of their rights to family planning services and receive full access to these services regardless of what plan they are enrolled in.

The advent of Medicaid managed care has had serious implications for organizations that provide reproductive health services and are not included in Medicaid managed care networks. Because of the lack of office-based obstetrician-gynecologists participating in Medicaid, low-income women have grown to rely heavily on family planning clinics or STD clinics for contraceptive services and STD testing and treatment.[30] These providers, who have been instrumental for decades in providing care to people for whom other caregivers are inaccessible, depend on Medicaid for their financial viability. However, many plans are reluctant to work with these providers. When the Kaiser Family Foundation surveyed a nationally representative sample of members of the American Association of Health Plans (then Group Health Association of America) in 1994, just 18 percent of managed care plans were interested in contracting out for reproductive health services, and only 9 percent had current contracts to do so. The majority of plans in the survey stated potential interest in contracting out for family planning and abortion services, with only a minority interested in contracting out services related to STDs, prenatal care, breast screening, pelvic exams, and Pap smears.[31]

Many of these traditional family providers have pushed for

various reproductive health services to be "carved out" of Medicaid managed care so that beneficiaries can seek these services from any qualified Medicaid provider, not just those "within-plan." In a survey of women's health centers, Weisman and colleagues found that only 39 percent of reproductive care providers had managed care contracts.[32] The freedom of choice provisions have made it possible for some traditional providers to continue to operate in a time when funds for family planning services are diminishing. However, these providers continue to find themselves financially pressed and are concerned about their continued ability to provide care to the millions of low-income women who lack coverage.[32]

Coordinating and Integrating Care

One of the hallmarks of managed care is care coordination. To the extent that a patient's reproductive health is linked to other facets of her health, and that the various aspects of her reproductive health are linked to each other, coordination of care is advantageous. A fractured health care system in which Medicaid managed care enrollees seek their reproductive health care outside of the plan may be at odds with this principle, unless the MCO and out-of-plan providers establish protocols to share information about patient care.

However, the sensitivity of some of the services involved—sterilization, abortion, contraception, screening and diagnosis for STDs, and infertility diagnosis and treatment—may lead to patients' desire for confidentiality from family members, employers, and even from their ongoing health care providers about the services they receive. While some managed care plans permit obstetrician-gynecologists to be primary care providers, or allow women to self refer to them, many plans allow generalist primary care providers to manage their patients' reproductive health care.

Even with their obstetrician-gynecologists, who are relatively accustomed to discussing sensitive reproductive issues, many women do not discuss issues that directly affect their reproductive health. A recent survey found that 30 percent of sexually active women who did not wish to become pregnant did not discuss birth control with their physicians at the time of their gynecological visit; neither the physician nor the patient raised the topic.[33] At women's first visits, obstetrician-gynecologists asked about birth control only 33 percent of the time, HIV and acquired immune deficiency syndrome (AIDS) 19 percent of the time, and STDs other than HIV/AIDS only 12 percent of the time.[34] It is likely that generalist primary care physicians are less willing than obstetrician-gynecologists to initiate conversation with their patients about these topics.

Finally, concern about confidentiality may compromise access to reproductive health services. For example, access to health care for teenagers is most often based on the insurance status of a parent. Needing the family insurance card may effectively reduce access to reproductive health services for a teen reluctant to share her health concerns. If a plan sends home an explanation of the benefits it provided to a teen, it may reveal to parents those services that the teen wished to keep confidential.

Adults can also be faced with these dilemmas if their insurance coverage is through their spouses or domestic partners. In general, patients' desires for confidentiality regarding reproductive health care also may be at odds with coordinating care.

Monitoring Care and Plan Accountability

As managed care becomes the dominant delivery system for providing care to low-income women on Medicaid, there is increasing pressure on states to assure that the care provided by MCOs meet quality standards. There are, however, a number of difficulties in assessing the quality of reproductive health care for Medicaid managed care beneficiaries that are related to measurement tools, data collection, and states' ability to use data to monitor care and gauge quality.

There are currently a number of initiatives underway to provide measures of the quality of care under managed care. One of the most prominent initiatives is the Health Plan Employer Data and Information Set (HEDIS). The most recent iteration, HEDIS 3.0, was developed, in part, to capture many of the dimensions of care that are relevant to the Medicaid population. The current HEDIS reporting set contains a number of reproductive health indicators. These include measures for breast and cervical cancer screening, a description of the plan's network of family planning providers (for use with Medicaid reporting only), and some indicators of the accessibility and availability of prenatal care and delivery services. However, the number of measures is very limited. Several measures are being evaluated for inclusion in a future HEDIS that would broaden the scope of mea-

surement of reproductive health services. These would include measures for chlamydia screening, follow-up treatment after abnormal Pap smears and mammograms, stage of breast cancer detection, HIV patient management, and counseling about hormone replacement therapy for women.[35] However, even this expanded testing set falls short of a comprehensive assessment of the quality of reproductive health care in a managed care plan. For example, counseling may be the most important element in preventing unplanned pregnancy, but it is difficult to demonstrate that counseling contributes to the prevention of unplanned pregnancy and to measure the quality of that counseling.[36] Measurement of the quality of reproductive health services will be an important area to develop.

Even if the science of measurement were adequate to assess the quality of reproductive health care, a number of logistical hurdles exist that are important to consider. Major challenges to assessing the quality of care lie in the ability of Medicaid MCOs to collect quality of care measures accurately as well as in the capacity of state agencies to use the data in a meaningful way. Not only has the growth of managed care changed how patients, providers, and plans interact with the health system, it has also created new responsibilities for state agencies. They must invest in training and the acquisition of new information systems to monitor care. One of the important lessons from states that have shifted to managed care is that they must have the infrastructure—including the technology and staff—to oversee the care that MCOs provide to Medicaid beneficiaries.[37] This infrastructure requires a critical investment of resources, which is increasingly difficult for state governments in the face of pressure to reduce staffing levels and administrative costs.

Finally, despite significant managed care enrollment in the Medicaid population, a disproportionate share of Medicaid beneficiaries continues to use traditional family planning providers for reproductive health care. Current Medicaid data systems cannot easily track these women's care or determine whether they obtained care that met existing standards. Concerns about confidentiality, problems with obtaining data on out-of-plan use and care coordination, and limitations on data collection systems make it difficult to collect basic data on the use of services.

Meeting the reproductive health care needs of low-income women in Medicaid managed care presents critical challenges at many levels. Populations new to managed care must learn to choose plans, select providers, negotiate for reproductive health services through their gatekeeper primary care providers (who may or may not be their obstetrician-gynecologists), and seek care only from health professionals affiliated with their plans, unless they are aware of out-of-plan options. Plans and health care providers must also recognize beneficiaries' need for supplemental services, such as language translation, child care, transportation assistance, and other social services that are beyond the realm of what has been traditionally viewed as medical care. Because of the vulnerability of the Medicaid population, Medicaid sometimes makes demands on MCOs that exceed those of the private sector. It is now incumbent on states to take on responsibilities beyond their

historical roles as payers of care. They must learn to be prudent purchasers of care, provide more oversight and monitoring of care, and develop and establish quality standards. This is especially challenging when state administrative budgets and staffs are shrinking.

Finally, as one strives to design a system to meet the reproductive health needs of women in Medicaid managed care, it is important to be cognizant of the considerable discontinuity in Medicaid coverage, because women on Medicaid today are often the very same women who are uninsured next month. Some 28 percent of women on Medicaid have been covered for less than two years, and two-thirds of women who leave the Medicaid program become uninsured.[38] These women have the same reproductive needs whether they have Medicaid coverage or not. This presents difficulties for MCOs because women are often not enrolled for a continuous period of time—perhaps decreasing incentives to provide preventive services that reap benefits to MCOs only in the long term. Discontinuous Medicaid coverage is also problematic for the traditional providers of reproductive health services. The growth of managed care threatens the very survival of the freestanding traditional providers upon whom women will still depend when their coverage runs out. In efforts to assure that Medicaid managed care best meets the needs of low-income women, it will be increasingly important to consider the needs of uninsured women as well. Regardless of insurance coverage or care arrangement, low-income women will continue to need access to a broad range of quality reproductive care services at an affordable price.

References

1. U.S. Department of Health and Human Services, Health Care Financing Administration, *Medicaid Managed Care Enrollment Report, Summary Statistics as of June 30, 1997. Baltimore, MD.:* Health Care Financing Administration, 1998.

2. Delbanco, S., and Smith, M.D. Reproductive Health and Managed Care—An Overview. *Western Journal of Medicine* 163 (supplement to no. 3) (1995): 1–6.

3. Kaiser Commission on Medicaid and the Uninsured. Unpublished estimate based on Urban Institute analysis of the March 1996 Current Population Survey, Bureau of the Census.

4. Henshaw, S.K. Unintended Pregnancy in the United States. *Family Planning Perspectives* 30, no. 1 (1998): 24–29, 46.

5. Jones, E.F., and Forrest, J.D. Contraceptive Failure Rates Based on the 1988 NSFG. *Family Planning Perspectives* 12, no. 1 (1992): 12–19.

6. Forrest, J.D., and Frost, J.J. The Family Planning Attitudes and Experiences of Low-Income Women. *Family Planning Perspectives* 28, no. 6 (1996): 246–255.

7. U.S. Department of Health and Human Services, Centers for Disease Control and Prevention. *Sexually Transmitted Disease Surveillance 1995.* Atlanta, GA: U.S. Department of Health and Human Services, Centers for Disease Control and Prevention, 1996.

8. Devesa, S.S., and Diamond, E.L. Association of Breast Cancer and Cervical Cancer Incidences with Income and Education Among Whites and Blacks. *Journal of the National Cancer Institute* 65, no. 3 (1990): 515–528.

9. Krieger, N. Social Class and the Black/White Crossover in the Age-Specific Incidence of Breast Cancer: A Study Linking Census-Derived Data to Population-Based Registry Records. *American Journal of Epidemiology* 131, no. 5 (1990): 804–814.

10. Ayanian, J.X., et al. The Relationship Between Health Insurance Coverage and Clinical Outcome Among Women with Breast Cancer. *The New England Journal of Medicine* 329, no. 5 (1993): 326–31.

11. Levine, R.E., and Tsoflias, L. *Publicly Supported Family Planning*

in the United States. Washington, D.C.: The Urban Institute and Child Trends, Inc., 1994.

12. The Alan Guttmacher Institute. *The Status of Major Abortion-Related Laws in the States.* New York: The Alan Guttmacher Institute, 1998.

13. Lyons, B., et al. Poverty, Access to Health Care, and Medicaid's Critical Role for Women. In *Women's Health, The Commonwealth Fund Survey,* ed. Falik, M.M., and Collins, K.S. Baltimore, MD: The Johns Hopkins University Press, 1996.

14. Frost, J.J., and Bolzan, M. The Provision of Public-Sector Services by Family Planning Agencies in 1995. *Family Planning Perspectives* 29, no. 1 (1997): 6–14.

15. U.S. Department of Health and Human Services, Health Care Financing Administration, Medicaid Bureau. *Medicaid Statistics, Program and Financial Statistics, Fiscal Year 1995.* Pub. No. 10129. Washington, D.C.: HCFA, 1996.

16. National Governors' Association. *State Medicaid Coverage of Pregnant Women and Children. MCH Update.* Washington, DC: National Governors' Association, 1997.

17. Salganicoff, A. *Access to Health Care for Low-Income Women: Impact of Medicaid and Private Insurance.* Presentation to the Restructuring Health Care for the Poor: Conference of the Kaiser Commonwealth Low-Income Coverage and Access Project. Washington, D.C., June 1997.

18. The Center for Reproductive Law and Policy. *Removing Barriers Improving Choices, A Case Study in Reproductive Health Services and Managed Care.* New York: The Center for Reproductive Law and Policy, Inc., 1996.

19. Donovan, P. *The Politics of Blame, Family Planning, Abortion and the Poor.* New York: The Alan Guttmacher Institute, 1995.

20. Kaiser Commission on the Future of Medicaid. Medicaid and Managed Care. *Medicaid Facts,* December 1997.

21. Rosenbaum, S., et al. Beyond the Freedom to Choose Medicaid, Managed Care, and Family Planning. *The Western Journal of Medicine* 163 (supplement to no. 3) (1995): 33–38.

22. Rosenbaum et al. Medicaid Managed Care and the Family Planning Free-Choice Option: Beyond the Freedom to Choose. *Journal of Health Policy, Policy Politics and Law* 22, no. 5 (1997): 1,191–1,214.

23. Murray, M. *Medicaid and Expanded Family Planning 1115 Waivers.* Working Paper of the U.S. Office of Management and Budget, 1997.

24. Armstead, R.C., and Gorman, J.K. Baby Love and Budget Relief: Some Promising Practices in Prenatal Managed Care in Medicaid. *JAMA* 50, no. 5 (1995): 178–181.

25. United States General Accounting Office. *Medicaid Prenatal Care: States Improve Access and Enhance Services, But Face New Challenges.* GAO/HEHS-94-152BR, Washington, D.C.: GAO, 1994.

26. Shulman, E., Et al. Primary Care Case Management and Birth Outcomes in the Iowa Medicaid Program. *American Journal of Public Health* 87, no. 1 (1997): 80–84.

27. Goldfarb, N., et al. Impact of a Mandatory Medicaid Case Management Program on Prenatal Care and Birth Outcomes: A Retrospective Analysis. *Medical Care* 29, no. 1 (1991): 64–71.

28. Rowland, D., et al. *Medicaid and Managed Care Lessons from the Literature.* Washington, D.C.: Kaiser Commission on the Future of Medicaid, 1995.

29. Rosenbaum, S., et al., *Negotiating the New Health System: A Nationwide Analysis of Medicaid Managed Care Contracts.* Washington, D.C.: George Washington University Center For Health Policy Research, February 1997.

30. Celum, C.L., et al. Where Would Clients Seek Care for STD Services Under Health Care Reform? Results of a STD Client Survey from Five Clinics. Eleventh Meeting of the International Society for STD Research, August 27–30, 1995. New Orleans, LA [abstract no. 101].

31. Bernstein, A.B., et al. Women's Reproductive Health Services in Health Maintenance Organizations. *Western Journal of Medicine* 163, supplement to no. 3 (1995): 15–18.

32. Weisman, C.S., et al. Women's Health Centers and Managed Care. *Women's Health Issues* 6, no. 5 (1996): 255–263.

33. Kaiser Family Foundation/Glamour National Survey/Princeton Survey Research Associates. 1997. *Survey of Women about Their Knowledge, Attitudes and Practices Regarding Reproductive Health.* Menlo Park, Ca.: Kaiser Family Foundation, 1997.

34. Kaiser Family Foundation/Glamour National Survey. *Talking about STDs with Health Professionals: Women's Experiences.* Menlo Park, Ca.: Kaiser Family Foundation, 1997.

35. National Committee for Quality Assurance. *HEDIS 3.0., Health Plan Employer Data & Information Set.* Washington, D.C.: National Committee for Quality Assurance, 1997.

36. McGlynn, E.A. Quality Assessment of Reproductive Health Services. *Western Journal of Medicine* 163 (supplement to no. 3) (1995): 19–27.

37. Gold, M., et al. Medicaid Managed Care: Lessons from Five States. *Health Affairs* 15, no. 3 (1996): 153–166.

38. Short, P.F. *Medicaid's Role in Insuring Low-Income Women.* New York: The Commonwealth Fund, 1996.

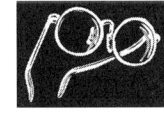 **Article Review Form at end of book.**

One of the prevention program's unforeseen benefits was the increase in _____. What kind of effect did this prevention program have on the hospital's physicians and patients?

Community Health Initiative Uses Casefinding, Intervention to Boost Prevention and Revenues

Disease management professionals know that if you screen a patient and find a problem early enough, you can significantly decrease disease risk and subsequent costs. But in the real world, often this routine care slips through the cracks.

Replicating the clinical and financial success of an aggressive program of prevention and risk screening in Waltham, MA, however, could jumpstart your hospital, clinic, or health plan and put prevention into practice.

The Winchester Hospital's Clinical Health Initiative has not only resulted in earlier diagnoses, according to its developers, it has also translated into significant risk pool savings and more revenue for both the hospital and local physician practices.

The program began modestly enough, focusing on only a single disease state. "When we began shifting to a prevention model back in 1992, we were shocked to discover a large num-

ber of undiagnosed diabetics in our community," says Kathleen Beyerman, RN, CNA, EdD, director of the Clinical Health Initiative.

In the program's early stages, Beyerman and her colleagues set out to write a health mapping report on diabetes. Unlike other traditional community health initiatives such as health fairs that focus strictly on identification and diagnosis, the initiative's long range goal was to prevent disease from occurring in the first place.

Almost all of the community's 350,000 residents had a primary care physician and knew their doctor by name. "This gave us a real opportunity to access information through the physicians," says Beyerman.

To gain access to medical records and begin the casefinding process, however, hospital officials first met with physicians to develop a memorandum of understanding. The agreement

called for strict confidentiality on the part of casefinders and special handling of any medical records with a confidential diagnosis such as HIV/AIDS.

Astounding Level of Undetected Risk

The physicians were "extremely receptive to the idea" of case review, says Beyerman. She hired two casefinders with a background in medical record review. They followed a software program that searched the records to identify certain diabetes risk factors by looking at patient age, history of gestational diabetes, family history, and other factors.

After identifying individuals at risk for diabetes, a letter and lab slip was sent to patients for testing by the hospital's lab, and results were returned to the doctor's office.

The results were startling. Of 5,486 records reviewed in the pilot phase of the program in

1996, 1,506 patients were found to be at risk. Subsequent lab testing revealed 42 new cases of diabetes and 136 previously diagnosed diabetics whose blood sugar readings were found to be not in control.

"This served as a real consciousness raising for us and the physicians. They had no system in place to call in a patient for routine lab work," Beyerman illustrates. Even though they had been diagnosed for diabetes, these 136 patients had not had an HbA1c test in the last 12 months.

The diabetes patients were immediately enrolled in a patient education program at the hospital and scheduled for routine tracking and follow-up. Each patient was seen for three follow-up visits, and some with more serious diabetes also received telephone monitoring.

At the completion of the follow-up program, medical records were again reviewed, revealing the following results:

- 75% of patients showed glycemic improvement;

- 60% of patients were monitored for blood sugar with results logged;

- 67% of patients had lost weight;

- 59% of patients reported taking medications;

- 72% of patients had started an exercise program.

Prevention Program Rolled Out

After the initial diabetes effort, Beyerman and her colleagues sought to apply a similar two-phase program of casefinding and prevention to all chronic disease states. "We felt that we had racks of medical records that were the train wrecks of tomor-row," says Beyerman. In retrospect, she alerts other providers of these common findings: many women have not seen a physician since they had their last baby, and many middle aged men have not seen a physician since childhood.

The Community Health Initiative piloted its "Putting Prevention into Practice" program to insure that potential health problems are caught at the earliest stage through compliance with recommended national screening guidelines, Beyerman says.

Now, before new patients arrive for a scheduled visit or exam, their charts are reviewed by an RN prevention specialist, who then creates a personal prevention plan showing recommended frequency and dates of screening tests and fills out lab slips for testing that should be completed. These screenings are based on a compiled list of national guidelines from the National Cancer Institute and the U.S. Preventive Service Task Force. (See screening protocols in Figure 1, page 192.)

The prevention specialist arranges with physician practices to use their office space to review cases. After reviewing the records of all new patients, the nurse begins a complete chart review in alphabetical order.

The prevention program hired registered nurses to do the case finding because of the wide variety of risk factors being addressed in the program roll-out. Nurses use the software program and their own expertise to identify at-risk patients, she adds.

If a record review turns up a patient needing a screening, a follow-up letter is sent from the physician's office advising the patient to make an appointment for the test.

If there is no response to the letter, the evening staff in the clinic will call and ask the patient to book an appointment. Each patient's preventive screenings are measured on a flow chart. (See female preventive care flow sheet in Figure 2 below.*)

After the initial case finding, a tickler system in the database generates letters to patients at the beginning of each month. For example, the letters notify patients when they need a follow-up screening such as an HbA1c test. Patients also receive a copy of their prevention care plan.

Clinical Results

As one example of this system's success, Beyerman says the number of Pap smears has more than doubled since the program began in late 1996. Other clinical benefits of the prevention into practice program have been equally substantial, and the initiative helps with HEDIS compliance as well, she points out. In one local practice, the first year in the program demonstrated the following results:

- More than 603 new diagnoses including skin cancer, hypertension, hypercholesterolemia, and hyperglycemia;

- More than 1700 additional patient visits over a 24-month period, with an average of 72 additional patient visits per month

Overall, just under 10,000 patients have been screened since the program began. More than 1,700 of these screenings resulted from follow-up letters generated by chart review of existing patients. The new diagnoses included:

- 133 patients with hypertension

- 16 patients with skin cancer

*Fig. 2 appears on page 193

Figure 1 Screening Protocols—Putting Prevention into Practice Pilot

Test	Interval	High Risk Interval	Standard	Determining Factors for High Risk
Physical Examination	For men, every 2 years if not at high risk: annually after age 40. For women, annually after age 20.	Annually		Previous occurrences of major illness or disease/chronic disease.
Blood Pressure	At least every two years and at every visit to a practitioner.	At least annually	American Academy of Family Physicians, American Heart Association	Diastolic blood pressure between 85 and 89 mm Hg, moderate or extreme obesity, first degree relative with hypertension, personal history of hypertension.
Blood Cholesterol	Once in young adulthood and every 5 years thereafter up to age 70.	Annually	American Academy of Family Physicians, American College of Physicians	2 or more CHD factors: HDL ≤ 35, LDL ≥ 160, family history of premature CHD, cigarette smoking, hypertension, diabetes mellitus, men over age 45 and women over age 55 or premature menopause without estrogen therapy.
Plasma Glucose	Baseline @ 40 years of age and every three years thereafter. If high risk, baseline at 30 years of age and every year thereafter.	Annually for adults with four or more risk factors	American Diabetes Association	Family history of diabetes, over age 40, 20% above recommended weight, ethnic background, gestational diabetic or women who delivered a baby over 9 pounds, persistent skin, yeast or urinary tract infection, hyperlipidemia, retinopathy, neuropathy, or nephropathy, vascular problems, hypertension, fatigue, blurred vision, thyroid disorders.
Skin Screen	Every 2 years for those age 20–39 and yearly after age 40.	Annually	American Cancer Society	Fair skinned, history of overexposure to the sun, family history of skin cancer.
Digital Rectal Examination	All patients annually starting at age 40.	Yearly at age 35	American Cancer Society	Family history of colorectal or adenomatous cancer, a personal history of adenomas or of ovarian, endometrial or breast cancer, personal history of ulcerative colitis, or inflammatory bowel disease.
Fecal Blood Occult	Annual test beginning at age 40.	Annually at age 35	American Cancer Society	History of one of the familial polyposis syndromes, familial cancer syndromes, colorectal cancer in first degree relatives or a personal history of ulcerative colitis, adenomatous polyps, or endometrial, ovarian or breast cancer.
Breast Examination	Annually at age 20.	Same	American Cancer Society	Breast cancer in first degree relative, estrogen replacement therapy.
Mammogram	Baseline sometime between ages 35–40 and annually after age 40.	Yearly after age 35	American Cancer Society, National Cancer Institute	Increased age, breast cancer in first degree relative, estrogen replacement therapy.
Pap Smear	Every 1 to 3 years at the onset of sexual activity or age 18—annually unless three or more consecutive years with negative pap smear results.	Annually until age 80 and then every three years thereafter	American Cancer Society, American Academy of Family Physicians, National Cancer Institute	Early age at first intercourse, multiple sex partners, smoker, family history.
Testicular Examination	Every 2 years from age 20–39 and annually beginning at age 40.	Annually	American Cancer Society	Males with a history of cryptorchidism, gonadal dysgenesis, Klinefelter's syndrome or in utero exposure to DES.

Check if Appropriate: Please note date(s) of discussion.

❑ Weight Control					❑ Work/Home			
❑ STD/HIV/AIDS					❑ Nutrition			
❑ Drug					❑ Tobacco			
☒ Family Planning	06/01/1998				☒ Exercise	06/01/1998		
❑ Testicular					❑ Stress			
☒ Seat Belts					❑ Parenting			
❑ Health Safety					❑ _____			
❑ _____					❑ _____			

					1998	1999	2000	2001	2002	2003	2004	2005	2006
		Freq			35	36	37	38	39	40	41	42	43
Physical Exam	❑	2	Date		06/01/98		×		×		×		×
			Results										
Blood Pressure	❑	2	Date		06/01/98		×		×		×		×
			Results										
Cholesterol	❑	5	Date		06/01/98					×			
			Results										
Plasma Glucose	❑		Date		06/01/03					×			×
			Results										
Skin Screen	❑	2	Date		06/01/98		×		×	×	×	×	×
			Results										
Rectal Exam	❑		Date		06/01/03					×	×	×	×
			Results										
Fecal Blood	❑		Date		06/01/03					×	×	×	×
			Results										
Vision	❑		Date										
			Results										
Mammography	❑	5	Date		06/01/98					×	×	×	×
			Results										
Breast Exam	❑	1	Date		06/01/98	×	×	×	×	×	×	×	×
			Results										
Pap Smear	❑	1	Date		06/01/98	×	×	×	×	×	×	×	×
			Results										

Suggested Result Codes: O=Ordered N=Result Normal A=Result Abnormal R=Refused E=Done Elsewhere X=Next Due Date

Tetanus	10	Date	01/01/1997										
		Results											
Pneumococcus		Date											
		Results											
Influenza	1	Date	01/12/1997										
		Results											
HepB		Date											
		Results											
Varicella		Date											
		Results											

Referral to	Date	Result
Diabetes Education Program		
Nutrition Education Program		
Smoking Cessation Counseling		

Figure 2 Female Preventive Care Flow Sheet

- 316 patients with elevated hypercholesterolemia
- 50 patients with diabetes (See Figure 3,* page 153.)

Financial Results

One of the prevention program's unforeseen benefits has been the sharp increase in revenues for both the hospital and physicians, says Beyerman. "This program prepares practices for a capitated environment while still managing a predominantly fee-for-service operation," she maintains.

Appropriately providing preventive care can assist physicians in lowering overall costs and man-

*Figure not included in this publication.

aging risk pools more effectively, she says. It also generates revenue for the hospital and for physicians due to the increase in visits. (See Figure 4 and 5,* above.)

In the pilot practice, for example, an additional $348,163 in physician procedures and visits were billed. These in turn generated an additional $298,617 in radiology and laboratory revenues for the hospital.

The program tracks and reports on its performance in a number of key areas, including the following:

- the number of letters sent to recall patient by practice;

*Figures not included in this publication.

- the number of patient visits generated by type;
- new diagnoses made as a result of the program by practice;
- physician revenue by procedure code (see sample physician report in Figure 6*);
- nutrition and diabetes counseling referrals;
- hospital lab and radiology revenue generated;
- physician satisfaction.

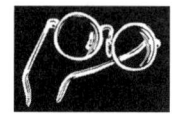 **Article Review Form at end of book.**

FAIR recommends five priority strategies to reduce and prevent barriers to reproductive health care for managed care enrollees. List three. How does lack of adequate information about reproductive health care coverage affect appropriate care?

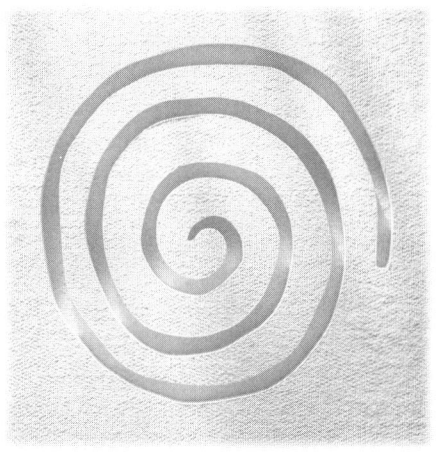

Removing Barriers and Improving Choices:

A Case Study in Reproductive Health Services and Managed Care

Shirley G. Gordon

Shirley G. Gordon, BS, RN, MS, is President, Gordon and Gordon Associates, Inc., in New York, New York. She was formerly Director of FAIR: Health Care and Reform, a project of the Center for Reproductive Law and Policy, a public interest law firm based in New York City.

Managed care contains inherent structural features that can create obstacles to time-sensitive, confidential reproductive health services. Such structural impediments often exacerbate the sociocultural barriers that have historically affected low-income women—the population that has been targeted for mandatory enrollment in Medicaid managed care plans in many states. This article recommends public policy strategies to overcome and prevent multiple barriers that were identified in a New York-based study in 1995, which focused on access to reproductive health services in managed care settings. This article also includes updated evidence supporting the study's findings and its relevance to other states.

Barriers to preventive health care can delay timely treatment and lead to greater health risks. Family planning and related reproductive health services are particularly time sensitive: A one-day lapse in contraception can result in an unintended pregnancy and potentially serious consequences. A woman with an unintended pregnancy is less likely to seek early prenatal care and is more likely to expose her fetus to harmful substances such as alcohol and tobacco. The child resulting from an unwanted conception is at greater risk of being born at low birth weight, of dying in his or her first year of life, of being abused, and of not having sufficient resources for healthy development. Mothers are at risk of depression, and both parents may suffer economic hardship or fail to reach educational and career

goals.[1] In terms of the human and societal costs of these lost opportunities, the full impact is incalculable.

Assuring unimpeded timely access to preventive and primary reproductive health care must be one of the highest priorities in any health care delivery system. This was the underlying premise of the FAIR Project,* which focused on access to family planning and related reproductive health services in managed care. The twin goals of the project were to identify sociocultural barriers to reproductive health services in managed care settings and then to develop a blueprint for public policy strategies to overcome

*FAIR stands for Focus on Access, Information and Reproductive Rights. The project was sponsored by the Center for Reproductive Law and Policy and funded, in large part, by Opening Doors: Reducing Sociocultural Barriers to Health Care, a national program jointly funded by the Robert Wood Johnson Foundation and the Kaiser Family Foundation.

these barriers. The objective was to ensure unimpeded access for all adult women and adolescents, whether they choose to, or are required to, enroll in managed care. Medicaid managed care became the centerpiece of the FAIR Project because of the nationwide trend to move into this system virtually all poor families headed by women. These women have a higher incidence of reproductive health-related problems. This article highlights key findings and recommendations detailed in *Removing Barriers, Improving Choices: A Case Study in Reproductive Health Services and Managed Care,* a 1996 report on the FAIR Project research that was conducted throughout 1995. Also included are findings of several more recent, related studies, which support many of the FAIR Project's findings and recommendations.

Project Design

Using New York State as a laboratory, the FAIR Project undertook qualitative research in 1995 to identify sociocultural barriers to reproductive health services in managed care settings. Between May and October, seven focus groups were conducted with 55 Medicaid managed care enrollees. These participants were primarily African American and Latina women, who were either adults or adolescents from urban and rural areas of New York (including women enrolled in the state's only religiously sponsored plan). The project also surveyed staff from family planning agencies to identify problems encountered by family planning clinic patients who were enrolled in commercial or Medicaid managed care plans. Responses from 52 providers at 32 clinics have been integrated in the report.

To validate the findings from these subjective research components, the project reviewed member handbooks from 23 Medicaid managed care plans, and examined public and private evaluations of New York's Medicaid managed care program. Further research confirmed the relevancy of project findings beyond New York. The project also conducted interviews with 16 leading policymakers and health care advocates in New York and gathered input from the FAIR Project advisory committee. These components formed the basis for project conclusions, public policy recommendations, and strategies to overcome barriers and improve access to reproductive health care.

Because of limitations of this qualitative study, caution must be used in drawing conclusions from the subjective observations of the focus group participants and survey respondents. The methodology does not permit measurement of the scope of the identified problems, the application of the findings to managed care plans other than those mentioned in the report, or even the application of findings to other enrollees in those same plans.

Barriers Identified in Focus Groups and Provider Survey

Impediments to timely care were identified by participants in both the focus groups and the provider survey. The predominant problems can be divided into three areas: communication, confidentiality, and appropriateness of care.

Communication

Complaints about inadequate, inappropriate, and inaccurate

communication were common throughout the state. Consumers reported never being informed prior to enrollment about coverage of reproductive health services or the self-referral option.[†] Women in the sectarian-sponsored plan said they were misled by the plan's marketers, who told them that the plan would offer more services than the traditional Medicaid program. It was not until they needed contraceptive or abortion services that they learned that the plan could not meet their full reproductive health care needs. These women all said they had not received a member handbook when they enrolled and had no knowledge of their right to go outside of the plan for contraception, abortion, and other confidential reproductive health services not covered by their plan. Although consumers in nonsectarian plans may have seen member handbooks, they also were often unaware of the self-referral option. Communication was also inadequate when enrollees sought information on sensitive sexual health issues. One young woman in Syracuse said that when she told her primary care doctor about a sex-related problem she was experiencing, his response was "That's none of my business." Other participants in this same focus group confirmed the primary care provider's discomfort when answering sex-related questions. One said, "That's what

[†]The self-referral option, also referred to in this article as direct access (applies to commercial plans) or free access (applies to Medicaid plans), is a New York state policy that permits enrollees to go directly to a reproductive health provider of their choice without prior approval of their primary care provider for family planning and related reproductive health services. Medicaid enrollees may self refer to providers in or out of the plan's network. Enrollees in commercial plans may only self refer to network providers.

I can't stand. You have to dig it out of them."

Other communication problems stemmed from the lack of interpreters on staff. Non-English speaking consumers often had to rely on a relative, other patient, or even custodial personnel to translate for the doctor their most personal reproductive health symptoms.

Confidentiality

Lack of interpreters can lead to a breach of patient confidentiality. So can a plan's procedures, such as calling a patient's home to remind her of an appointment for contraception or abortion or sending notices to adult policyholders of all medical services that were provided to their dependents, including reproductive health services that adolescents expected to be kept confidential. These were two of the problems the FAIR Project learned about through the provider survey.

Complaints about lack of confidentiality and privacy were heard from enrollees in every focus group. Most common were expressions of anger over people walking in and out of the examining room while patients were "up in stirrups" receiving pelvic exams. These patients said it made them feel as if they didn't exist.

Appropriateness of Care

While enrollees generally were not often aware of what care was inappropriate, it was clear to focus group facilitators and survey respondents that there were many examples of care that did not meet quality care benchmarks for obstetrics and gynecology. Many focus group participants said they had not been informed about birth control options even though they were sexually active;

they were not counseled on safe sex practices to prevent human immunodeficiency virus (HIV) infection even though they were at high risk; or they were not given full options counseling following a positive pregnancy test. All participants in one group said their primary care doctor never had given them a pelvic exam even though they had been enrolled in that plan for more than a year. Providers responding to the survey gave examples of care that did not meet generally accepted standards of practice. For example, a woman who was 28 weeks pregnant could not be scheduled for a prenatal care appointment for two months. A rural woman who wanted an abortion was scheduled for an appointment 20 weeks from the date she requested it. A woman in a New York City plan, who asked for an abortion referral, received a copy of the plan's extensive directory of providers and was told that it was her responsibility to find one who could do the procedure. One woman on Medicaid who was three months pregnant could not be scheduled for her first prenatal appointment for three weeks. When she asked for an appointment sooner, she was told that she had waited this long "so a few more weeks wouldn't matter." She disenrolled from that plan and obtained an appointment that same week from a nearby freestanding prenatal care clinic. If this woman had been in a mandatory enrollment program, she would essentially have been "locked" into her plan's provider network because these services are not covered by the free access policy.

Two other examples from the focus groups underscore inappropriate care that can increase health risks for patients: A

woman who was on Depo-Provera had experienced a hemorrhage that required immediate attention. After she had called her plan's member services line twice—and was told they would call her right back, but did not—she went directly to the plan's hospital emergency department. The woman was told she needed a dilation and curettage (D&C), but would first have to obtain a referral from her primary care provider. Because it was a weekend and her primary care doctor would not be available for two more days, the woman went to the nearest hospital emergency department, even though the hospital was not in her plan. She had the D&C that night, but her plan subsequently refused to cover the costs.

The following example highlights the negative impact of diminished access to the full range of reproductive health services in sectarian-sponsored plans. One focus group participant told of her primary care provider refusing to give her contraception. After she had asked for it twice, the provider told her that he couldn't give it to her because her plan was sponsored by a Catholic hospital. The doctor failed to refer this woman elsewhere for the service or advise her that Medicaid would cover the service if she self referred to another provider. This single mother of two, who was on Medicaid, was five months pregnant at the time of the focus group and blamed her unintended pregnancy on that doctor not giving her birth control when she had requested it.

Although most focus group participants had not filed complaints, changed plans, or switched primary care providers, they clearly articulated their dissatisfaction with the reproductive health services and lack of information provided by their plans. For many, the barriers they faced created not only a reluctance or inability to seek timely care, but also an unwillingness to provide to their physicians full information about their lifestyles and sexual practices, request information about sexual health concerns, or comply with their provider's care plan. Three women underscored this in one of the Brooklyn focus groups by emphatically telling the facilitator that they would never go back to their plan for a Pap smear because their primary care doctor had treated them so disrespectfully.

Supporting Evidence

Because qualitative research is often dismissed as too subjective, the FAIR Project report incorporates objective documentation to validate many of the barriers perceived by the participants in the focus groups and provider survey. These barriers include the following:

• *Lack of adequate information about reproductive health coverage and free access.* Both FAIR Project's own review of member handbooks and evaluations by state and city agencies validated the inadequacy of information that prospective and current enrollees received about reproductive health services and the free access option. The 1995 handbook review found that 83 percent prominently stated that all services must be obtained directly through the plan, or only through a referral from the plan except in cases of life-threatening emergencies. A typical handbook provided information about the free access option six pages after enrollees were instructed to

stay in the plan. Furthermore, most of the handbooks were written at a tenth-grade reading level,[2] whereas the state recommends that materials be written at a fourth-grade level for the Medicaid population.

An Office of Public Advocate of the City of New York study conducted in November 1995 found that plans routinely distribute "vague, false, potentially misleading or inadequate information to prospective enrollees." The Advocate's office concluded that "some plans . . . create confusion by failing to explain the law regarding family planning services . . . [or explanations are] placed out of context . . . [and/or] worded in a technical manner."[3] A state department of social services marketing review of five major Medicaid managed care plans in New York City confirmed confusion among enrollees about family planning services. The department's report revealed that only 26 to 36 percent of enrollees of these plans were aware of the free access policy. The report stated that the enrollee's level of knowledge about this option was among the lowest recorded on any question asked in the survey.[4]

• *Lack of access.* A 1995 undercover investigation by the New York State Department of Health validated the severe access barriers experienced by consumers. Posing as consumers, department staff called 18 of the largest plans in New York City. They asked to see doctors for such basic services as prenatal care. In 13 of the 18 plans, the investigators had so much trouble getting an initial appointment that the New York

State Department of Health cited them for providing substandard care.[5]

• *Gaps in appropriate care.* A 1994 New York State Department of Social Services compliance review of the only Medicaid mandatory enrollment program underscored the gaps in gynecological care. It compared gynecological services provided to adult women in managed care plans to a control group of adult women on Medicaid who used fee-for-service providers [who are generally obstetrics-gynecology (OB-GYN) physicians or family planning clinics]. The study found that women in managed care received fewer Pap smears, gonorrhea tests, and breast exams.[6]

Updated Evidence Supports Findings

Since completion of the FAIR Project report in June 1996, there have been several studies related to Medicaid managed care and reproductive health that support many of the FAIR Project findings and recommendations. These include the following:

• *Knowledge Gap: What Medicaid Beneficiaries Understand—And What They Don't About Managed Care.* This New York City-based study, in which the Community Services Society interviewed 400 Medicaid beneficiaries in the South Bronx and Harlem between February and March of 1996, confirms FAIR's findings about the lack of information and understanding among consumers about how managed care works and how to obtain care within that system. The authors conclude that one-time education and dense handbooks are not good.

More education is needed to prepare beneficiaries for managed care.[7]

- *Don't Ask, They Won't Tell: The Quality of Adolescent Health Screening in Five Practice Settings.* This December 1996 study underscores FAIR's conclusion that practitioners who have less experience with adolescent reproductive health may be less qualified to provide appropriate education and services to sexually active youth. The authors found that non–teen-focused practice settings typically failed to screen for sociobehavioral health risks, regardless of the patient's age or gender. The authors said this suggested that primary care providers may still be reluctant or ill prepared to address social and behavioral etiologies that underlie the major causes of adolescent morbidity and mortality. If pertinent screening questions are not asked, they concluded, appropriate services cannot be offered to those who need them.[8]

- *Delivery of STD/HIV Preventive Services to Adolescents by Primary Care Physicians.* This 1996 California-based survey examined the extent of sexually transmitted disease (STD) preventive care delivered to adolescents by primary care physicians. It provides further evidence that not all primary care doctors who routinely see adolescents provide them with a high level of sexual health-related preventive care. The study found that 41 percent of all surveyed physicians screen all of their patients to determine if they are sexually active, and 31 percent furnish all adolescent patients with information about STDs, including HIV. Only 4 percent provide condoms to all of their sexually active patients. OB-GYN and female physicians are more likely to provide STD preventive care.[9]

- *Survey of Women about Their Knowledge, Attitudes, and Practices Regarding Their Reproductive Health.* This February 1997 study, sponsored by *Glamour* magazine and the Kaiser Family Foundation, supports FAIR's conclusion that non–OB-GYN physicians as gatekeepers may adversely impact access to and quality of reproductive health care. The survey found that women who see a gynecologist are more likely to have discussed birth control at their last visit—or had an HIV or STD test performed at some point than are women who use another health professional for their routine care or who do not have a regular provider for this care.[10]

- *Do MCOs Inform Members About the Free Access and Direct Access Laws?* This 1997 study by Planned Parenthood of New York City (PPNYC), confirms FAIR's finding of confusion and misinformation among managed care staff about the state's policies on the ability of managed care enrollees to self refer for certain reproductive health services. PPNYC staff and volunteers made 226 calls to 22 managed care plans in New York City to determine the accuracy of information given to callers on free access for Medicaid managed care members and direct access for all others. While answers were correct about free access 54 percent of the time, the most common incorrect response was insisting that enrollees had to go to their primary care provider for reproductive health services.[11]

- *The Transition to Managed Care: Experiences of Planned Parenthood Patients.* This 1997 study by PPNYC, detailed in this issue, confirms FAIR's finding that appropriate physical examinations or information may not be provided to members by their primary care practitioners even though they may be enrolled in their current plan for over a year. Of Planned Parenthood patients enrolled in Medicaid managed care who had visits to their primary care providers, two thirds had never discussed STDs and more than one third had never discussed contraception.[12]

- *Reforming State Medicaid Programs.* This 1997 study by Mathematica Policy Research assessed Medicaid programs in the states of Hawaii, Tennessee, and Rhode Island after the first year of implementation of their federally approved mandatory managed care programs (all had Section 1115 waivers). The study confirms FAIR's conclusion about the need to build in more time for planning, implementing, and evaluating such programs prior to initiating them. Relevant conclusions included: procedures for enrolling pregnant women and newborns should be modified to avoid snags that threaten access to care; more consumer education about their choices and how managed care works is needed; and special arrangements may be needed to help safety-net hospitals continue serving vulnerable populations as they transition to managed care. The authors noted that an array of problems resulted from rapid implementation and that none of the states had produced final encounter data for the first year, even 18 months after startup. This limited their ability to monitor the performance of managed care organizations (MCOs).[13]

- *Health Plans Join in Call for National Standards.* In September of 1997, three major non-profit health maintenance organizations (HMOs) joined two national consumer groups in calling for more regulation of managed health care. It was their view that all health plans should be subject to "legally enforceable national standards." Such standards, they said, are essential to restore confidence in the health care system, which has been eroded by reports from many HMO patients that they have had difficulty getting the care they need. The "statement of principles for consumer protection" was issued by Kaiser Permanente, HIP of New York, and the Group Health Cooperative of Puget Sound. The consumer groups were Families USA and the American Association of Retired Persons (AARP). Among the standards proposed that are similar to those recommended by FAIR are: direct access for women to OB-GYN providers; freedom to see outside doctors at no additional cost if the plan does not have a doctor with appropriate training and expertise; and coverage by plans for emergency care in any situation that a prudent lay person would regard as an emergency.[14]

Contributing Factors: A Baseline for Building Strategies

Understanding the genesis of a problem is a crucial bridge to de-veloping effective strategies. The FAIR Project's research, which included a search of the literature and interviews with policymakers, helped to identify factors that may have contributed to the barriers faced by women and adolescents enrolled in managed care plans. These barriers include the range of sociocultural impediments to access that have long been present in the fee-for-service system as well as "structural" barriers that are unique to managed care. The structural barriers, a spin-off of features that have been built into managed care to reduce overutilization and control costs, often compound and exacerbate the long-standing sociocultural impediments, especially for low-income women and adolescents seeking confidential reproductive health services. A pattern that clearly emerged in this study was that the confluence of these sociocultural and structural barriers may become obstacles that not only jeopardize the health of these vulnerable individuals, but also may strip them of their ability to control their own lives. For example, a woman in a religiously sponsored plan who took the initiative to prevent HIV infection by requesting condoms from her primary care doctor was told that condoms were not available through that plan. The sociocultural and structural factors that the FAIR Project found to be most directly compromising of access to quality reproductive health care in managed care settings are summarized below.

Sociocultural Influences

Lack of child care, public transportation, geographically accessible services, culturally competent and respectful staff, interpreters, and easy-to-understand and culturally appropriate information are all factors that contributed to the identified barriers. The age of the patient, where he or she lived, and gender differences between a provider and the patient also affected access and usage of services. More nebulous influences included the patient's sense of control over his or her own life, and the patient's relationship with and perspective of others who do not share his or her beliefs and background. Each of these factors, or a combination thereof, could have played a role in determining which providers or services an enrollee ultimately used, whether timely care was provided, whether the enrollee would comply with a treatment regime, whether the enrollee would be assertive or file a complaint if unhappy with services or providers, and whom the enrollee would trust.

Structural Influences

Features that contributed to diminished access to reproductive health care included: benefit packages with restricted coverage for reproductive health services; enrollment practices and member handbooks that failed to provide full and understandable disclosure about a plan's limited services; and gatekeepers with minimal experience in managing sexual and reproductive health problems, especially in adolescents. Other factors were inflexible rules that may breach confidentiality, such as notification to policyholders (usually a parent) of services provided to dependents, or calls to a patient's home to remind her of an appointment. Closed provider networks also were problematic because they virtually "lock in" enrollees who do not have financial resources to pay for services outside of the plan. The bureaucratic "red tape"—exemplified by the intimidating rules and procedures as well as imposing member handbooks that consumers never had to deal with in the fee-for-service system—played a role as well. This "red tape" may account for a heightened perception reported among Medicaid enrollees of being treated insensitively and disrespectfully by managed care staff. Also significant was the absence of state-required practice standards and performance measures for assessing the quality of family planning and STD-related services provided by plans. This failure may have resulted in these important preventive services being relegated to a lower priority by most plans—even Medicaid plans that disproportionately enroll women of reproductive age who are at higher health risk.

Political Climate

The political climate at the time of the FAIR Project study significantly contributed to the access barriers in the Medicaid managed care program and cannot be ignored. A new governor had taken office in January 1995 promising to press for mandatory managed care enrollment for most Medicaid-eligible individuals. The managed care industry responded swiftly with a massive marketing and enrollment effort to position their plans for the vastly expanded program. With inadequate time for building primary care capacity or mechanisms for monitoring enrollment practices, the system seemed to be in chaos by the summer of 1995. Complaints from consumers and advocates about overaggressive managed care plans or fraudulent marketing and enrollment tactics by managed care plans led the New York State Health Commissioner to

suspend direct enrollment of Medicaid recipients by plans in New York City.[15]

FAIR's focus groups and provider surveys were conducted during the spring and fall of that year. The environment in New York City, and uncertainties in the rest of the state about the direction of the Medicaid managed care program, contributed to confusion among both consumers and managed care staff about managed care policies. It may also have led to the misinformation that plan staff often provided to potential enrollees and enrollees regarding reproductive health care.

Recommendations

The FAIR Project recommends five priority strategies to reduce and prevent barriers to reproductive health care for managed care enrollees: (1) enacting statutory protections, (2) monitoring compliance, (3) building service capacity, (4) educating the public and enrollees, and (5) forming partnerships among the entities with a major stake in managed care. These strategies, briefly highlighted here in order of importance, are applicable to both Medicaid and commercial managed care enrollees, unless otherwise noted.

Enacting Statutory Protections

At a minimum, these protections should require the following:

- full disclosure to all potential and current enrollees of any limitations on reproductive health services or referrals

- full disclosure of any financial or other incentives (including "gag orders") that would

diminish an enrollee's information about, or access to, reproductive health care

- strict confidentiality for patients when identifying information related to any reproductive health service

- comprehensive reproductive health services in the benefit package

- free access policy that permits enrollees to self refer, in or out of plan, to a provider of their choice for family planning and other reproductive health services

- external monitoring of managed care plans to assess compliance with laws, regulations, and professional standards that are relevant to reproductive health care

- formal linkage between each plan and a reproductive health care "safety-net" provider to assure maximum opportunity for Medicaid enrollees to obtain timely, confidential, and appropriate reproductive health care

- accessible providers who are qualified to meet the full reproductive health needs of women and adolescents

- choice of plans to allow women to enroll in a plan that covers the full range of reproductive health services

- independent state ombudsperson who can be reached through a toll-free telephone number

- culturally appropriate and easy-to-understand member handbooks with a clear, unambiguous explanation of the free access policy and scope of services

- consumer advisory board for each plan

- demonstrated capacity by each plan to develop, implement, and monitor cultural and linguistic services appropriate for the needs of the enrolled population, as a condition of approval

- user-friendly complaint procedure for enrollees

- significant penalties for a plan's noncompliance with relevant laws and policies

Monitoring Compliance

The state must establish an effective mechanism for monitoring compliance with all statutory and regulatory requirements related to managed care. The state also must enforce the law. Two avenues are recommended for monitoring compliance with reproductive health-related laws, policies, and standards: through state regulators and through reproductive health care providers.

State regulators should work with reproductive health care advocates and providers to develop best practice guidelines for managed care plans as well as effective strategies for monitoring compliance. Community-based reproductive health providers also can play an important role by gathering information on barriers directly from their patients who are enrolled in managed care and by bringing any concerns to the attention of the managed care plan's member services department, or the state regulators when warranted.

Building Service Capacity

States must designate funding to build the capacity and capability of both MCOs and community-based "safety-net" providers to meet the needs of low-income and uninsured populations. At a minimum, funds should be earmarked for technical assistance to reproductive health and other "safety-net" providers to assist them in obtaining managed care contracts; fiscal incentives for Medicaid managed care plans to encourage them to contract with "safety-net" providers; and recruitment, training, and retention of primary care providers in underserved areas as well as primary care training for practitioners who now specialize in reproductive health services, so that they can be gatekeepers. Fiscal incentives are needed to encourage managed care plans to hire staff who reflect the racial composition and sociocultural characteristics of the community served. Subsidies for reproductive health and other community-based "safety-net" providers will enable them to maintain services to the growing number of uninsured individuals.

Educating the Public and Enrollees

States must develop effective educational mechanisms to ensure that prospective and current enrollees understand their rights and responsibilities under managed care. This includes an awareness of questions to ask in choosing a plan and a primary care provider and knowledge of how to obtain the full range of reproductive health care services in or out of plan. Enrollees also should know how to obtain care after hours and how to resolve any problems that arise in obtaining needed services. A "readiness process" for enrollees should be developed by the state. Contracts also should be offered to family planning clinics and other community-based providers to encourage them to help educate their Medicaid clients who are prospective or current enrollees of managed care about how managed care works. Reproductive health care providers who have gained the trust of women and adolescents in their communities are seen as a credible source of information; they can facilitate access and promote a smooth transition for enrollees into managed care.

Forming Partnerships with Major Stakeholders

Policymakers, reproductive health care providers, and women's health advocates are critical players in health care reform. Other major stakeholders who must be engaged include regulators, employees, employers and other purchasers, HMOs and other insurers, and organizations that accredit HMOs and hospitals.

Advocates need to ensure that each of these stakeholders understands the benefits of family planning and other reproductive health services. They should understand that these are essential preventive and primary care services that not only will improve women's health, but also prevent high costs and lost productivity associated with unintended pregnancies and reproductive-related illness. All stakeholders should be encouraged to use their leverage—especially purchasers, who have the greatest clout—to ensure that comprehensive, quality reproductive health care is provided by every managed care plan. States should develop and implement protective laws and policies as well as offer fiscal incentives to encourage plans to remove barriers to reproductive health services. MCOs must take responsibility for improving their efforts to inform enrollees about the free access policy and must be more vigilant about identifying, offering, providing, or arranging timely, appropriate, and quality reproductive health care. Traditional "safety-net" providers, particularly those with experience in providing family planning and reproductive health care services to low-income and diverse populations, should help educate their patients and coordinate with managed care plans to ensure comprehensive care.

To realize the potential of managed care—and simultaneously enable enrollees to obtain time-sensitive, confidential reproductive health care—strong statutory protections must be enacted, as well as effective mechanism for monitoring compliance and enforcement of the law. Furthermore, to adequately address the comprehensive health needs of all consumers, all interested parties must cooperatively work to identify and reduce sociocultural and structural barriers to health care, to prepare consumers for effective participation in managed care, and to strengthen both managed care and community-based health and social services networks.

References

1. Institute of Medicine. *The Best Intentions: Unintended Pregnancy and the Well-being of Children and Families.* Washington, D.C.: National Academy Press, 1995.
2. Center for Reproductive Law and Policy. *Removing Barriers, Improving Choices: A Case Study in Reproductive Health Services and Managed Care,* New York: Center for Reproductive Law and Policy, 1996.
3. Office of the Public Advocate for the City of New York. *Managed Confusion: How HMO Marketing Materials are Tricking The Elderly and The Poor,* 1995.
4. Office of Quality Assurance and Audit, Metropolitan Regional Office, New York State Department of Social Services, *MHS Marketing Review. HIP Marketing Review, Oxford Marketing Review, Metropolitan Marketing Review, U.S. Healthcare Marketing Review.* 1994–1995.
5. Havemann, J. New York Finds Bumps on the Road to HMOs: 13 Plans Fail to Meet Standards in State Probe. *The Washington Post.* December 19, 1995, p. A22.
6. Office of Quality Assurance and Audit, Metropolitan Regional Office, New York State. Department of Social Services. *Southwest Brooklyn Managed Care Program Compliance Review of the Freedom of Choice Waiver Requirements Issues By the Health Care Financing Administration of the United States Department of Health and Human Services.* 1994.
7. Community Service Society of New York. *Knowledge Gap: What Medicaid Beneficiaries Understand—And What They Don't About Managed Care. A Survey of Medicaid Recipients in the South Bronx and Harlem.* New York: Community Service Society of New York, 1996.
8. Blum, R.W., et al. Don't Ask, They Won't Tell: The Quality of Adolescent Health Screening in Five Practice Settings. *American Journal of Public Health* 86, no. 12 (1996: 1767–1772).
9. Millstein, S.G., et al. Delivery of STD/HIV Preventive Services to Adolescents by Primary Care Physicians. *Journal of Adolescent Health* 19 (1996): 249–257.
10. Kaiser Family Foundation. *The Glamour, Kaiser Family Foundation, Princeton Survey Research Associates Survey Women about their Knowledge, Attitudes and Practices Regarding their Reproductive Health.* Menlo Park, CA: Kaiser Family Foundation, 1997.
11. Planned Parenthood of New York City. Do Managed Care Organizations Inform Members About Free Access and Direct Access Laws? *Reproductive Health and Managed Care Policy Series. Report 1.* New York: Planned Parenthood of New York City, 1997.
12. Planned Parenthood of New York City. The Transition to Managed Care: Experiences of Planned Parenthood Patients. *Reproductive Health and Managed Care Policy Series, Report 2.* New York: Planned Parenthood of New York City, 1997.
13. Mathmatica Policy Research, Inc. *Reforming State Medicaid Programs. First-Year Implementation Experience from Three States.* Princeton, NJ: 1997.
14. Pear, R. 3 Big Health Plans Join in Call for National Standards. *New York Times.* September 25, 1997, p. A 28.
15. Fein, EB. New York Stops Forcing the Poor Into Managed Care. *New York Times.* September 29, 1995, p. A 1.

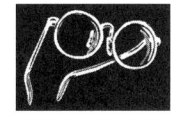

Article Review Form at end of book.

A health-promoting hospital promotes patients' health by continuously _____, thus reducing the risks involved in hospital stays and interventions. A health-promoting hospital is a "healthy organization." Explain.

Health-Promoting Hospitals

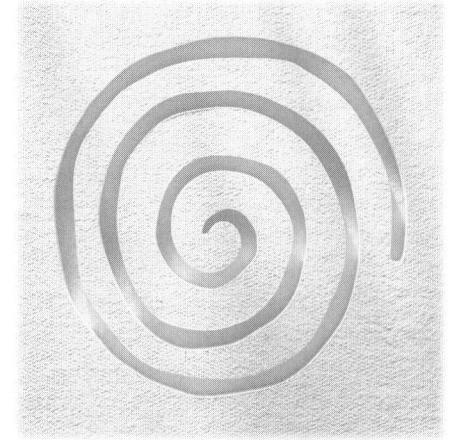

Juergen Pelikan, Hubert Lobnig, and Karl Krajic

Professor Juergen M. Pelikan is Director, Dr. Hubert Lobnig and Dr. Karl Krajic are both Senior Scientists at the Ludwig Boltzmann Institute for the Sociology of Health and Medicine, WHO Collaborating Centre for Hospitals and Health Promotion, Universitatsstrasse 7/2, 1010 Vienna, Austria. E-mail: hph.soc-gruwi@univie.ac.at

Abstract

The health-promoting hospital concept was started in 1988 by a group at the WHO regional office. Since then several directives have been issued and many hospitals, especially in Europe, have become health-promoting hospitals. The goals and objectives, and the strategies of such hospitals are discussed.

Started in 1988, the Health-Promoting Hospitals initiative has now proved to be not only a vision but a concrete development strategy for hospitals of all types and sizes, in widely varying health care systems, mainly in Europe.

What role can the health care services play in supporting people to adopt healthy lifestyles and make their living environments more health-promoting? Medical services are usually busy providing curative care, and many health professionals are already overworked. A growing population of elderly people, new diseases and epidemics, as well as technological innovation in diagnosis and treatment, already face health workers with more than enough challenges and opportunities for taking appropriate and useful professional action. The idea of health promotion is not to add to this burden but to ease it, and to improve the chances of effectiveness.

The Ottawa Charter for Health Promotion, issued in November 1986, focuses on political and intersectoral action for health but also asks for a reorientation of the health care sector itself towards health promotion. Actually putting this proposition into effect took some time to get started.

In 1988, a working group in the WHO Regional Office for Europe recommended focusing on the hospital as the hub of the modem medical and health care system—a centre providing education, training and professional standards.

Later that year, WHO initiated a first demonstration project called "Health and Hospital" at the Rudolfstiftung Hospital in Vienna, Austria.

During the next eight years, 12 sub-projects, mainly using existing know-how from health promotion and organizational development, were planned and carried out with the aim of improving the health of patients, hospital staff and the population in the community. The project also aimed at improving the overall organization of the hospital by focusing on effectiveness, quality, flexibility, staff commitment and becoming "a learning organization."

Evaluation showed that most of the measures taken were successful. For example, the health of patients was promoted by reducing hospital infections through establishing a professional hygiene team. An educational programme became part of the standard treatment for diabetics. The quality of nursing services was improved by changing to team nursing on many wards. Staff satisfaction increased as a result of personnel development projects, and this was reflected in a reduction of staff turnover. The cooperative culture of the hospital changed significantly: all levels of staff actively participated in project groups composed of members from different units, professions and levels of the hierarchy. Opening the hospital towards the local community, on the other hand, proved more difficult for a big inner-city hospital without a defined catchment area.

The Budapest Declaration

The "Budapest Declaration on Health-promoting Hospitals," worked out at a WHO meeting in 1991 by a multi-professional European group, presented a model for health-promoting hospitals. Since then, many hospitals and other partners in Europe, as well as Australia, Canada and some other countries, have got involved. In 1993, the model was extended to 20 hospitals in 11 European countries, and pilot projects were started. All but one of the 20 hospitals have been successful in initiating health-promoting processes and maintaining them for four years.

By early 1997, 150 subprojects, planned according to local needs and available resources, had been documented. The majority were aimed at improving the health of patients, but almost half included activities aimed at improving the health of staff and of the population in the community, and at helping the hospital as a whole to develop into a "healthy organization." Most of these subprojects were carried out within the normal hospital budget, relying to a large extent on voluntary work contributed by staff. Only 13 of them have had to be cancelled, and

most of the others are now part of normal hospital routine. Detailed reports on these activities were presented at the fifth International Conference on Health-Promoting Hospitals, which was held in Vienna, from 16 to 19 April, 1997. The conference was organized by WHO in cooperation with the European Union and other partners, and was attended by 315 participants from 33 countries.

In 1995, a European Project of National and Regional Networks of Health-Promoting Hospitals (HPH) was initiated, and since then HPH networks have been set up in 15 European countries, as well as in Australia and Canada, with an increasing number of hospitals participating. The HPH network is being coordinated by WHO and the Ludwig Boltzmann Institute for the Sociology of Health and Medicine, Vienna (sponsored by the Austrian Federal Ministry of Health).

What Is a Health-Promoting Hospital?

When people first hear about "health-promoting hospitals," there are usually two types of reaction. The first is: "Of course every hospital fights illness and is thus health-promoting in itself—what else should it do?" The second is almost the opposite: "Hospitals are full of sick and dying people. What a strange place to choose for health promotion!" The following points try to clear up these misconceptions by mentioning some of the more important characteristics of such a hospital.

- A health-promoting hospital does not have to change its main functions, which in industrialized countries consist

of combining "high tech" with "high touch" in caring for patients, coordinating different professions and specialties, managing crises and emotional stress, and performing reliably for 24 hours a day and 365 days a year. But such a hospital expands the scope of these activities and tries to keep them in a constructive longerterm perspective.

- A health-promoting hospital promotes patients' health by continuously improving and developing services, thus reducing the risks involved in hospital stays and interventions. It improves patients' well-being by providing services in a humane, caring way in a health-promoting physical environment. Such a hospital also uses episodes of acute illness or injury as windows of opportunity to promote health, for instance by providing or organizing rehabilitation, and empowering patients to protect themselves against disease, cope with chronic illness, or make better use of primary health care services. Resources are allocated according to the potential health gain to be derived from the service in question.

- A health-promoting hospital pays attention to the health of its staff. Awareness of biological, chemical, psychosocial and other risks involved in hospital work leads to policies and measures aimed at reducing these risks and helping staff to fulfill their own health potential.

- A health-promoting hospital modifies its services to reduce risks for the community stemming from hazardous wastes such as radioactive, pharmaceutical and biological materials. It networks with the relevant local services and associations to build alliances for continuous care and health promotion, thus becoming an agent for health development in the community.

- A health-promoting hospital is a "healthy organization," which means it has effective management, active staff participation and an overall organizational culture which is "people-oriented." It uses effective organizational development techniques such as project management, mission statements, quality management, expert support for change processes, and re-engineering of wards and functional units.

Health-promoting hospitals have already proved to be not only a vision but a concrete development strategy. The concept is being applied in hospitals of all types and sizes and in widely varying health care systems. By taking a health promotion approach many hospitals have been discovering new opportunities for effective action and new ways to solve difficult problems. Rather than facing them with a new challenge, health promotion is providing them with fresh ways to tackle existing challenges.

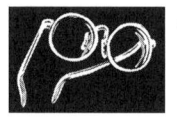 **Article Review Form at end of book.**

WiseGuide Wrap-Up

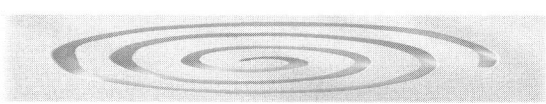

- From Medicaid to managed care, beneficiaries will face some difficulties in attaining reproductive health care services such as family planning, abortion, and STD treatment as the switch is made across the country.

- Prevention programs that strive to decrease risks also have the

potential to diagnose patients earlier and to increase revenue for hospitals and physician practices.

- The FAIR Project findings indicate that obstacles to receiving reproductive health care services in a managed care system need to be addressed and overcome. Barriers

identified are communication, confidentiality, and appropriateness of care.

- A health-promoting hospital promotes healthy lifestyles among patients, staff, and community members, without changing its main functions.

R.E.A.L. Sites

This list provides a print preview of typical **Coursewise** R.E.A.L. sites. (There are over 100 such sites at the **Courselinks**™ site.) The danger in printing URLs is that web sites can change overnight. As we went to press, these sites were functional using the URLs provided. If you come across one that isn't, please let us know via email to: webmaster@coursewise.com. Use your Passport to access the most current list of R.E.A.L. sites at the **Courselinks** site.

Site name: Centre for Health Information and Promotion

URL: http://www.sickkids.on.ca/chip/default.asp

Why is it R.E.A.L.? This site profiles this hospital's attempts at making the hospitals and communities healthier and safer.

Key topics: child safety, various educational campaigns, health messages

Try this: Learn more about folic acid and its effect on childbirth and diseases.

Site name: World Health Day

URL: http://www.aawhworldhealth.org/whealth.htm

Why is it R.E.A.L.? This page is an informative site on the World Health Day established by the World Health Organization.

Key topics: investing in the future, supporting safe motherhood

Try this: Learn the ten themes of safe motherhood.

Site name: Southern Illinois Healthcare

URL: http://www.sih.net/

Why is it R.E.A.L.? This site provides information on the SIH system and its services. It also lists facility and physician information.

Key topics: services, facilities, career opportunities

Try this: Select Services and then select Community Education Programs. Examine the list of programs available at the facility of your choice.

Site name: Health Promotions

URL: http://www.it-warehouse.com/kah/healthpro.htm

Why is it R.E.A.L.? This page profiles and lists the Karachi Adventist Hospital's Health Promotion Department. It also includes some very interesting links to similar hospitals and organizations.

Key topics: health programs and services offered, news and events

Try this: Read the Mission, Vision and Values Statement by clicking on the "profile" button. What are the major differences among each statement?

section

6

Learning Objectives

- To review four successful collaborative projects

- To examine the association between risk factors and medical expenditures

- To review what we as health educators know, what we have done in our short history, what we must do if we are to continue to play a meaningful role in society, and what we need to do in the future

- To study a comprehensive curriculum that addresses social and emotional development through community support

- To examine the first five years of the Baton Rouge Health Forum and gain insight into what makes a successful collaboration

Collaborative Projects

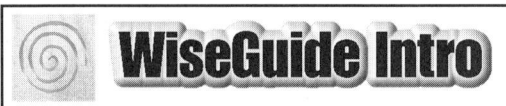 **WiseGuide Intro**

When conducting an Internet search for the key word *collaboration,* one can expect nearly a million hits, depending on which search engine used. A random glance proves that collaboration is the single key to many successful projects. From solving the Y2K problems to addressing school needs, *collaboration* is the buzzword that will carry into the twenty-first century.

As community health education prepares for the new millennium, collaboration will continue to be the key to successful programming. In an age of budget cuts, personnel shortages, and increasing health concerns, no single agency, facility, or system can single-handedly conquer the task of positive outcome–based community health-education programming.

In this section, we will look at a sample of successful collaborative projects. It is important to note that many of the featured articles in prior sections also represent collaborative efforts.

R. William Whitmer (HERO), Ron Z. Goetzel (MEDSTAT Group), and David R. Anderson (StayWell Company) present "The HERO Study on Risks and Costs: Research Findings." This research represents a first step in the process: the examination of the association between ten modifiable risk factors and individual health care expenditures in a working population. HERO is a not-for-profit coalition of organizations with specific interests in health promotion, disease management, and health-related productivity research.

John R. Seffrin (American Cancer Society) presents the 1997 AAHE Scholar Address at the AAHPERD convention in St. Louis entitled "Premises, Promises and Potential Payoffs of Responsible Health Education." This speech examines what we as health educators know: what we have done in our short history, what we must do if we are to continue to play a meaningful role in society, and how it should be done. Collaboration with other organizations in the social, governmental, and private sectors are highlighted.

Roger P. Weissberg (University of Illinois at Chicago), Timothy P. Shriver (Special Olympics International), Sharmistha Bose (Collaborative for the Advancement of Social and Emotional Learning), and Karol DeFalco (New Haven Public Schools) present "Creating a Districtwide Social Development Project." In the New Haven, Connecticut, public schools, these authors have found that sustained efforts to enhance children's social and emotional development can help students become knowledgeable, responsible, and caring citizens. Collaboration is the key to their success.

Virginia M. Pearson (Baton Rouge Health Forum) presents "Five Years of Collaboration: Baton Rouge Health Forum Focuses on Community Needs." This article highlights the accomplishments of a five-year collaborative effort known as the Greater Baton Rouge Health Forum. After five years, hindsight is occasionally rocky, but no organizations have left the forum. The successes and challenges are reviewed.

Questions

Reading 29. What is HERO? The report suggests that greater emphasis needs to be placed on correctable psychosocial risks than on many of the risks that have historically been center stage. Explain.

Reading 30. What must be done in order to promote health education to its rightful and necessary place in the overall health care system? Discuss the three alternatives Seffrin suggests for dealing with social morbidity, excessive health care costs, and premature mortality within our society

Reading 31. To prevent social and health problems among our young people, policy makers have urged us to _____. Describe the positive approach adapted by the New Haven public schools.

Reading 32. What was the first project addressed by the Baton Rouge Health Forum? The key to successful partnerships is _____. Explain.

What is HERO? The report suggests that greater emphasis needs to be placed on correctable psychosocial risks than on many of the risks that have historically been center stage. Explain.

The HERO Study on Risks and Costs:

Research Findings

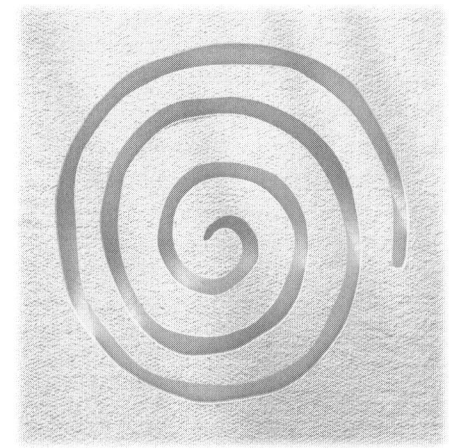

R. William Whitmer, MBA

President and CEO—HERO

Ron Z. Goetzel, Ph.D.

Vice President, Consulting and National Practice—The MEDSTAT Group

David R. Anderson, Ph.D.

Vice President, Programs and Services—The StayWell Company

Overview of Study

One of the most frequent health promotion frustrations deals with economics. Questions about the association between risk factors and medical expenditures are often asked, but are seldom answered. While there is substantial peer-reviewed data on the impact of risk factors on morbidity and mortality,[1,2] there is little on the relationship between health risks and individual costs.[3,4,5]

This study reports on an effort to address this research void. To do so, a multi-employer database of over 45,000 employees was created. Ten modifiable risk factors were evaluated, as independent variables, for their asso-ciation with health care expenditures. The overall intent was to prioritize the economic impact so that health promotion providers and users of these services may have an idea of the relative potential for cost savings if specific risks are controlled or eliminated.

Why is interest in research on the economic impact of risk factors at an all time high? Reports indicate that for the first time, health care costs exceeded the $1 trillion barrier in 1996.,[6] Such expenditures amount to $2.7 billion spent daily on disease care[7] or $3,759 spent for every man, woman and child each year.[8] Even though annual increases in health care costs have moderated over the past several years,[9] some experts believe that annual increases will escalate in the near future.[10] The per capita cost and the potential for substantial annual increases have caused employers, hospitals, physicians, health maintenance organizations (HMO), medical insurers, health promotion providers and others to have increased interest in containment of medical costs. One approach to cost control is to improve health habits, thus reducing the incidence of preventable illnesses and their associated costs. To do so, more needs to be learned about the relationship between modifiable risk factors and individual health care expenditures. Once this is understood, it could provide the economic rationale to research, develop and deliver specific intervention programs that reduce population risk and consequently lower health care expenditures. This research represents a first step in this process—the examination of the association between ten modifiable risk factors, and individual health care expenditures in a working population.

Even though the importance of risk factor oriented economic data is obvious, the reason it has not been done is often little understood. To address this situation, it is important to recognize there are different approaches to prevention. Public health and clinical preventive services include such things as: water purification, sanitation, inoculations, pap tests, mammograms and the like. Over the years, the effectiveness and economic rationale for many of these activities have been thoroughly researched and documented. Behavioral-based prevention, defined often as lifestyle or risk factor reduction activity, is where there is a clear void in economic impact research. Why the dichotomy?

One reason may be that the public health and medical communities have been in existence and operational for many decades. Organizations responsible for research in these areas such as the Centers for Disease Control and Prevention (CDC) and the National Institutes of Health (NIH) are well organized, staffed with highly competent scientists and well funded. By comparison, the behavioral-oriented health promotion discipline is relatively new, being operational for about 25 years. It is small and fragmented with inadequate funding for sophisticated, prospective, randomized and controlled research trials. This does not suggest lack of interest in health promotion economic research, but a lack of organization or strategic research planning for the overall discipline. What may be needed is a central facilitator organization that can bring together, over time, the key organizations and individuals (scientists, research populations and funders) required to discuss, develop, initiate and implement a national health promotion research agenda. Several years ago, the Health Enhancement Research Organization (HERO)[11] accepted this challenge.

The Study Database

HERO is a not-for-profit coalition of organizations with specific interests in health promotion, dis-

ease management and health related productivity research. It has been operational for nearly three years. Among HERO's sustaining partners are: hospital systems, HMOs, health insurers, employers, health care consultants, health promotion providers and groups such as The American Heart Association, The American Diabetes Association, The American Dietetic Association, The Health Project and the National Business Coalition on Health. Also on the HERO Board of Directors, in an ex-officio status, are individuals from the Centers for Disease Control and Prevention (CDC), the Department of Health and Human Services–Office of Disease Prevention and Health Promotion (HHS-ODPHP) and the National Aeronautic and Space Administration (NASA). These organizations work together to create a system of research synergy, the overall objective being to ultimately shift the health care paradigm from a system involved almost exclusively with diagnosis and treatment to one that emphasizes prevention. In order to accomplish this, high quality, reproducible health promotion research is required.

The first step in this process was for HERO to create a multiple-employer research database. This was accomplished through collaboration among HERO, the StayWell Company and The MEDSTAT Group, both of which are HERO sustaining partners, and six large employers: Chevron Corporation, Health Trust, Inc., Hoffman–La Roche, Marriott Corporation and the states of Michigan and Tennessee.

The HERO health promotion research database includes 46,026 employees who completed a com-

mon health risk appraisal (HRA), the StayWell Health Path(r) and were enrolled in a fee-for-service, self-insured health care plan for the study period of 1990 to 1996. Approximately 12,000 of these employees completed two or more HRAs during this time. Inclusion criteria for the study were: active employees, age 18 to 64 at the time of the first HRA, who had at least six months of medical plan eligibility after the first HRA was completed.

The HERO database was created by connecting the HRA data set with the medical claims data set and the eligibility data set. Including the eligibility data permitted the inclusion of study subjects who have no medical claims. The confidentiality of individuals was maintained by scrambling personal identifiers across all data sources. The merging of these data sets yielded 113,963 person years experience. One of the previously largest research database of this kind is the Control Data-Milliman Robertson database, which includes about 15,000 study subjects and provides approximately 40,000 person years experience.[12]

Creation of the HERO database could have a major impact on the future of health promotion and disease prevention research. It is amenable to the creation of numerous longitudinal research studies that examine the association or impact of single risk factors, risk factor combinations, risk factor change, selected chronic diseases and demographics on: medical costs, diagnosis, treatments, procedures, outcomes, hospitalization or any other parameter usually recorded in a typical fee-for-service medical claims database. A consortium of 22 HERO sustaining partners funded the creation of the database.

The Research Focus

During the two years it took to get HERO organized and operating, dozens of employers, hospitals, HMOs, health care insurers, health promotion providers, consultants and others were asked their opinions about what kind of health promotion research should be done first. The majority indicated the impact of risk factors on health care costs was the most important research topic. The second most frequently requested research was to determine the most effective intervention methods and techniques for permanent lifestyle change and risk elimination.

Based on this information, the same group of 22 HERO sustaining partners funded a research effort, using the HERO database to address the following question: Do those at high risk have greater health care costs than those at lower risk? On the surface, this may appear to be a rhetorical question. For several decades, health promotion providers and those who purchase services and programs have empirically assumed that high risk equals greater medical expenses. However, little has been reported in the peer-reviewed literature to define the relationship. There is a particular lack of data that evaluates specific risk factors as independent variables and prioritizes the economic impact of various risks within a single group of study subjects.

A second research question addresses multiple risk factors: Do those with specific high risk factor combinations have greater medical expenditures than those at lower risk? Three models were crated to examine this question: a psychosocial risk model, a stroke risk model and a cardiovascular disease risk model.

Description of Methods

Most published risk factor–medical care cost research has not attempted to adjust for the influence of other risk factors or demographics. For example, if smoking is investigated for its impact on morbidity, mortality or medical expenditures, the smoker may be obese, have hypertension, and consume excessive amounts of alcohol. All these risks have an impact on research outcomes, but are seldom accounted for. This makes it difficult to evaluate the specific impact of smoking. In order to address this problem and control for confounding factors, a retrospective, two-stage multi-variate analyses, including logistic and linear regression models were used. This permits the examination of specific risk factors as independent variables, thus eliminating the impact of other existing risks. In addition to adjusting for specific risk factors, other potentially confounding factors adjusted for were: gender, age, education level, race, type of job, employer and the number of months that employees were followed after the first HRA was completed. In so doing, financial impact data are reported in two ways: *unadjusted,* which reflects the influence of all related health risks, and *adjusted,* which indicates the independent cost impact of the risk factor being evaluated with the influence of all other specific risks removed. When considering the peer-reviewed literature, Yen, et al. are the only other researchers to use a multivariate approach on individual data, but their sample sizes were substantially smaller than reported here.[13]

Data from the first HRA were used to classify study subjects in terms of risks for poor health outcomes. Ten risks were examined. Six were self-reported and four were based on biometric measurements. The self-reported standards were: *physical activity*—no vigorous exercise during a typical week;[14,15,16] *alcohol consumption*—five or more drinks per day on two or more days per week;[17] *nutrition*—based on reported intake of total fat/saturated fat, fruits, vegetables/complex carbohydrates, salt, lean meat and low-fat dairy products;[18] *tobacco use*—(two categories) current and former users (i.e., pipe, cigar, snuff/smokeless tobacco); *stress*—reported "my life is extremely stressful" and "I am not at all effective in dealing with stress;"[19] *depression*—reported they "feel depressed most of the time;"[20,21] *body weight*—30% or more above or 20% or more below the midpoint of frame-adjusted desirable weight according to height.[22]

In addition, biomedical screening for high risks were: *cholesterol* levels of 240 mg/dl or higher; *systolic blood pressure* 160 mg Hg or higher, and/or diastolic blood pressure of 100 mg Hg or higher: and fasting *blood glucose* levels of 115 mg/liter or higher.[23]

In summary, models were crated to predict total health care costs for individuals who were found to be at high risk. These expenditures were compared with the expenditures of persons at lower levels of risk. The difference between the high and lower risk individuals were calculated. This calculation was done on an unadjusted and adjusted basis. This research study has been peer reviewed and published in greater detail elsewhere.[24] Portions of the published study are reproduced here with written permission.

Results

It was found that 46,026 study subjects met the inclusion criterion and were followed for up to three years after the completion of the first HRA. Table 1 provides descriptive statistics relative to the frequency of risks, age, gender, race and job type. Poor exercise habits was the most prevalent risk factor and self-reported depression the least reported. Those in the 35 to 44 year old group accounted for over 40 percent of the study subjects. About 60 percent of the study population were men. Over 80 percent were white, with approximately half having professional or managerial job responsibilities.

With regard to economic impact, those at high risk were compared to those at lower risk, adjusting for covariates via the regression analyses. Table 2 shows that employees who self-reported being persistently depressed (n=997, 2.2% of the study sample) had adjusted health care expenditures 70.2% higher than those who reported not being depressed. Those reporting uncontrolled stress (n=8,518, 18.7%) had adjusted health care expenditures 46.3% higher than those who reported less difficulty with stress. Those with high blood glucose (n=2,271, 4.9%) had adjusted health care expenditures 34.8% higher than those with normal blood sugar. Table 2 also shows that the other risk factors, in order of descending impact on individual health care cost were: being significantly over weight or underweight, tobacco use, high blood pressure, and lack of exercise.

For most risk factors, unadjusted percentage differences in expenditures were much different (usually higher) than adjusted

Table 1 Descriptive Statistics

Measure	Value	Study Sample (n=46,026) Count	Percent
Risk Category	Poor Exercise	14,908	32.4%
	Former Tobacco User	14,329	31.1%
	Poor Nutritional Habits	9,278	20.2%
	Extreme High or Low Weight	9,197	20.0%
	Current Tobacco User	8,797	19.1%
	High Cholesterol	8,641	18.8%
	High Stress	8,518	18.5%
	High Blood Glucose	2,271	4.9%
	High Blood Pressure	1,827	4.0%
	Excessive Alcohol Use	1,723	3.7%
	Depression	997	2.2%
Age Group	18–34	8,830	19.2%
	35–44	18,696	40.6%
	45–54	12,805	27.8%
	55–64	5,695	12.4%
Gender	Female	19,335	42.0%
	Male	26,691	58.0%
Race	White	38,220	83.0%
	African-American	4,259	9.3%
	Hispanic	1,653	3.6%
	Asian	1,300	2.8%
	Native-American	362	0.8%
	Other	232	0.5%
Job Type	Professional or Managerial	25,739	55.9%
	Sales	442	1.0%
	Laborer, Clerical, Technician	19,845	43.1%

percentages, which illustrates the need for the multivariate approach for controlling for confounding variables (Table 2). There was a dichotomy between the adjusted and unadjusted data relative to high cholesterol levels (n=8,641, 17.7%). Based on unadjusted data, health care costs were 16.9% greater than those with normal cholesterol levels, however, when adjusted, health care costs were 0.8% lower.

In the case of alcohol consumption and nutrition it was found that those at high risk had lower health care expenditures than those at lower risk. Those at

high risk for health problems due to alcohol (n=1,723, 3.7%) had adjusted health care expenditures 3.0% lower than those at lower risk. In the case of nutrition, those who reported poor nutritional habits (n=9,278, 20.2%) had adjusted health care expenditures 9.2% lower than those who reported good nutritional habits.

Investigating multiple risk factors is important. For those at risk, having two or more risks is more common than a single risk. It has been estimated that for those at risk, the average number of risks is 2.1.25. For this reason, three models were created in

Table 2	Percentage Differences in Mean Annual Medical Expenditures for High Risk vs. Lower Risk Employees, with and without Independent Variable Adjustment					
Risk Measure	**Risk Level**	**Sample Size**	**Unadjusted Means***	**% Difference Without Adjustment**	**% Difference As Independent Variable**
Depression	High Risk	997	$3,189.01	89.90%	70.24%
	Lower Risk	44,701	$1,679.31	—	—
Stress Level	High Risk	8,518	$2,287.40	44.88%	46.35%
	Low Risk	36,833	$1,578.86	—	—
Blood Glucose	High Risk	2,271	$2,597.99	53.67%	34.76%
	Low Risk	35,994	$1,690.60	—	—
Body Weight	High Risk	9,197	$2,317.53	47.56%	21.41%
	Low Risk	36,782	$1,570.59	—	—
Tobacco	Current User	8,797	$1,949.66	29.69%	14.46%
	Former User	14,329	$1,872.66	24.57%	19.74%
	Never Used	22,237	$1,503.32	—	—
Blood Pressure	High Risk	1,827	$2,122.79	23.71%	11.65%
	Low Risk	43,295	$1,715.89	—	—
Exercise Habits	High Risk	14,908	$2,011.06	28.31%	10.35%
	Low Risk	30,680	$1,567.35	—	—
Cholesterol	High Risk	8,641	$1,962.35	16.92%	(−0.79%)
	Low Risk	35,986	$1,678.38	—	—
Excessive Alcohol	High Risk	1,723	$1,430.72	(−17.12%)	(−3.01%)
	Low Risk	43,991	$1,726.22	—	—
Nutritional Habits	High Risk	9,278	$1,498.24	(−15.46%)	(−9.25%)
		37,709	$1,772.31	—	—

*In 1996 dollars

order to determine the association between certain risk factor combinations and medical expenditures. One model is psychosocial in nature and includes all study subjects who reported being persistently depressed and experiencing uncontrolled stress. Table 3 shows for these employees, annual health care costs were 147 percent higher than for those who reported being neither stressed or depressed. The second is a stroke model that includes those who had high blood pressure, high cholesterol and reported being a current smoker and had self-reported uncontrolled stress. These employees had annual health care costs 85 percent greater when compared to those with none of these risk factors. The heart disease model was made up of those who had high blood pressure, high blood glucose, high cholesterol, were seriously over/underweight, and reported poor exercise habits, high stress and being a former or current tobacco user. When study subjects with all these risks were compared to those with none, the annual medical expenditures were 228 percent greater.

Health care expenditures were incurred by 72 percent of the employees during the study period. On a person-year basis, expenditures ranged from $0 to $130,014, with an average value of $1,712. The median value was $353.

Discussion of Results

Because of the changing health care delivery environment, health promotion providers, employers, managed care organizations, health insurers, individual physicians, those interested in disease management and others, have become increasingly interested in learning how health risks affect expenditures.[26] For several decades, health promotion efforts have usually been directed toward risk factors such as smoking, lack of physical activity, excess alcohol, proper nutrition, obesity and blood pressure. Within the past decade increasing interest has been directed toward the risk factors of

| Table 3 | Annual Medical Expenditures (in 1995 dollars) for Those with and without Selected Multiple Risk Factors, Assuming Average Values for Other Risk Categories and Covariates |

| Coexisting Multiple Risk Factors Leading To: | Medical Expenditures for Those: | | |
	With Multiple Risk Factors	Without Any of These Risk Factors	Risk Factors
High risk for heart disease	$3,804	$1,158	228%
High risk for stroke	$2,349	$1,272	85%
High risk for psychosocial problems	$3,368	$1,363	147%

elevated cholesterol and blood pressure levels. This research suggests that three correctable conditions that have not received as much attention (depression, stress, high blood glucose) are even more costly. Those that have empirically received the greatest attention and effort are mid-line or lower in regard to cost impact.

Few health promotion programs concentrate on screening for depression. A significant number of widely used HRAs have no questions directed toward depression screening. Those that do, usually have no more than two or three. Some health care plans, instead of being proactive in the aggressive diagnosis and management of depression, seek to cut back on the diagnosis and treatment of mental and nervous diseases. This research suggests that the art of health promotion may be enhanced by a greater emphasis of worksite depression screening and a more realistic approach to quality diagnosis and treatment.

Screening for excess stress and its management have been part of health promotion programs for a number of years, but some practitioners tend to side-step the issue because stress is considered as nebulous as depres-

sion. It's difficult to detect and even more of a challenge to manage. It is different from smoking, obesity, physical fitness and cholesterol levels. In these cases, there are specific starting and end points. Success or failure are fairly easy to measure. With stress, end points are not as accessible. Based on this research, more attention to screening for excess stress and appropriate follow-up are recommended.

In this study, among those who self-reported depression or stress, it is interesting to note that only 2.2 percent feel they are depressed at the time of the survey while 18.5 percent (n=8,518) reported uncontrolled stress. The percent reporting depression is about one-third of those that are considered as being depressed on a national level.[27] This difference could reflect denial or lack of understanding between the two conditions on the part of individuals.

Those study subjects with elevated blood glucose were associated with the third highest medical costs. While many health promotion programs routinely screen for blood glucose, some do not provide rigorous follow-up and clinical and/or behavioral intervention. Attention to this risk factor is recommended and may enhance the art of health promo-

tion. Several large health maintenance organizations (HMO) have recently reported on the economic payback of aggressive and well-designed blood glucose monitoring and treatment programs.[28]

Elevated blood cholesterol was found to be equivocal when examined as an independent variable. The reason may be that it takes years, perhaps decades, for high cholesterol levels to manifest itself in the form of clinical disease. The study period may not be sufficient for this to occur. It was found that poor nutritional habits were associated with lower health care expenditures. This may be explained by the fact that the impact of poor nutrition habits on expenditures was made after already accounting for the impacts related to cholesterol levels, blood glucose levels, blood pressure, unhealthy weight, and other factors that may be related to poor nutritional habits. Clearly, those with poor eating habits had lower health care expenditures than those with good eating habits. This is contrary to the vast body of existing nutrition research. There may be several explanations for this finding. First, the impact of all other risks usually associated with poor eating habits (obesity, high cholesterol, hypertension, high blood glucose, etc.) have been eliminated through the adjustment process. Put another way, with the exception of poor heating habits, these study subjects were risk free. There is also the question of the validity of nutrition questions used in HRAs. Thirdly, this is self-reported data which is understood not to be as valid as keeping a detailed food diary.

With regard to excess alcohol consumption, other studies have also found that heavy drinkers do not necessarily incur greater health care costs. One explanation may be that those who abuse alcohol often fail to seek care for their health problems.[10]

In summary, it is suggested that risk factors that have been center stage in the world of health promotion, in several cases, are not necessarily those associated with the greatest health care costs. Greater emphasis on correctable psychosocial risks is hereby recommended.

Some Limitations of the Study

This research represents an important step forward in applying rigorous statistical methods to an investigation of the relationships between widely accepted risk factors and medical expenditures in a working population.

There are, however, limitations to the study. First, decisions to complete the HRA were voluntary therefore, the study sample may not represent the general working population. Second, some of the analyses used self-reported data on health behaviors, therefore, some of the risk factor measures may be subject to errors in judgment, which in turn, would bias the regression model coefficients toward zero. Finally, claims data were examined for up to three years after the first HRA was taken, but the long-term implications of high-risk behavior may take longer to observe.

Conclusion

This study suggests that within a large, multi-employer, multi-site, group of private and public sector employees that completed an HRA, a significantly higher level of individual health care expenditures was associated with high

risk for seven of the ten risk factors evaluated. The risk factors have been prioritized according to their impact on individual health care expenditures. High risks related to self-reported depression, self-reported stress and high blood glucose were associated with the greatest medical expenditures. High expenditures were also associated with inappropriate body weight, tobacco use, high blood pressure and poor exercise habits. Since there are little data available on the association between risk factors and medical expenses, it is anticipated that this study will be useful to those who desire to research, develop and deliver health-promoting intervention programs aimed at reducing health risks and their consequent health expenditures.

References

1. U.S. Centers for Disease Control and Prevention. Estimated national spending on prevention—United States, 1988. *Morbidity and Mortality Weekly Report* 1992; 41:529–531.
2. Amler RW, Dull HB (eds.). Closing the gap: The burden of unnecessary illness. *American Journal of Preventive Medicine* 1987; 3 (Sup 5).
3. Yen LT, Edington DW, Witting P. Associations between health risk appraisal scores and employee medical claims costs in a manufacturing company. *American Journal of Health Promotion* 1991; 6:46–54.
4. Yen LT, Edington DW, Witting P. Corporate medical claim cost distributions and factors associated with high-cost status. *Journal of Occupational Medicine* 1994; 36:505–515.
5. Bertera RL. The effects of behavioral risks on absenteeism and health-care costs in the workplace. *Journal of Occupational Medicine* 1991; 33(11):1119–1124.
6. National Health Spending Trends in 1996. *Health Affairs.* January/February 1997, 137.
7. Whitmer RW. The need for research in health promotion, disease prevention and demand management. *Employee Health Benefits* 1996; 6:24–30.
8. U.S. Chamber of Commerce. Survey Data from Benefit Year 1996; 243.
9. DataWatch. The latest breakdown on benefit dollars. *Business & Health.* February 1998; 64.
10. Hefty Increases Predicted for Medical Costs. *Wall Street Journal.* November 26, 1997; 1.
11. Whitmer RW, Dundon MW. The Health Enhancement Research Organization (HERO). *American Journal of Health Promotion* 1997: 11(6):388–393.
12. Milliman & Robertson, Inc. and Control Data. Health risks and behavior: The impact on medical costs. 1987; p. 24.
13. Yen LT, Edington DW, Whitting P. Predictions of prospective medical claims and absenteeism costs for 1,284 hourly workers from a manufacturing company. *Journal of Occupational Medicine,* 1988; 30(2):106–112.
14. American College of Sports Medicine. Position stand on the recommended quantity and quality of exercise for developing and maintaining cardiorespiratory and muscular fitness in healthy adults. *Med Sci Sports Exerc.* 1990; 22:265–274.
15. American Heart Association. Recommendations of the Nutrition Committee, 1983.
16. Pate RR, Pratt M, Blair SN, et al. Physical activity and public health: A recommendation from the Centers for Disease Control and Prevention and the American College of Sports Medicine. JAMA 1995; 273:402–407.
17. National Institute on Alcohol Abuse and Alcoholism. Alcohol Alert: Moderate Drinking. U.S. Department of Health and Human Services. Publication No. 16, PH 315; April 1992.
18. U.S. Department of Agriculture. Nutrition and Your Health: Dietary Guidelines for Americans, Third Edition. Home and Garden Bulletin No. 232, 1990.
19. Lazarus RS. Psychological Stress and Coping Process. New York, NY: McGraw-Hill, 1996.
20. Burnam MA, Wells KB, Leake B, Landsverk J. Development of a brief screening instrument for detecting depressive disorders. *Medical Care* 1988; 26: 775–789.

21. Stoudemire A, et al. Depression. In: Amler RW, Dull HB, eds., Closing the Gap: The Burden of Unnecessary Illness. New York, NY: Oxford University Press, 1987.
22. Metropolitan Life Insurance Company. 1983 Metropolitan height and weight tables. Statistical Bulletin of the Metropolitan Life Insurance Company, 1983; 64 (January–June): 3.
23. American Diabetes Association. Screening for Diabetes, Diabetes Care, 1997; 20(1):522–523.
24. Goetzel RZ, Anderson DH, Whitmer RW. The relationship between modifiable health risks and health care expenditures: an analysis of the multi-employer HERO health risk and cost database. *Journal of Occupational and Environmental Medicine.* (40)(10) October 1998; 1–12.
25. U.S. Centers for Disease Control and Prevention. Risk Factor distribution. *Healthy People 2000,* 1991; 605–606.
26. Heaney CA, Goetzel RZ. A review of health-related outcomes of multi-component worksite health promotion programs. *American Journal of Health Promotion* 1997; 11(4):290–308.
27. Kessler, RL, Underwood, L. Measuring Stress. Oxford University Press, New York, N.Y. 1992; 114.
28. The Expert Committee on the Diagnosis and Classification of Diabetes Mellitus. *Diabetes Care.* 1997; 20:1183–1197.

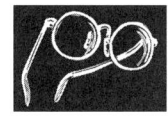 **Article Review Form at end of book.**

What must be done in order to promote health education to its rightful and necessary place in the overall health care system? Discuss the three alternatives Seffrin suggests for dealing with social morbidity, excessive health care costs, and premature mortality within our society.

Premises, Promises and Potential Payoffs of Responsible Health Education

John R. Seffrin

John R. Seffrin is Chief Executive Officer of the American Cancer Society, Inc., Atlanta, GA 30329–4251.

As we are about to complete a millennium and the century during which the field of health education was born, it seems appropriate to consider where we are in our mission of assuring a health-educated populace. As I proceed, I will try to be brief about the past and the present so that I can focus on what I feel needs to happen in the immediate future if we are to realize our professional dreams in the new decade and century. More specifically, I will consider the following four topics of interest: what we as health educators know, what we have done in our short history, what we must do if we are to continue to play a meaningful role in society, and how I believe we should do it.

What We Know

First, what we know. By this I mean what have we learned about human health that is certain and incontrovertible. While we have thousands of studies, some good and some not so good, I submit that we still don't really know all that much, certainly not as much as we would like, if we define "what we know" as that which we can attest to with near or absolute certainty.

When considering this situation, I'm reminded of a line from Robert Frost's "A Masque of Reason" that reads, "We don't know, don't we?" Although the phrase is purposefully discordant, it is both grammatically correct and discouragingly accurate far too much of the time. So often in life and in our profession, we are forced to move forward, not really knowing with any real certainty what is right or best.

This sometimes painful and always humbling fact notwithstanding, we must focus on what we do know and then muster the courage to move ahead. Indeed, in many ways our profession has made real progress over the years. When done well, research in the fields of health education, epidemiology, and public health has been able to provide us with some of the most interesting and valuable knowledge we have today. It has generated the sort of information that can make a profound difference in the health and wellbeing of our nation. With this in mind, I would like to share with you data from the American Cancer Society's Cancer Prevention Study-II (CPS-II), which I believe is an excellent example of how well-designed and carefully conducted research can have a real impact on our current understanding and future decisions.

This article is reprinted with permission from the *JOURNAL OF HEALTH EDUCATION,* September/October, 1997. The *JOURNAL OF HEALTH EDUCATION* is a publication of the American Alliance for Health, Physical Education, Recreation and Dance, 1900 Association Drive, Reston, Virginia 20191.

American Cancer Society Cancer Prevention Study II

The American Cancer Society's CPS-II is the largest prospective epidemiological study ever undertaken in the history of public health. We are following, and have since 1982, 1.2 million Americans until they die in order to learn more about cancer causes and prevention. The data I am presenting here is based on a subset of the overall CPS II cohort that contains over half-million Americans who were all judged to be healthy at the time they entered the study and had verifiable status regarding their smoking history.

This huge data set is aggregated in this particular way for the first time and has not been seen before by any professional group or the public at large.

Methods

Our analytic cohort included 200,000 men and 350,000 women recruited by the American Cancer Society's volunteers. Although all regions of the country were represented and a wide range of people were included, this cohort is largely made up of white, married, middle class adults (Table 1).

In considering these individuals, we looked at four important lifestyle behaviors—smoking, not exercising, lower vegetable and fruit intake, and obesity—which were found to be directly related to increased mortality during the prime of life, ages 35 to 69. Specifically, we measured death rates from all cancers, vascular disease, and all causes of death combined, controlling for age, education, race, and the four behavioral characteristics. From the multivariate adjusted death rate,

Table I	Characteristics of Individuals in This Analysis	
Men		**Women**
200,000 men		350,000 women
Average age 55		Average age 54
95% white		95% white
34% high school or less		40% high school or less
39% college graduates		28% college graduates
36% never smokers		57% never smokers
30% current smokers		23% current cigarette smokers
No major disease reported at baseline		No major disease reported at baseline

we calculated the absolute probability, or risk, of dying between ages 35 to 69. Thus, we were able to compare how each of the four factors affected mortality individually as well as when they were combined. This led to a number of interesting findings.

Results

Nearly 16,000 deaths were experienced in the cohort, 8,972 men and 7,069 women. The number of deaths by disease category and for all causes combined and the actual death rates per 100,000 appear in Table 2.

These figures were in line with our expectations, but when we considered the ways in which lifestyle behaviors affected death rates, we found some very interesting and significant relationships, the most dramatic of which involve smoking. Consider Figures 1a and 1b* (In these and the following figures, only deaths from all causes will be considered; the data for deaths from cancers and vascular diseases follow similar patterns).

As you can see, a woman who smokes is more than twice as likely to die before her 70th birthday. The same holds true for men. What is remarkable about these findings is not the fact that smok-

*Figures not included in this publication.

ing affects mortality but the magnitude with which it does. None of the other lifestyle behaviors we looked at had as pronounced an effect on mortality rates.

Please also note the "stairstep phenomenon." Never smoking is best, but quitting certainly helps. In fact, when smokers quit, their risk decreases slowly but significantly, and over time can return to near normal levels. To date, smoking cessation is the only behavior change in adulthood that has proven to reduce one's risk of dying prematurely.

When it comes to exercise, we see another interesting pattern. Heavy exercise is associated with the lowest mortality risk (Figures 2a and 2b).*

Again, the findings tend to confirm earlier suspicions and are particularly significant for men. Men who do not exercise are more than twice as likely to die in mid-life. In fact, not exercising at all can increase a man's chances of dying prematurely to more than one in three, assuming the relation is causal. This is a rather shocking statistic and should serve as a wake-up call to all those who believe physical activity is optional for good health.

Perhaps our most important finding was that exercise and smoking, when taken together

*Figures not included in this publication.

| Table 2 | Number of Deaths and Multivariate Adjusted Death Rate per 100,000 (CPS II, 1982–1988) |

Men			Women		
	Deaths	Death Rate		Deaths	Death Rate
All causes combined	8972	703.8	All causes combined	7069	325.5
All cancers	3552	278.6	All cancers	3334	153.5
All vascular diseases	3279	257.2	All vascular diseases	2174	100.1

without regard for any other behaviors, yield the most significant and dramatic differences in dying prematurely (Figures 3a and 3b).*

The results are clear and uncompromising. As a woman, if you never smoke and you exercise regularly, you are only one-third as likely to die in mid-life as your smoking, non-exercising counterpart. That's a fairly remarkable statistic—one that's worth noting again and again. Consider, as well, the following inverse relationship. A smoking male who does not exercise has nearly a 40 percent chance of dying in mid-life. Not very good odds, especially when you're gambling with your life.

Our other results were also quite interesting. When we examined vegetable and fruit intake, we found a gradual increase in mortality risk as consumption decreases (Figures 4a and 4b).*

As you can see, both men and women in the highest category, which is closest to the "5-a-day" group, experienced the lowest mortality risk. In fact, the highest consumers of fruits and vegetables had only a 15 percent absolute risk of dying between ages 35 to 69, compared to almost 20 percent in the lowest group.

And when we looked at body mass index, the ratio of weight (in kilograms) to height (in meters squared), we found a

*Figures not included in this publication.

gradual but definite increase in mortality rates as body weight deviates from optimal (Figures 5a and 5b).*

For both men and women, being either underweight or overweight led to an increased risk of death. (It's important to note that some of the increase in mortality seen with underweight individuals may be accounted for by sickness. That is, people who are not well often lose weight, and some of these individuals eventually die.)

Figures 6a and 6b* show what the other three behaviors combined add to the mortality risk by smoking status.

Whether one is a present smoker or a former smoker or has never smoked at all, the other three factors (diet, weight, exercise) add to or reduce your mortality risk depending on your lifestyle. As the risk behavior factors add up, the mortality risk increases dramatically.

Epidemiologic Conclusions

While these findings are quite significant in themselves, it is important to point out that since our analytic cohort was made up largely of white, married, middle-class adults, the results may actually underestimate the actual adverse impact on mortality of the

*Figures not included in this publication.

four risk factors. Nevertheless, our CPS II data lead us to the following important conclusions, which we believe hold true for all people:

1. Each risk factor (smoking, not exercising, lower vegetable and fruit intake, and being overweight or obese) contributes independently to poorer survival, and these risks compound each other.

2. Each step in the right direction improves the survival odds; that is, moderate exercise is better than no exercise, but heavy exercise is best.

Our findings are in many ways similar to those reported by Michael McGinnis and Bill Foege in their review of U.S. mortality rates emphasizing tobacco and diet. Table 3 summarizes their findings.

All these data, along with volumes of other reports, lead us to what we know to be true. Simply stated, if no more research were to be done forever more, we would be on safe ground to assert that: One's personal lifestyle is of profound and overriding importance in determining one's health status and one's chances for a full and complete life.

This is what we know.

What We've Done

Next, I would like to consider briefly what we have done—by this I mean, what we as health educators have accomplished thus far in the history of our profession. Obviously, giving this issue its just treatment would take much more space than I am allotted here, and for this reason, I will confine my remarks to those pertinent historical events that have most shaped our profession.

Early in this century, the term health education gradually began

Table 3 Actual Causes of All U.S. Deaths

Cause	Percent
Tobacco	19%
Diet/activity patterns	14%
Alcohol	5%
Microbial agents	4%
Toxic agents	3%
Firearms	2%
Sexual behavior	1%
Motor vehicles	1%
Illicit use of drugs	<1%

McGinnis, J.M., & Foege, W.H. *Journal of the American Medical Association, 270*(18), p. 2208.

to replace hygiene, and in 1922 the first health educator received a baccalaureate degree in this field. Over the next three decades, both undergraduate and graduate programs in health education began to develop in a number of institutions of higher learning, and by 1950, 38 colleges and universities had developed a health education major (Means, 353).

Once doctoral degree programs were developed, scholars naturally began to conduct studies aimed at determining how best to make health education work. Unfortunately, these studies didn't always tell us if our efforts were leading to real outcome differences, and to make matters worse, few of them were replicable. It took some time before we learned how to develop and conduct research in ways that would provide us with information we could really put to use.

However, due to efforts beginning primarily in the 1980s, we now have a growing body of knowledge about what seems to be effective and what isn't. Thanks to the work of individuals like Parcell, Perry, Botvin, Vincent, Kolbe, Kirby, Green, Gold, and a good many others, and with the assistance of our professional associations and the Division of Adolescent and School Health at our nation's

Centers for Disease Control and Prevention, we can assert today that well-designed and well-supported health education programs can work.

In fact, quite frequently they *do* work, and that is more, often *much* more, than we can say about the medical interventions and public policy initiatives that often are used in an attempt to change unacceptably high-risk behaviors. We know, for example, that affecting smoking cessation through health education is far less expensive than treating the illness of the smoker who gets lung cancer, but the value of health education is not so much in its economic benefits as it is in ability to save lives. Richard Peto has suggested that if we could reduce by just 15 percent the number of children who take up smoking by implementing comprehensive school health education, we could save 50,000 lives a year early in the next century. And if we could reduce this number even further through a broad range of initiatives, we could save even more. In fact, researchers at the American Cancer Society believe that if we could reduce cigarette smoking in young people (under age 20) by 60 percent over the next 10 years (1998–2007), about 3,000,000 more young people would never become smokers, and of these be-

tween 750,000 and 1,500,000 would be saved from dying prematurely of diseases caused by smoking (Endnote 1).

Obviously, we still have a long way to go before we fully understand all that is needed to make our interventions as efficacious as possible. Nevertheless, we must start where we are, and quite frankly, where we are is the best place we've ever been. We can now say with confidence, backed by objective measures, that well-designed and well-supported health education can help alleviate a number of social ills. It can reduce unwanted teenage pregnancies, childhood addiction to tobacco, unnecessary dental caries, and at the same time, it can improve dietary practices, exercise patterns, and feelings of self-worth (Endnote 2).

Of course, like anything else, health education is more valuable when done right. At a minimum, it is important that our future health education efforts be comprehensive, coordinated, and concentrated. However, achieving these goals will require a serious commitment on our part. It will take substantial funding to develop the necessary infrastructure and, at the same time, to integrate our health education programs into existing systems, including our schools, the workplace, the media, the health care industry, and others. If we do this, there is no doubt that health education can make a profound difference in our society.

What Must Be Done— Making Health Education a National Priority

This, then, brings me to the next issue—what must be done in order to promote health education to its rightful and necessary place in the overall health care system. It is my belief that we will never realize our full potential until we make health education a national priority. Moreover, if we sincerely believe in health education's importance to human welfare and the future of our nation, then it is incumbent upon each of us to promote this goal as aggressively as possible.

Allow me to illustrate just how important this is. Consider, if you will, the following startling facts:

- 71.3 percent of students have tried cigarette smoking.

- Virtually all new tobacco addicts are children.

- Nearly 1/3 of students first drink alcohol—other than a few sips—before age 13.

- 21.7 percent of students rarely or never use safety belts.

- Of students who are sexually active, one-fourth used alcohol or drugs at last sexual intercourse.

- The U.S. has the highest teenage pregnancy rates in the industrialized world.

- Last year people went to jail at nearly twice the rate they did 10 years ago.

- We now have more people in prison than any other country in the world.

- Only 61 serious crimes are prevented for every $1 million spent incarcerating repeat offenders, while 258 are prevented for every $1 million spent on high-school graduation incentives.

- We now spend seven tax dollars per prisoner each day for every two dollars spent on a U.S. public school student.

- When it comes to literacy, the United States is now 38th among all countries of the world.

- The nation's social wellbeing has fallen to its lowest point in 25 years, and children and young people are suffering most.

- One in five of our children is poor.

- The gap between rich and poor children is greater here than in any other industrialized country.

- The gap between the "haves" and "have nots" correlates strikingly with increased mortality rates.

- Only 23 percent of federal spending on entitlements goes to programs for the poor; however, 93 percent of budget cuts to entitlements made by the 104th Congress will come from those programs (Endnote 3).

In a very real sense, all these facts—and tragically, many more like them—constitute a true health-education challenge, if not an outright crisis, and yet we very rarely hear any of these issues raised among our current crop of pundits and policy makers. In an age when budget cutting and tax breaks are all the rage, I fear there is little interest in such matters.

As I have stated previously, I am not asserting that health education is a panacea, but I do confess to being a true believer in what it can do if and when it becomes a national priority. Sometimes, it's helpful to turn things on their head in order to see them from a different perspective. Let me place it before you this way: If we believe that social morbidities, excess health care costs, and premature mortal-

ity are problems our society must eventually deal with, then we can simply outline the alternatives. I submit there are three:

One is to do nothing. We have done a lot of that, it seems to me, and I can't see that it helps much. On the contrary, the health of our children has declined significantly under this policy of neglect. In fact, the current adolescent population is far less healthy than their parents as the same age (*Code Blue*). Nevertheless, we should recognize that doing nothing is a very real option and that not to act is a decision, too.

A second option is to legislate human behavior—the "thou shalt not" approach, accompanied by sanctions and censures. Certainly, this is an option to be considered and one that can sometimes work, especially when combined with education as in the case of drunk driving. However, in general, this approach is only second best at best, and it's often unacceptable to the public, not without good reason. After all, we are a democratic country that puts a premium on personal freedom. The fewer laws necessary, the better. I, like many Americans, still cherish the fact that I can decide for myself whether or not to engage in behaviors that some might consider risky—hang gliding, rock climbing, dessert with dinner, a drink with friends. That is what freedom is really all about—the freedom of one's values, the freedom of one's intellect, the freedom of one's education, and the freedom of one's right to choose.

If neither of the above options is very attractive, then it seems to me that aggressive health education is the solution. Not only has it shown promise in rather impressive pilot projects, but its basic underpinnings are consonant with preserving the right of people to choose for themselves once they've been provided with the facts and helped to develop the skills to analyze the risks and rewards inherent in their decisions.

Since all of us in the profession care deeply about health education, I suspect we will all agree that making health education a national priority is a good thing. However, agreeing that it is a good idea and actually making it happen are two very different propositions, and this leads me to the last issue I wish to address: How can we achieve this goal? How can we make health education a national priority?

How We Should Do It

I believe we as health educators can make health education a national priority if, and only if, we accomplish four critical goals. First of all, we must begin to see our role large. Not only do we need to identify and address the health education needs of children, adults, parents, and others, but we must also identify and address those of stakeholders, opinion leaders, and policy makers. It is my understanding that the current Speaker of the House is very interested in diabetes control, in part, because he has been health-educated by the Centers for Disease Control and Prevention that 27 percent of all Medicare costs annually are incurred to treat persons with uncontrolled diabetes. This is just the sort of opportunity for health education that we must seek out and exploit if we are to advance our beliefs beyond the academy. It is not enough to teach the next generation of policy makers. We must teach the current generation as well.

Initially, this new role may feel uncomfortable. We may not always know how to proceed, but this will change with time and practice. There are countless ways and places to intervene throughout our communities and society as a whole and these will become more and more evident as we begin to focus on them (see Figure 7).*

Whether we address the proximal or more distant causes of preventable disease and premature mortality, it is possible to envision innumerable opportunities for health education. Remember the poignant words of John W. Gardner: "Life offers us endless opportunities often disguised as insoluble problems . . . and our job as change agents and leaders is, in essence, to redefine the unacceptable."

In addition to seeing our role large, we must begin rethinking our relationships with others. We can no longer limit our interactions to members of a close-knit academic society. It is not enough to write and speak and hope that others will follow in our footsteps. To make a real difference, we must be willing to collaborate with a broad range of individuals and organizations.

Let me share one or two examples of what I mean with you. The American Cancer Society has begun to collaborate more and more with other organizations in the social, governmental, and private sectors, and these new collaborations have unquestionably helped us further our mission. We now have a cause-marketing partnership with SmithKline Beecham pharmaceutical company in order to reach smokers with messages about, and assistance with, quitting through use of nicotine replace-

*Figure not included in this publication.

ment. This partnership has allowed us to reach millions of smokers—more than ever before—and at the same time, to promote our Great American Smokeout. Over the course of the first year of our partnership, our smoking cessation message was propelled with some $10 million of media support—about $2 million during our November Smokeout time frame alone. Such public exposure would never be possible without the help of the private sector.

Another exciting example of the American Cancer Society's new policy of engagement is our recent collaboration with MTV to develop television spots targeted at young teens. As I sat in my office on a summer weekend last year, I laughed out loud as I read the proposed script for these two spots. They are clever, witty, and perfectly suited for their intended audience. It's quite unlikely that the American Cancer Society could have developed either of these spots as effectively without the help of MTV, which has the best data I've seen anywhere on the attitudes, beliefs, and preferences of young Americans. Both spots eventually became finalists in the 1996 Emmy Awards competition (Endnote 4).

In addition to these efforts, we must strive for greater professional solidarity so that we can develop a better consensus among ourselves and a common message to all other professional groups and the at-large public. At present, we spend far too much time debating details within the profession, and as a result, we lose the opportunity to communicate to others who we are and what we are about.

We must unify our professional organizations as quickly as possible and then empower them to work together to standardize professional preparation, accreditation, and certification. While I'm proud of the progress we have made to date, we must redouble our efforts until it is clear to everyone that we have our house in order and that all credentialed professional health educators are competent, regardless of the institution they come from.

Having spent three decades in higher education and having chaired two academic departments, as well as far too many curriculum committees, I can assure you that I understand the concept of academic freedom. But concerns about academic freedom, local autonomy, regional traditions, and experiential biases do not have to be at variance with the development of solid standards ensuring the basic competence of all health educators. Indeed, to be truly effective, they must reinforce each other. We need better standards for professional preparation, better standards for program accreditation, and better standards for graduate-level credentialing. With no intention of being harsh or judgmental, may I respectfully suggest that we can't expect others to take us seriously until we are willing to take ourselves seriously enough to reach agreement on what constitutes acceptable standards for professional preparation at all levels.

Finally, if we are really serious about making health education a national priority, we must be willing to act as advocates for our cause. As one looks over the past decade at other changes in public attitude, public support, and public policy, it is painfully obvious that the squeaky wheel gets the grease. Last year, the amount of federal research funds allocated for AIDS was significantly higher than that spent on Alzheimer's. Obviously, both causes could and should receive more funding, but these levels were set, I submit, not on the basis of need, but as a function of influence. Those who are interested in funding AIDS research are simply better at getting their message out.

Before leaving my position at Indiana University, I would often tell my graduate students that being an advocate was a part of being a competent and effective health educator. After all, we are about changing what is into what ought to be. Now more than ever we must continue to promote our causes. We must advocate to make health education a nationwide priority at every level of society if we wish to succeed, and we must do so with all the vigor and tenacity we can muster. Unless and until we are willing to make this commitment, health education will not realize its full potential.

In conclusion, I believe it is the best of times and the worst of times for our profession. It is the worst of times because the health problems facing us today have never been more pressing, difficult, or complex, and the prospect of new funding for social programs, including health education interventions, is poor.

And yet in many ways, it is the best of times. We've learned a lot during the 20th century, including a great deal about what does and doesn't work in health education. We now know absolutely that one's circumstances and chosen lifestyle are vitally important in determining one's health and one's prospects for self-actualization, and we have found creative and effective ways to help people make enlightened choices to promote their own quality of life.

Indeed, we have every reason to hope. Whenever our nation has set a goal, it has had an uncanny record of achieving it. Whether it's putting a man on the moon, driving Sadaam Hussein from Kuwait, or rescuing the Savings and Loan industry, whenever we establish a true priority, we eventually get it done. Mission accomplished.

My colleagues, the polling data are clear: our public has never been more interested in health nor more concerned about health care. Isn't it time for us to capitalize on this real public need and natural human interest? Isn't it time we make health education a true national priority? As Robert Kennedy once said, "Some men see things as they are and ask why? I dream of things that never were and ask why not?"

Means, R. K. (1962). *A history of health education*. Philadelphia: Lea and Febiger.

National Association of State Boards of Education. (1990). *Code blue: Uniting for healthier youth*. Alexandria, VA.

Peto, R. Personal comment.

Endnotes

(1) These projections were made by Clark Health, Phyllis Wingo, and Michael Thun on June 7, 1997. They assume (1) a 10 year linear reduction in youth smoking from 30 percent in 1997 to 12 percent in 2007, and (2) linear growth of the total U.S. population from 267,900,000 in 1997 to 295,900,000 in 2007 and of the 15–19 year age group from 17,900,000 to 19,700,000.
The 1,500,000 lives-saved projection assumes that all young people who smoke regularly continue to do so as adults, and the 750,000 projection, that half do not continue smoking.

(2) The following studies are among the many that show the effectiveness of health education:

Iverson, D.C., & Sheer, J.K. (1982). School-based cancer education programs: An opportunity to affect the national cancer problem. *Health Values: Achieving High Level Wellness, 6,* 27–35.

Kolbe, L.J. (1985). Why school health education? An empirical point of view. *Health Education, 16,* 116–120.

Metropolitan Life Foundation, Louis Harris and Associates, Inc. (1988). *Health: You've got to be taught. An evaluation of comprehensive health education in American public schools.* New York: Metropolitan Life Foundation, Louis Harris and Associates, Inc.

Vincent, M.L., Clearie, A.F., & Schlucter, M.D. (1987). Reducing adolescent pregnancy through school and community-based education. *Journal of the American Medical Association, 257,* 3328–3386.

(3) A number of these items are based on information contained in the "Youth Risk Behavior Surveillance—United States, 1995" conducted by Laura Kann, Charles W. Warren, et al. (1966). *Journal of School Health, 66*(10).

The following brief citations are in the same order as the facts above: *Journal of School Health.* December, 1996; American Cancer Society. *Cancer Risk Report,* 1996; *Journal of School Health.* December, 1996; *Journal of School Health.* December 1996; Alan Guttmacher Institute. "Risk and Realities of Early Childbearing Worldwide," 1997; *USA Today,* January 20, 1997; U.S. Justice Department; *Harper's Magazine.* February, 1997; *Harper's Magazine.* September 1996; PBS, "Breakfast with Random House." March 15, 1997; *New York Times,* October 14, 1996; UNICEF, "The Progress of Nations"; *British Medical Journal.* April, 1996; UNICEF, "The Progress of Nations"; *Harper's Magazine.* February, 1997.

(4) To receive a copy of the ads produced by MTV and ACS, please contact Nathan Grey or Cathy Swaney at the American Cancer Society, 1599 Clifton Road, NE, Atlanta, GA 30329–4251.

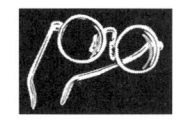 **Article Review Form at end of book.**

To prevent social and health problems among our young people, policy makers have urged us to _____. Describe the positive approach adapted by the New Haven public schools.

Creating a Districtwide Social Development Project

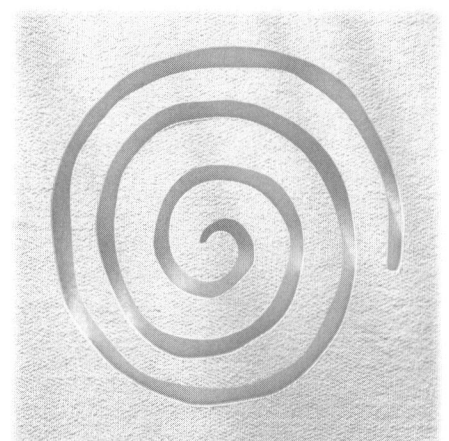

In New Haven, Connecticut, educators take the social and emotional development of their students seriously through comprehensive curriculums that have built-in community support.

Roger P. Weissberg, Timothy P. Shriver, Sharmistha Bose, and Karol DeFalco

Roger P. Weissberg is Professor of Psychology at the University of Illinois at Chicago, Senior Researcher for the Mid-Atlantic Regional Laboratory for Student Success, and Executive Director of the Collaborative for the Advancement of Social and Emotional Learning (CASEL). Timothy P. Shriver is President of Special Olympics International, Washington, D.C., and the former Supervisor of the Department of Social Development for the New Haven, Connecticut, Public Schools. Sharmistha Bose is a senior research associate for CASEL. Karol DeFalco is a facilitator for Social Development, New Haven Public Schools.

To prevent social and health problems among our young people, policymakers have urged us to fight a war on drugs, a war on AIDS, and a war on violence. Using war as a model for prevention, however, is misguided (Shriver and Weissberg 1996). Although single-issue campaigns—even isolated "character education" programs—are well-intentioned, they have so far yielded only limited success.

In the New Haven, Connecticut, public schools, we have found that *sustained* efforts to enhance children's social and emotional development can help students become knowledgeable, responsible, and caring citizens (Elias et al. in press). This positive approach promotes competence—and it prevents many high-risk behaviors. For the past 10 years, we have continued to develop this program and have enhanced students' academic performance, social competence, and health.

Task Force Findings

In 1987, the superintendent convened a task force—including educators, parents, students, community leaders, university researchers, and human service providers—to assess the high-risk behaviors of students that lead to drug use, teen pregnancy, AIDS, delinquency, truancy, and school failure. Through in-depth surveys, the task force found that a significant proportion of New Haven's high school students engaged in behaviors that jeopardized their academic performance, health, and safety.

Concerns about the social and health-related behaviors of youth are not limited to urban areas like New Haven. For example, in 1995 the Centers for Disease Control and Prevention conducted a national survey of high school students. In this survey, 30 percent of the students indicated that they engaged in binge drinking and 18 percent smoked marijuana.

Another survey finding: 50 percent of high schoolers indicated that they had already had sexual intercourse, and almost 20 percent reported having four or more partners. These data show that many students across the United States are experiencing social, emotional, and health problems and are not succeeding in school.

The New Haven task force noted that the same students experienced several problems simultaneously—problems that seemed to have common roots, such as poor problem-solving and communication skills; antisocial attitudes about fighting and education; limited constructive after-school opportunities; and a lack of guidance and monitoring by adults who are positive role models. The task force recommended that New Haven create a comprehensive K-12 social development curriculum to address these needs.

The Social Development Project

The superintendent and board of education established a district-level Department of Social Development—with a supervisor and staff of facilitators—that coordinated all prevention and health-promotion initiatives. The department ensured broad, representative, ongoing involvement by school staff, parents, and community members in establishing coordinated social and emotional education opportunities for all students—in regular, special, and bilingual education.

The goals are to educate knowledgeable, responsible, and caring students who acquire a set of basic skills, values, and work habits for a lifetime of meaningful work and constructive citizenship. Other goals include helping students develop positive self-

concepts and helping them learn to live safe, legal, and healthy lives.

Curriculum objectives and content. Curriculum committees at all grade levels developed a K–12 scope and sequence for the Social Development curriculum. The committees established student learning objectives at each grade level and then undertook a comprehensive review process to find and adapt appropriate programs. Throughout the process, the committees considered federal standards, state mandates, and the priorities of local educators, parents, community members, and students; and they obtained the support of university psychologists.

Over a period of five years, New Haven phased in the new curriculum, with 25–50 hours of instruction at each grade. The curriculum emphasizes the following:

- Self-monitoring, problem solving, conflict resolution, and communication skills.

- Values such as personal responsibility and respect for self and others.

- Content about health, culture, interpersonal relationships, and careers.

Each school's team—as representative as the task force—plans new initiatives and ensures support by all segments of the school community. The department also encourages everyone in the school community to plan extracurricular educational, health-promotion, and recreational activities for students.

Professional development. The Department of Social Development established profes-

The curriculum focuses on self-monitoring, problem solving, conflict resolution, and communication skills.

sional development programs to support and train teachers, administrators, and pupil personnel staff who implement these programs. Master teachers and coaches are the core of this effort, as they help coordinate classroom instruction with school and community programming. In this ongoing program, teachers bring their successes and challenges back to the group (see fig. 1).

Program evaluation. Finally, the department designed monitoring and evaluation strategies to assess the effectiveness of the program and to identify ways to improve it. Collaborating with university researchers, the department evaluated the process and outcomes, incorporating the perspectives of teachers, students, administrators, and parents.

These evaluations document that the project has been well received and has improved the attitudes and behaviors of students. For example, research has demonstrated positive effects on students' problem-solving skills, attitudes about conflict, impulse control, social behavior, delinquency, and substance use (Weissberg et al. 1997, Caplan et al. 1992, Kasprow et al. 1991).

Recommendations

The New Haven Social development Project, like many other ambitious innovations, has achieved exciting successes and frustrating setbacks. We have found several principles that may help other districts establish similar systemwide programs:

- School-based prevention programs should embrace a broad conceptualization of health and positive youth development, addressing children's social, emotional, and physical health through coordinated programming.

- Programs should offer developmentally appropriate, planned, sequential K–12 classroom instruction, using culturally relevant information and materials.

- Effective prevention involves teaching methods that ensure active student engagement, emphasize positive behavior change, and improve student-adult communication. Students are more likely to benefit when they are encouraged to apply skills to real-life situations and to learn effective communication skills.

- Peers, parents, the school, and community members should work together to reinforce classroom instruction.

- Team members must design programs that are acceptable to and reach students at risk, including students already engaging in risky behaviors. Classroom instruction must be better coordinated with social, mental health, and health services that are provided to high-risk youth.

- Districts must develop systemwide practices and infrastructures to support social and emotional development programs.

As educators, we have the determination and knowledge to address the urgent needs of our young people. Unfortunately, many widely used and heavily marketed programs have poor or inconsistent evaluation results and only emphasize single issues (Dusenbury and Falco 1997). Preventive efforts work when

comprehensive, systemic supports exist (Dryfoos 1997).

Healthy social and emotional learning goes beyond the prevention of specific negative outcomes. We need to abandon piecemeal approaches to prevention; we must provide supportive, creative, and caring learning environments to nurture the healthy development of children.

References

Caplan, M., R.P. Weissberg, J.S. Grober, P.J. Sivo, D. Grady, and C. Jacoby. (1992). "Social Competence Promotion with Inner-City and Suburban Young Adolescents: Effects on Social Adjustment and Alcohol Use." *Journal of Clinical and Consulting Psychology* 60, 1: 56–63.

Centers for Disease Control and Prevention. (March 24, 1995). "CDC Surveillance Summaries." *Morbidity and Mortality Weekly Review* 44 (SS-1): 1–56.

Dryfoos, J.G. (1997). "The Prevalence of Problem Behaviors: Implications for Programs." In *Healthy Children 2010: Enhancing Children's Wellness*, edited by R.P. Weissberg, T.P. Gullotta, R.L. Hampton, B.A. Ryan, and G.R. Adams. Thousand Oaks, Calif.: Sage.

Dusenbury, L.A., and M. Falco. (1997). "School-Based Drug Abuse Prevention Strategies: From Research

to Policy and Practice." In *Healthy Children 2010: Enhancing Children's Wellness*, edited by R.P. Weissberg, T.P. Gullotta. R.L. Hampton, B.A. Ryan, and G.R. Adams. Thousand Oaks, Calif.: Sage.

Elias, M.J., J.E. Zins, R.P. Weissberg, K.S. Frey, M.T. Greenberg, N.M. Haynes, R. Kessler, M.E. Schwab-Stone, and T.P. Shriver. (in press). *Fostering Knowledgeable, Responsible, and Caring Students: Social and Emotional Education Strategies.* Alexandria, Va.: ASCD.

Kasprow, W.J., R.P. Weissberg, C.K. Voyce, A.S. Jackson, T. Fontana, M.W. Arthur, E. Borman, N. Mormorstein, J. Zeisz, T.P. Shriver, K. DeFalco, W. Elder, and M. Kavanaugh. (1991). *New Haven Public Schools Social Development Project: 1990–91 Evaluation Report.* New Haven: New Haven Public Schools.

Shriver, T.P., and R.P. Weissberg. (May 15, 1996). "No New Wars!" *Education Week* 15, 34: 33, 37.

Weissberg, R.P., H.A. Barton, and T.P. Shriver. (1997). "The Social-Competence Promotion Program for Young Adolescents." In *Primary Prevention Exemplars: The Lela Rowland Awards*, edited by G.W. Albee and T.P. Gullotta. Newbury Park, Calif.: Sage.

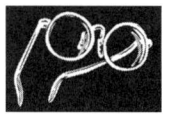

Article Review Form at end of book.

What was the first project addressed by the Baton Rouge Health Forum? The key to successful partnerships is _____. Explain.

Five Years of Collaboration:

Baton Rouge Health Forum Focuses on Community Needs

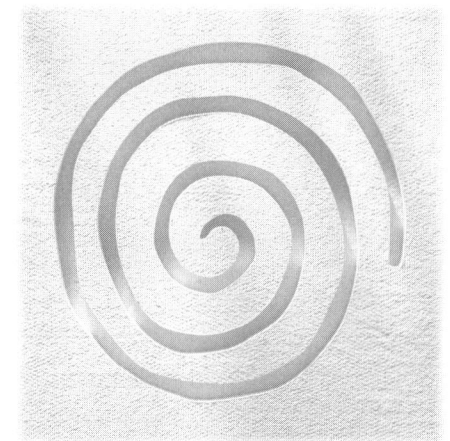

Virginia M. Pearson

Virginia Pearson is executive director, Baton Rouge Health Forum, Baton Rouge, LA.

Five years ago in Baton Rouge, Bob Davidge, president/CEO of Our Lady of the Lake Regional Medical Center, a member of the Franciscan Missionaries of Our Lady Health System, invited other Baton Rouge hospital executives to a breakfast meeting to discuss conducting a jointly sponsored community-needs assessment. All the CEOs agreed to participate to the extent of their organizations' ability. The assessment process took six months, and at its conclusion the group decided to continue their monthly meetings. As a consultant, I had led the assessment process. The group retained me as executive director to help them find ways they could continue working together.

Thus was born the Baton Rouge Health Forum (BRHF) (see Box). The forum's members now include the local charity hospital, the local Columbia/HCA affiliate,

the largest privately owned hospital in Louisiana, and the two largest competitors. The members represent for-profit, not-for-profit, large, small, specialty, and general acute care facilities. The East Baton Rouge Parish Medical Society is also a member and keeps local physicians in the loop. The society's president is a member of the forum's Executive Committee.

BRHF's first project evolved because of Louisiana's requirement that high school students take a semester-long course on health prior to graduation. The high school teachers tapped to teach this course (primarily physical education teachers) were scrambling to find resources, and the school system contacted a couple of the larger hospitals for help. The director of the BRHF proposed putting together a resource manual with information from all the forum members, and the schools eagerly accepted.

The manual, inexpensively produced in conjunction with the community education and mar-

keting staff from each of the forum hospitals, lists, by topic, all the presentations the hospitals offer to the community. As they put the information together, the committee's members realized that they could use the information for all ages, so they coded each topic for age appropriateness. Teachers could hardly get their hands on these manuals fast enough, and each public and parochial school received at least two copies. Copies of the manual, which was created in 1994, are still being requested.

Coordinating Efforts

This year, the BRHF will conduct seven free community screenings, at which people can be tested for colorectal, skin, and prostate cancer; high blood pressure; and depression. The advertisement for these screenings lists information for each forum member, and the news release, printed on BRHF letterhead, also emphasizes the collaborative nature of the screenings.

Mission Statement: Greater Baton Rouge Health Forum

The mission of the Greater Baton Rouge Health Forum is to improve the health status of the Greater Baton Rouge community by:

1. Identifying and prioritizing community health needs through an ongoing process and through community partnerships.

2. Coordinating and leveraging the resources and influence of its member institutions to bring them to bear on improving community health.

For the past three years, BRHF has provided free hepatitis B inoculations for every fifth grader in four parishes. More than 10,000 inoculations were administered during the 1997–98 school year, and almost 70 percent of the target population received the three-dose regimen. The BRHF hospitals coordinate nurses and medical supplies, and the vaccine is donated as part of the national Vaccines for Children program. This program, which has received national attention, is scheduled to run through 2002.

> **One way to facilitate group trust is to begin with relatively small and easily achievable projects. Their success will support further efforts.**

Sickle Cell Anemia Program

BRHF hospitals are also collaborating on a program to enhance the lives of local sickle cell anemia sufferers, and to change emergency room protocols. In April 1998 an Atlanta physician presented a program on sickle cell management and potential new therapies to more than 200 area healthcare professionals, and in May Southern University presented a program on the dietary needs of the sickle cell patient for dietitians and nurses. This program will be presented again in the spring of 1999.

Each hospital will present a program on a specific topic for sickle cell patients and their caregivers and families. One program will be presented each month for the next six months, and then the programs will be evaluated and a new six-month schedule outlined. The local and state sickle cell anemia associations participate in and endorse this program, and other communities have expressed interest in adapting the program for their own needs. Louisiana's Department of Health and Hospitals has received federal funding for a sickle cell initiative and will consult the BRHF to determine the best way to utilize these funds to reduce patient stays and enhance the quality of life for sickle cell sufferers. All this progress is due to the fact that nurses from two BRHF hospitals, Our Lady of the Lake and Baton Rouge General, sat down together to discuss ways to improve quality of care. The president of the medical society brought their idea to the BRHF Executive Committee and it was adopted by all the hospital CEOs.

Mutual Trust Is Key

In a partnership of this nature, building trust is imperative. This takes time, but one way to facilitate group trust is to begin with relatively small and easily achievable projects, so that their success supports and encourages the group's further efforts.

Potential problem areas involve questions of ownership, equality, and leadership. All the partners must feel they have input in the projects, from the choice of undertakings throughout their execution. Each partner must also feel that its voice carries as much weight as the others'. Finally, the partnership's steering committee must be composed of the member organizations' top leaders—the CEOs or their equivalent. Delegating this responsibility can undermine success.

After five years, the forum's members can look back on significant accomplishments. The road is occasionally rocky, but no organization has left the forum, and three have joined the original group. Building and keeping mutual trust has been key to BRHF's success, and it will be key in the future.

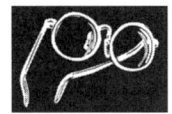 **Article Review Form at end of book.**

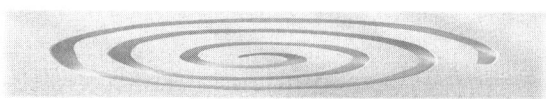

WiseGuide Wrap-Up

- The association between risk factors and medical expenditures suggests that greater emphasis needs to be placed on correctable psychosocial risks than on many of the risks that have historically been center stage.

- To be positioned for success, we must unify our professional organizations and empower them to work collaboratively to standardize professional preparation, accreditation, and certification.

- School-based prevention programs should embrace a broad conceptualization of health and positive youth development, addressing children's social, emotional, and physical health through coordinated programming.

- Preventive efforts work when comprehensive, systematic supports exist.

- For successful collaboration, all partners must feel they have input in the projects, from the choice of undertaking throughout their execution. Each partner must also feel that its voice carries as much weight as the others'.

R.E.A.L. Sites

This list provides a print preview of typical **Coursewise** R.E.A.L. sites. (There are over 100 such sites at the **Courselinks**™ site.) The danger in printing URLs is that web sites can change overnight. As we went to press, these sites were functional using the URLs provided. If you come across one that isn't, please let us know via email to: webmaster@coursewise.com. Use your Passport to access the most current list of R.E.A.L. sites at the **Courselinks** site.

Site name: The Cochrane Collaboration

URL: http://www.cochrane.de/

Why is it R.E.A.L.? The Cochrane Collaboration is an international not-for-profit organization. Its aim is to make up-to-date, accurate information about the effects of health care readily available worldwide.

Key topics: collaboration, health care

Try this: Select Help for Newcomers, then Chronology, and review the timeline. Note the increasing collaborative efforts from 1972 to the present.

Site name: HERO

URL: http://www.the-hero.org

Why is it R.E.A.L.? HERO facilitates collaboration between sustaining partners in order to identify research needs, to create protocols, and to provide or secure funding.

Key topics: collaboration, health care

Try this: Select HERO Operations and Partners and review the list of national partners.

Site name: WHO Collaboration

URL: http://www.wits.ac.za/wits/fac/med/comhealth/collabor.htm

Why is it R.E.A.L.? This site provides information relating to the 1995 World Health Organization–designated Department of Community Health, the National Urbanization and Health Research Program of the MRC, and the Health, Housing and Urbanization Directorate of the Greater Johannesburg Transitional Metropolitan Council, a WHO Collaborating Centre for Urban Health.

Key topics: collaboration, health, community health, urban health

Try this: Select The Units. Examine the list of programs and the collaborative nature of each.

Index

Names and page numbers in **bold** type indicate authors and their articles.
Page numbers followed by *t* indicate tables. Page numbers followed by *n* indicate notes.

fruit consumption, 39, 59–62, 219
funding, health services, 27–28, 141, 145
future health concerns, *Parade* respondents, 4–5
future of public health, 2, 24–25, 26–32
The Future of Public Health [Institute of Medicine (IOM)], 27, 171

G-8 Summit, 19
Gadow, Patricia, 122, **138**
Gandhi, Mahatma, 31
Gardner, John W., 223
GATT (General Agreement on Tariffs and Trade), 23
gender
    health condition, 3–4
    health promotion programs, 88, 92
    healthy workplace attributes, 75, 76*t*
    HERO study, 213
    smoking, 166, 168–70
General Agreement on Tariffs and Trade (GATT), 23
General Agreement on Trade in Services, 18
General Motors (GM), 116
genetics revolution, 28
Glamour (magazine), 199
globalization of public health
    altruism *vs.* self-interest, 2, 21–25
    economy, 28–29
    opportunities and threats, 1, 17–20
    public health, 18, 19*t*
glucose, blood, 212–15
GM (General Motors), 116
Goetzel, Ron Z., 208, **210**
Gold, Robert, 39, **50**
Goldberg, R.A., 153
Gordon, Shirley, 179, **195**
Gorenflo, Grace, 122, **138**
Gorman, D.M., 122, **152**
government
    changing role of, 29
    health care reform, 102
    health education as priority, 221–23
    health responsibility to citizens, 126
    lack of federal health leadership, 134
    statutory protections, FAIR Project, 201–3
Grant, M., 46, 47
grass-roots groups, 153
Great American Smokeout, 223
Green, L.W., 8
Gregg, M., 167
Grosch, James, 69, **83**
Group Health Cooperative of Puget Sound, 200

Hales, Dianne, 1, **3**
Handler, Arden S., 122, **124**
Hanlon, J.J., 127
Harris, Kari Jo, 39, **59**
Harris Poll, 14, 15*t*, 16, 27
Hartwell, T.D., 106
Hartwell, Tyler, 69, **105**
Hawaii Public Health Association (HPHA), 30
HCFA (Health Care Financing Administration), 145
head lice, 57
Healey, Bernard, 123, **166**
The Healing of America (Williamson), 29

health
    American condition of, 3–6
    defined, 1, 111
    See also specific topics
Health Affairs (Fielding and Rice), 96
health and global change, 19*t*
Health Care Financing Administration (HCFA), 145, 184
health education. *See* education, health
Health Enhancement Research Organization (HERO) study, 208, 210–16
health maintenance organization (HMO), 96, 200
Health Plan Employer Data and Information Set (HEDIS), 187
Health Security Act, 128
Health Trust, Inc., 211
Healthcare Demand and Disease Management, 179, 190
Health-Promoting Hospitals, defined, 205–7
Healthy Communities [(Institute of Medicine (IOM)], 171–73
Healthy People 2000, 83, 85
Healthy People: National Health Promotion and Disease Prevention Objectives for the Year 2000, 7, 8, 9
healthy workplace attributes, 73–78, 79*t*, 80
hearing screening, 56
heart disease, 3
HEDIS (Health Plan Employer Data and Information Set), 187
HERO (Health Enhancement Research Organization) study, 208, 210–16
high blood pressure, 3, 212–15
high school students, 41–49, 226
high-risk populations. *See* at-risk populations
Hill, H., 154
HIV (human immunodeficiency virus), 67, 139, 182, 199
HMO (health maintenance organization), 96, 200
Hoffman-La Roche, 211
Holder, H.D., 155
Holman, C.D'Arcy, 69, **71**
Holmes, T.H., 113
Hoopes, D., 36
hospital-based promotion, 179
    community health initiatives and casefinding, 190–94
    at health-promoting hospitals, 204–6
    reproductive health and managed care, 181–88, 195–203
    host in community-based intervention program, 155–57
HPHA (Hawaii Public Health Association), 30
Human Genome Project, 28
human immunodeficiency virus (HIV), 67, 139, 182, 199
Humphrey, Hubert, 30
Hurty, John, 31
hypertension, 3, 212–15

IDPH (Illinois Department of Public Health), 146–47
Illinois, 133, 134*t*, 144–51
Illinois Department of Public Health (IDPH), 146–47
immigrant unemployment, 115
immunizations, 95

incarceration of youth, 222
individual method studies, unemployment, 112, 114, 117
industrial factors and healthy workplace attributes, 71–81
industrial group and health promotion programs, 89*t*, 90
information issues, 28, 30, 198
Institute of Medicine (IOM)
    and globalization, 24, 27
    Healthy Communities, 171–73
    measurement of public health practice, 124–36
    smoking, 166–67
insurance and managed care, 4, 5
interactive participation programs for drug prevention, 43, 44, 48
internal *vs.* external employee assistance programs (EAPs), 106–7, 108*t*, 109
international public health law, 23*t*
International Union for Health Promotion and Education, 72–81
interventions
    available in school based health programs, 52
    community-based, 155–61
    improve fruit and vegetable consumption, 60
    peer-led drug prevention, 41–49
    for unemployment, 114–17
    See also worksite health promotion

jail and youth, 222
Jalleh, Geoffrey, 69, **71**
JAMA (Journal of the American Medical Association), 36
JCAHO (Joint Commission on the Accreditation of Health Care Organizations), 133
Jernigan, D.H., 153
Johnson, C.A., 157
Johnson, Judy, 39, **59**
Johnston, L.D., 47
Joint Commission on the Accreditation of Health Care Organizations (JCAHO), 133
Jones, Michael C., 122, **144**
Journal of Health Education, 7*n*, 50*n*, 64*n*
Journal of Occupational Medicine, 97
Journal of Public Health Management, 181*n*
Journal of Public Health Management Practice, 138*n*, 144*n* 195*n*
Journal of School Health, 41*n*, 65
Journal of the American Medical Association (JAMA), 36
junior high, 39, 48
Just Say No campaign, 155

Kaiser Family Foundation, 186, 199
Kaiser Permanente, 39, 54–58, 200
Kandel, D.B., 160
Kansas LEAN School Health Project, 39, 59–62
Karachi Adventist Hospital Promotions Page (R.E.A.L. site), 207
W.K. Kellogg Foundation, 172
Kierkegaard, Sören, 31
Kimmell, Patti, 122, **144**
Kingery, Paul M., 96
Klitzner, M., 161
knowledge gap about managed care, 198–99
Koop, C.E., 22

Krajic, Karl, 204
Kramer, N.A., 127
Kreuter, M.W., 10

Landrum, Laura B., 122, **144**
law enforcement, community-based prevention, 158–59
Lay Opportunities-Collaborative Outreach Screening Team (LO-COST), 48
leadership
    and APHA, 135
    and credentialing, 11
    future of public health, 26–32, 31–32
    lack of federal, 134
    peer-led drug prevention programs, 42–43, 44*t*
    tuberculosis and LHDs, 141
LEAN School Health Project, Kansas, 39, 59–62
learning problems, 57
Lenfant, Claude, 3
Levi, Lennart, 70, **110**
Levy, Barry, 2, **26**
LHDs. *See* local health departments (LHDs)
lice, 57
listening and improving public health, 30
Lobnig, Hubert, **204**
local health departments (LHDs)
    Centers for Disease Control (CDC), 128, 134, 139
    historical perspectives on, 125–29
    Medicaid, 146–47, 149–51
    tuberculosis and managed care, 138–43
local media and community-based prevention, 158–59
LO-COST (Lay Opportunities-Collaborative Outreach Screening Team), 48
Louis Harris and Associates, Inc., 14, 15*t*, 16, 27
Loustaunau, Martha, 2, 33, **36**
Luebke, J.K., 11
Lumpkin, John R., 122, **144**

Majumdar, B., 36
managed care
    community *vs.* marketplace, 171–73
    cost-effectiveness of programs, 94–95, 96–97, 103
    as insurance, 4, 5
    reproductive health and Medicaid, 179, 181–88, 195–203
    tuberculosis and Medicaid, 139–43
managed care organizations (MCOs)
    Medicaid and reproductive health, 184–85
    school integration of health care, 54–58
    tuberculosis and local health departments (LHDs), 138–43
Managed Care Plus (MC+), 139–40
management and health care, 84, 89*t*, 92
mandated health care and MCOs, 55–58
Mantoux skin testing, 56
marijuana. *See* alcohol, tobacco, and other drugs (ATOD)
market issues, 52, 97, 171–73
Marriott Corporation, 211
Mason, J.O., 9
mass media and community-based prevention, 158–59
MC+ (Managed Care Plus), 139–40

McGinnis, Michael, 219
MCOs. *See* managed care organizations (MCOs)
measurement of public health practice, 124–30, 131–32*t*, 133–35
mechanism for unemployment, 111–12
media, 22, 158–59
Medicaid
    core responsiblities and Illinois LHDs, 144–51
    and Medicare as health care, 5
    reproductive health and managed care, 181–88
    state reform, 199–200
    tuberculosis and managed care, 139–43
medication, 4
medicine, modern *vs.* folk, 34–35
MediPass, 139–40
MEDSTAT Group, 211
mental health issues
    depression and anxiety, 3, 6, 212–15
    help sought from, 4
    referrals, 57
    and unemployment, 113–14, 116
meta-analysis, efficacy of peer-led drug prevention, 42–45
Metropolitan Insurance Company, 96
metropolitan *vs.* rural location, healthy workplace attributes, 76–77, 79*t*
Michigan, 211
Michigan Electronic Library (R.E.A.L. site), 38
Michigan Prevention Research Center, 116
middle school, 39, 48
Midwestern Prevention Project (MPP), 156–57
Miller, C.A., 127
Mills, C. Wright, 35
Minnesota, 157, 158
minorities, 9, 110
Missouri, 139–40
models
    biomedical model, 34
    Clarion University teacher health education model, 64–67
    community health assessment, 174–77
    community public health model, 155
    ecological model of workplace health promotion, 71
    peer-led drug prevention, 45–47
    PRECEDE planning model, 8
    preservice teacher health-education emphasis model, 40
    Stepped Approach Model of Service Delivery, 48
    worksite health promotion model, 39, 50–53
Moody, Conny Mueller, 122, **144**
Morbidity and Mortality Weekly Report, 1, 13*n*
mortality, 113, 166, 219
Mosher, J.F., 153
Mountain, —, 129
MPP (Midwestern Prevention Project), 156–57
multiculturalism, 33–36
Murphy, Lawrence, 69, **83**
Myers, B.A., 127

NACCHO (National Association of County and City Health Officials), 128–29, 133*t*

Nader, Philip, 39, **54**
Nakajima, Hiroshi, 20
National 5 A Day for Better Health, 39, 59–62
National Association of County and City Health Officials (NACCHO), 128–29, 133*t*, 139, 141
National Cancer Institute, 95
National Center for Health Statistics, 84
National Commission for Health Education Credentialing, 7, 11
National Health and Medical Research Council, 80
National Health Education Standards: Acheiving Health Literacy, 7, 8
National Health Information Center (R.E.A.L. site), 121
National Health Interview Survey (NHIS), 84, 90–92
National Health Objectives, 134
National Institute on Drug Abuse, 43
National Institutes of Health (NIH), 211
National Peer Helpers Association (NPHA), 42, 45, 47, 48
national survey, public opinion on health issues, 14, 15*t*, 16
National Survey of Worksite Health Promotion Activities (NSWHPA), 83–84, 90–91
National Survey of Worksites and Employee Assistance Programs (NSWEAP), 105
New York, 179, 195–203
NGOs (nongovernmental organizations), 29
NHIS (National Health Interview Survey), 84, 90–92
nicotine, 167
NIH (National Institutes of Health), 211
1997 Tobacco or Health: Global Status Report, 22
nongovernmental organizations (NGOs), 29
non-interactive programs, peer-led drug prevention, 43, 44
NPHA (National Peer Helpers Association), 42, 45, 47, 48
NSWEAP (National Survey of Worksites and Employee Assistance Programs), 105
NSWHPA (National Survey of Worksite Health Promotion Activities), 83–84, 90–91
nutrition
    among high school students, 65
    CPS II, 219
    fruit and vegetable consumption, 59–62
    as healthy workplace attribute, 73–78, 79*t*, 80
    HERO study, 212–15
    teacher education, 67
    unemployment, 113

obesity, 4
Objective 8.14, Local Health Departments (LHD), 128, 133
occupational group, health promotion programs, 89–90
Oldfield, Angela, 122, **144**
OLF (out of the labor force), 111
O'Malley, P.M., 47
opportunities to public health, 27–30
organizational characteristics, health promotion programs, 89–90, 92–93
O'Rourke, T.W., 12

Ottawa Charter for Health Promotion, 204–6
out of the labor force (OLF), 111
overweight, 3, 4, 212–15

Parade survey, 1, 3–6
participation in worksite health programs, 83–93
partnership development and improving public health, 30–31
Partnership for a Drug-Free America, 156
PATCH (Planned Approach to Community Health), 8, 10
PCCM (primary care case management), 184
Pearson, Virginia M., 123, **174,** 208, **229**
peer-led intervention, youth substance abuse reduction, 41–49
Pelikan, Juergen, 204
Pelletier, Kenneth, 69, **94**
Pennsylvania, 64–67, 167–70
Pentz, M.A., 157
performance of public health, measurement of, 125
Perry, C.L., 46, 47
personal-individual approach, community-based prevention, 156
Petersen, Martin, 69, **83**
PHF (Public Health Foundation), 129
PHP (prepaid health plan), 184
PHPPO (Public Health Practice Program Office), 139
PHS (Public Health Service), 128, 134, 135
physical examination, 3, 5, 57
physician, satisfaction with primary care, 5
Pierce, A., 113
Planned Approach to Community Health (PATCH), 8, 10
Planned Parenthood of New York City (PPNYC), 199
Point of Service (POS), 96
policy implication, globalization, 19–20
policy recommendation, peer-led drug prevention, 45
political issues and program advocacy, 10
population
    changes in United States', 28
    cultural diversity, 34
    demographic shifts, 9
    diversity and health education, 2, 33–36
    medically underserved, 54
    See also at-risk population
POS (Point of Service), 96
PPNYC (Planned Parenthood of New York City), 199
PPO (Preferred Provider Organization), 96
practitioners, professional, 7–12, 33–36
PRC (Prevention Research Center), 159–60
PRECEDE planning model, 8
Preferred Provider Organization (PPO), 96
pregnancy, 182, 222
prepaid health plan (PHP), 184
prescription drugs, 4
preservice teacher health-education emphasis model, 40
Preventing Tobacco Use Among Young People (Surgeon General), 167
prevention
    community-based, 158–59, 166–70, 179, 190–94
    CPS-II, 218–20
    of drug abuse, 41–49, 152–62

Healthy People, 7, 8, 9
    in workplace, 71–81, 83–93, 94–103
Prevention Research Center (PRC), 159–60
primary care case management (PCCM), 184
primary prevention as cost-effective, 95
principle development between school staff and MCOs, 55–56
priorities, health service survey, 13, 14*t*
private vs. public sector health promotion, 76–77, 79*t*, 83–84, 90–91
problems, top ten health, 3
profession, health education as, 1, 7–12, 26–32, 33–36
Programmatic Standards National Peer Helpers Association (NPHA), 42, 45, 47, 48
programs, health. *See specific programs*
project coordinator for school-MCO collaboration, 56
Project Northland, 157, 158
promotion, health. *See specific topics*
protocols, infrastructure for school-MCO collaboration, 56
PSA (public service announcement), 155–56
Public Health: What It Is and How It Works (Turnock), 172
Public Health Foundation (PHF), 129
public health issues
    actions to take, 30–31
    community model, 154, 155
    defined, 26–27
    improving, 124–36
    opinion on, 13–16
    public *vs.* private sector health promotion, 76–77, 79t, 83–84, 90–91
    revenues, 14, 15*t*, 179, 190–94
    See also specific topics
Public Health Practice Program Office (PHPPO), 139
Public Health Reporting System, 129
Public Health Service (PHS), 128, 134, 135
public school-based promotion.
    See school-based programs
public service announcement (PSA), 155–56
public *vs.* private sector health promotion, 76–77, 79*t*, 83–84, 90–91

race, 92, 110, 213
Rahe, R.H., 113
R.E.A.L. sites, 38, 68, 121, 178, 207, 231
refugees, tuberculosis and Medicaid, 139
relativity, cultural, 35
relocation, 115
reporting, community assessment, 175–77
reproductive health and Medicaid managed care, 179, 181–88, 195–203
research knowledge and community-based prevention, 154
research methodology
    Australian workplace health promotion, 72–77
    California survey - public opinion on public health, 13–14, 15*t*
    CPS-II, 218–20
    efficacy of peer-led drug preventions programs, 42–45
    employee assistance programs (EAPs), 105–7, 108*t*, 109
    FAIR Project, 179, 195–203
    globalization, 21–24
    HERO study, 208, 210–16

Medicaid and Illinois LHDs, 146–47, 149–51
    National 5 A Day for Better Health, 59–61
    school-managed care collaboration, 56–57
    social development project, 227–28
    tobacco use by children, 167–69
    unemployment and health, 112–14, 114–17
    worksite health promotion programs, 84–91
revenue for public health, 14, 15*t*, 179, 190–94
Rice, Thomas, 96
Richards, Thomas B., 122, **138**
Richter, Kimber, 39, **59**
risks to health
    alcohol, tobacco and other drugs (ATOD), 152–53
    degree of undetected, 190–94
    HERO study, 208, 210–16
    transnationalization of, 2, 21–25
    See also at-risk population
Robert Wood Johnson Foundation, 103, 135
Roe vs. Wade, 186
Roemer, M. and R., 18
Room, R., 153
Rosenbaum, S., 185
Rosenbluth, Jason M., 96
rural *vs.* metropolitan location, healthy workplace attributes, 76–77, 79*t*

safety net, 112, 116, 203
Salganicoff, Alina, 179, **181**
San Diego, California, 54–58
SBHPM (School Based Health Promotion Model), 50–53
School Based Health Promotion Model (SBHPM), 50–53
School Health Innovative Programs (SHIP), 55–58
school-based programs, 39–40
    credentialing, 11
    fruit and vegetable consumption, 59–62
    health crisis in, 64–67
    PATCH, 8
    peer-led substance abuse prevention, 41–49
    and political issues, 10
    School Health Innovative Programs (SHIP), 55–58
    social development project, creation of, 208, 226–28
    worksite health promotion model for, 50–53
school-leavers and unemployment, 114, 115
Schroeder, Steven A., 103
Schultz, Jerry, 39, **59**
Sciacca, John, 39, **41**
Scott, L.A., 48
screening
    adolescent health, 199
    community health initiatives, 190–91, 192–93*t*, 194
    for drug prevention, 48
    in health promotion programs, 85, 87*t*, 88–92
    reproductive health, 183
seat belts and youth, 222
Seffrin, John R., 208, **218**
self-interest, at country level, 24
self-medication, 6

self-referral option, 196*n*
self-reported data, 106, 109
settings for community health programs, 9
sexual activity, 5–6, 65, 222, 226–27
sexually transmitted disease (STD), 181, 199
   See also reproductive health
Shea, S., 155
SHIP (School Health Innovative Programs),
   55–58
Shriver, Timothy P., 208, **226**
skills-training, community-based, 156–57
skin cancer, 3
small worksites, healthy workplace
   attributes, 81
Smith, Steven, 26
SmithKline Beecham, 223
smoking
   blue-collar workers, 81
   Centers for Disease Control (CDC), 166
   cessation programs, 85, 86, 87t, 88–92
   CPS II, 219, 220
   as crisis, 166–67
   Parade survey, 5
   restriction, as healthy workplace
      attribute, 72–78, 79t, 80
   workplace restrictions on, 72
   youth, 41–49, 65, 222
   See also alcohol, tobacco, and other
      drugs (ATOD)
Sobel, J.L., 156
Sobo, E., 36
social contagion, unemployment as, 112, 115
social development project, creation of, 208,
   226–28
social marketing, school-based health, 52
social safety net, 112, 116, 203
Social Security Act, 184
social services, tuberculosis and LHDs, 142
social-political approach to community-
   based prevention, 156
societal fabric, changes in, 29
sociocultural influences as barrier to care, 200
sociodemographic factors, healthy
   workplace attribute, 75–76, 77t, 81
Southern Illinois Healthcare (R.E.A.L.
   site), 207
Southwestern Bell Corporation, 96
stages of health care market, 97
stakeholders and statutory protections,
   FAIR Project, 202–3
statistics, program cost-effectiveness, 97
statutory protections, FAIR Project, 201–3
StayWell Company, 211
STD (sexually transmitted disease), 181, 199
Stepped Approach Model of Service
   Delivery, 48
sterilization, 4
Stratton, H., 43
stress, 6, 113, 212–15
stress buffering mechanisms, 114–15
stress-buster training, teachers, 227
structural barriers, 200–201
Studnicki, J., 133
substance abuse. *See* alcohol, tobacco,
   and other drugs (ATOD)
suicide and unemployment, 113
sun protection as healthy workplace
   attribute, 74–78, 79t, 80
Supplemental Security Income (SSI), 182
Surgeon General, 167

Surgeon General of United States, 167
surveys
   managed care barriers, 196–98
   National Health Interview Survey
      (NHIS), 84, 90–92
   national survey, public opinion on
      health issues, 14, 15t, 16
   National Survey of Worksite Health
      Promotion Activities (NSWHPA),
      83–84, 90–91
   National Survey of Worksites and
      Employee Assistance Programs
      (NSWEAP), 105
   Parade survey, 1, 3–6, 3*n*
   Youth Risk Behavior Survey (1989),
      64–65
Swiger, Holly, 39, **54**

TANF (Temporary Assistance for Needy
   Families), 182*n*
Taras, Howard, 39, 54
Taylor, H., 13
Taylor, Zachary, 122, **138**
TB (tuberculosis), 56, 138–43
teachers
   fruit and vegetable consumption, 61–62
   social development project, 227, 228
   teacher health education model, 64–67
   time spent on health topics, 65
   See also education, health
Temporary Assistance for Needy Families
   (TANF), 182*n*
TennCare, 139–40
Tennessee, 139–40, 211
Terris, M., 127
tobacco
   community-based approaches, 152–62
   CPS II, 219
   and global action, 22
   HERO study, 212–14
   peer-led prevention, 41–49
   and unemployment, 113
   Youth Risk Behavior Survey (1989), 65
   See also alcohol, tobacco, and other
      drugs (ATOD)
Tobacco or Health: Global Status Report
   (1997), 22
Tobler, Nancy, 39, **41**, 43, 44, 45
trade liberalization and public health
   globalization, 17, 18–20
trade unions
   and health-promoting workplace, 39,
      83–93
   healthy workplace attributes, 77, 78t,
      80–81
training and credentialing, 11
transnationalization of health risks, 2, 21–25
   See also globalization
treatment, inappropriate, 95–96
trust, school staff and MCOs, 55–56
tuberculosis (TB), 56, 138–43
Turnock, Bernard J., 122, **124, 144,** 172
type I error, 112
Type II error, 45, 48
Type III error, 45, 48

underemployment, 115
unemployement, 70, 110–17
unionized workplace and healthy
   workplace attributes, 71–81

United Nations' International Bill of
   Human Rights, 35
United States (U.S.)
   health opinion, 1, 13–16
   health promotion activities in, 72
   and LHDs, 145
   measurement of public health practice,
      124–36
   Public Health Service, 83
   public opinion on public health, 13–16
   Surgeon General, 167

values
   cultural relativity, 35
   future of public health, 26–32, 31
   and health programs, 9
vegetable consumption, 39, 59–62, 219
Videto, Donna M., 1, **7**
vigilance, global, 23–24
violence and unemployment, 114
vision for future of public health, 26–32, 31
vision screening, 56
Volpe, Welty & Company, 96

Wallack, L., 156, 159
Wallerstein, N., 154
weight, as problem, 3, 4
Weisman, C.S., 186
Weissberg, Roger P., 208, **226**
welfare reform and public health future, 27
well-being and unemployment, 114
Western Australian Health Promotion
   Foundation, 72, 73
white-collar workers, 74–77
The Whitehouse (R.E.A.L. site), 38
Whitmer, R. William, 208, **210**
WHO (World Health Organization), 17*n*,
   20, 21*n*, 22, 179, 204–6
Wilhelmsen, B.U., 45
Williamson, Marianne, 29
Winslow, C.E.A., 125, 135, 172
Wojtowicz, Greg, 39, **50**
women's reproductive health, 179, 181–88,
   195–203
   See also gender
worksite health promotion, 69–70
   availability and participation factors,
      83–93
   cost-effectiveness review, 94–103
   employee assistance programs (EAP),
      105–9
   in public schools, 39, 50–53
   trade unions and industrial factors,
      71–81
   unemployment, 110–17
World Health Day (R.E.A.L. site), 207
World Health Organization (WHO), 17*n*,
   20, 21*n*, 22, 179, 204–6, 231
World Trade Organization (WTO), 23
WTO (World Trade Organization), 23

Yach, Derek, 1, **17, 21**
youth, peer-led drug prevention, 41–49
Youth Risk Behavior Surveillance System
   (YRBSS) (R.E.A.L. site), 68
Youth Risk Behavior Survey (1989), 64–65
YRBSS (Youth Risk Behavior Surveillance
   System) (R.E.A.L. site), 68

Zarkin, Gary, 69, **105**

Putting it in *Perspectives*
-Review Form-

Your name:_____   Date: _____

Reading title: _____

Summarize: Provide a one-sentence summary of this reading: _____
_____
_____
_____

Follow the Thinking: How does the author back the main premise of the reading? Are the facts/opinions appropriately supported by research or available data? Is the author's thinking logical?

_____
_____
_____
_____
_____
_____

Develop a Context (answer one or both questions): How does this reading contrast or complement your professor's lecture treatment of the subject matter? How does this reading compare to your textbook's coverage?

_____
_____
_____
_____
_____
_____

Question Authority: Explain why you agree/disagree with the author's main premise.

_____
_____
_____
_____
_____
_____

COPY ME! Copy this form as needed. This form is also available at http://www.coursewise.com
Click on: *Perspectives*.